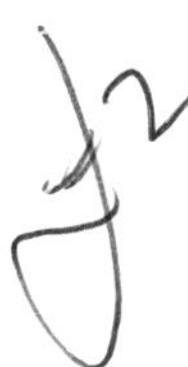

AF201735

Preterm Birth

Prevention and Management

To all pregnant women and their babies

Preterm Birth

Prevention and Management

EDITED BY

Vincenzo Berghella

Director, Maternal-Fetal Medicine;
Professor, Obstetrics and Gynecology,
Thomas Jefferson University,
Philadelphia
USA

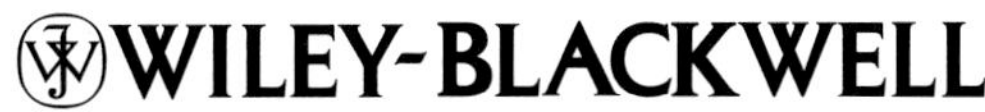

A John Wiley & Sons, Ltd., Publication

This edition first published 2010, © 2010 by Blackwell Publishing Ltd

Blackwell Publishing was acquired by John Wiley & Sons in February 2007. Blackwell's publishing program has been merged with Wiley's global Scientific, Technical and Medical business to form Wiley-Blackwell.

Registered office: John Wiley & Sons Ltd, The Atrium, Southern Gate, Chichester, West Sussex, PO19 8SQ, UK

Editorial offices: 9600 Garsington Road, Oxford, OX4 2DQ, UK
The Atrium, Southern Gate, Chichester, West Sussex, PO19 8SQ, UK
111 River Street, Hoboken, NJ 07030-5774, USA

For details of our global editorial offices, for customer services and for information about how to apply for permission to reuse the copyright material in this book please see our website at www.wiley.com/wiley-blackwell

Library of Congress Cataloging-in-Publication Data
Preterm birth : prevention and management / [edited by] Vincenzo Berghella.
p. ; cm.
Includes bibliographical references and index.
ISBN 978-1-4051-9290-3
1. Premature labor. I. Berghella, Vincenzo.
[DNLM: 1. Premature Birth–prevention & control. WQ 330 P91965 2010]
RG649.P 747 2010
618.3'97–dc22
2009030110

ISBN: 978-1-4051-9290-3

A catalogue record for this book is available from the British Library.

Set in 9.5 on 13 pt Meridien by Toppan Best-set Premedia Limited

Printed and bound in Singapore by Fabulous Printers Pte Ltd

1 2010

Contents

List of Contributors

Jason K. Baxter MD, MSCP
Director, Division of Research; Assistant Professor, Division of Maternal-Fetal Medicine, Department of Obstetrics and Gynecology, Thomas Jefferson University, Philadelphia, USA.

Vincenzo Berghella MD, FACOG
Director, Division of Maternal-Fetal Medicine; Director, Maternal-Fetal Medicine Fellowship Program; Professor, Obstetrics and Gynecology, Thomas Jefferson University, Philadelphia, USA.

Andrew M. Bisits MBBS, FRANZCOG, MMedStats
Director of Obstetrics, Acting Clinical Director, Division of Obstetrics and Gynaecology, John Hunter Hospital, NSW, Australia.

Maria Bisulli MD
Department of Obstetrics and Gynecology, St. Orsola Malpighi Hospital, University of Bologna, Bologna, Italy

Yair Blumenfeld MD
Clinical Assistant Professor, Division of Maternal-Fetal Medicine, Department of Obstetrics and Gynecology, Stanford University Medical Center, California, USA.

Suneet P. Chauhan MD
Aurora Sinai Medical Center, Milwaukee, Wisconsin, USA.

Frank A. Chervenak MD, MMM
Given Foundation Professor and Chairman, Department of Obstetrics and Gynecology, Weill Cornell Medical College, New York Presbyterian Hospital, New York, USA.

Shobhna A. Desai MD
Clinical Associate Professor of Pediatrics, Director, Children's Rehabilitation Unit, Director, Special Banies' Follow up Program, Division of Neonatology, Nemours Pediatrics, Thomas Jefferson University, Philadelphia, USA.

Dana Figueroa MD
Fellow and Clinical Instructor, Division of Maternal-Fetal Medicine, and Center for Women's Reproductive Health, The University of Alabama at Birmingham, Alabama, USA.

Robert L. Goldenberg MD
Professor, Department of Obstetrics and Gynecology, Drexel University College of Medicine, Philadelphia, USA.

Francesca Gotsch MD
Visiting Fellow, Perinatology Research Branch, *Eunice Kennedy Shriver* National Institute to Child Health and Human Development, National Institutes of Health, Michigan, USA.

Edward J. Hayes MD, MSCP
Perinatologist, Division of Maternal-Fetal Medicine, The Women's Center at Aurora Bay Care Medical Center, Wisconsin, USA.

Nancy W. Hendrix MD
Fellow, Division of Maternal-Fetal Medicine; Clinical Instructor, Department of Obstetrics and Gynecology, Thomas Jefferson University, Philadelphia, USA.

Eric J. Hodgson MD
Clinical Instructor and Fellow, Division of Maternal-Fetal Medicine, Department of Obstetrics, Gynecology and Reproductive Sciences, Yale University School of Medicine, Connecticut, USA.

Jay D. Iams MD
Frederick P. Zuspan Professor and Endowed Chair, Division of Maternal-Fetal Medicine, Department of Obstetrics and Gynecology, The Ohio State University Medical Center, Ohio, USA.

Priyadarshini Koduri MD
Fellow, Division of Maternal-Fetal Medicine; Clinical Instructor, Department of Obstetrics and Gynecology, Thomas Jefferson University, Philadelphia, USA.

Juan Pedro Kusanovic MD
Assistant Professor, Department of Obstetrics and Gynecology, Wayne State University, Perinatology Research Branch, *Eunice Kennedy Shriver* National Institute of Child Health and Human Development, National Institutes of Health, Michigan, USA.

Janet E. Larson MD
Chief, Division of Neonatology, Nemours Pediatrics, Thomas Jefferson University, Philadelphia, USA.

Charles J. Lockwood MD
The Anita O'Keefe Young Professor of Women's Health and Chair, Department of Obstetrics, Gynecology and Reproductive Sciences, Yale University School of Medicine, Connecticut, USA.

Shali Mazaki-Tovi MD
Fellow, Division of Maternal-Fetal Medicine, Department of Obstetrics and Gynecology, Wayne State University, Perinatology Research Branch, *Eunice Kennedy Shriver* National Institute of Child Health and Human Development, National Institutes of Health, Michigan, USA.

Elizabeth M. McClure MEd.
Department of Epidemiology, University of North Carolina School of Public Health, and Department of Statistics and Epidemiology, Research Triangle Institute, North Carolina, USA.

Laurence B. McCullough PhD
Dalton Tomlin Chair in Medical Ethics and Health Policy, Center for Medical Ethics and Health Policy, Baylor College of Medicine, Texas, USA.

William McNett MD
Associate Professor, Pediatrics; Division Chief, Department of Pediatrics, Nemours Pediatrics, Thomas Jefferson University, Philadelphia, USA.

Mario Merialdi MD, PhD, MPH
Coordinator, Improving Maternal and Perinatal Health (MPH), Department of Reproductive Health and Research, World Health Organization, Geneva, Switzerland.

Brian M. Mercer MD, FRCSC, FACOG
Professor, Reproductive Biology, Case Western Reserve University; Vice-Chair, Director of Obstetrics and Maternal-Fetal Medicine, Department of Obstetrics and Gynecology, MetroHealth Medical Center, Ohio, USA.

Kellie E. Murphy MD, MSc, FACOG, FRCSC
Associate Professor, University of Toronto, Mount Sinai Hospital, Toronto, Ontario, Canada.

Amen Ness MD, MSCP
Clinical Assistant Professor, Division of Maternal-Fetal Medicine, Department of Obstetrics and Gynecology, Stanford University Medical Center, California, USA.

Leonardo Pereira MD, MCR
Assistant Professor, Director Division of Maternal-Fetal Medicine, Oregon Health and Science University, Oregon, USA.

Timothy J. Rafael MD
Fellow, Division of Maternal-Fetal Medicine; Clinical Instructor, Department of Obstetrics and Gynecology, Thomas Jefferson University, Jefferson Medical College, Philadelphia, USA.

Jennifer Harris Requejo PhD, MA, MHS
Assistant Scientist, Institute for International Programs, Johns Hopkins Bloomberg School of Public Health, Maryland, USA; Technical Consultant, Partnership for Maternal, Newborn and Child Health and Department of Reproductive Health and Research, World Health Organization, Geneva, Switzerland.

Roberto Romero MD
Chief, Perinatology Research Branch, *Eunice Kennedy Shriver* National Institute to Child Health and Human Development, National Institutes of Health; Program Director of Obstetrics and Perinatology, Intramural Division, NICHD, NIH, DHHS; Professor of Molecular Obstetrics and Genetics, Center for Molecular Medicine and Genetics, Wayne State University; Professor of Epidemiology, Michigan State University. Wayne State University/Hutzel Women's Hospital, Michigan, USA.

Dwight J. Rouse MD, MSPH
Professor, Director, Center for Women's Reproductive Health, The University of Alabama at Birmingham, Alabama, USA.

Neil S. Seligman MD
Fellow, Division of Maternal-Fetal Medicine; Clinical Instructor, Department of Obstetrics and Gynecology, Thomas Jefferson University, Jefferson Medical College, Philadelphia, USA.

Hyagriv N. Simhan, MD, MSCR
Associate Professor and Chief, Division of Maternal-Fetal Medicine, Department of Obstetrics, Gynecology and Reproductive Sciences, University of Pittsburgh School of Medicine, Pittsburgh, USA.

Julia I. Smith BSc (Hons), MMedStats
Biostatistician, Mothers and Babies Research Centre, University of Newcastle, NSW, Australia.

Roger Smith MB, BS (Hons), PhD
Director, Mothers and Babies Research Centre and Endocrine Unit, John Hunter Faculty of Health/School of Medicine and Public Health, University of Newcastle, NSW, Australia.

Catherine Y. Spong MD
Chief, Pregnancy and Perinatology Branch, *Eunice Kennedy Shriver* National Institute of Child Health and Human Development, National Institutes of Health, Maryland, USA.

Joyce F. Sung MD
Fellow, Division of Maternal-Fetal Medicine, Department of Obstetrics and Gynecology, Stanford University Medical Center, California, USA.

Heidi L. Thorson MD
Fellow and Clinical Instructor in Maternal-Fetal Medicine and Medical Genetics, Department of Obstetrics, Gynecology and Reproductive Sciences, University of Pittsburgh School of Medicine, Pittsburgh, USA.

Jorge E. Tolosa MD, MSCE
Associate Professor of Obstetrics and Gynecology, Division of Maternal-Fetal Medicine, Department of Obstetrics and Gynecology, Oregon Health and Science University, Oregon, USA.

Jeroen P. Vanderhoeven MD
Department of Obstetrics and Gynecology, Oregon Health and Sciences University, Oregon, USA.

Definitions

Definitions regarding prematurity vary in different publications, but the ones most commonly accepted and used in trials, as well as this book, are:

Cervical insufficiency (CI) (formerly called incompetence, and defined as recurrent painless dilatation leading to second trimester losses): prior preterm birth(s) and/or second trimester loss(es) *and* cervical shortening or dilatation before 24 weeks in the current pregnancy

Infant: from birth until 1 year of life (so includes neonatal period)

Neonate: from birth until 28 days of life

Perinatal: includes fetal period (from 20 weeks until birth), and neonatal period (from birth until 28 days)

Pregnancy loss (PL): loss of pregnancy from conception to <20 weeks. The term spontaneous abortion is equivalent, but should be avoided since women associate negative feeling with this term. Miscarriage is a lay term for PL. Second trimester PL (a.k.a. Second trimester loss — STL): birth between 14 0/7 and 19 6/7 weeks

Preterm birth (PTB): birth between 20 0/7 and 36 6/7 weeks

Very early PTB: birth between 20 0/7 and 23 6/7 weeks

Early PTB: birth between 24 0/7 and 31 6/7 weeks

Late PTB: birth between 32 0/7 and 36 6/7 weeks

Preterm labor (PTL): uterine contractions (≥6/60 min) and documented cervical change in presence of either transvaginal ultrasound (TVU) cervical length (CL) < 20 mm, *or* TVU CL 20–30 mm and positive fetal fibronectin with intact membranes at 20–36 6/7weeks

Preterm premature rupture of membranes (PPROM): vaginal pooling, nitrazine and/or ferning at 16–36 6/7 weeks

- before the limit of viability (currently <23 weeks' gestation)
- remote from term (23–31 weeks' gestation)
- near term (32–36 weeks' gestation)

Viability: the ability of the fetus to exist *ex utero* with full technological support as needed

Abbreviations

ART Assisted reproductive technologies
BPD Broncho-pulmonary dysplasia
BMI Body mass index
CDC Center for Disease Control
CL Cervical length
DES Diethylstilbestrol
FDA Federal Drug Administration
FFN Fetal fibronectin
FLM Fetal lung maturity
GA Gestational age
GBS Group B streptococcus
HSV Herpes simplex virus
IUGR Intrauterine growth restriction
IVH Intra-ventricular hemorrhage
LBW Low-birth weight (infants)
NA Not available
NEC Necrotizing enterocolitis
NIH National Institute of Health
NRFS Non reassuring fetal status
NRFHR Non-reassuring fetal heart rate
PID Pelvic inflammatory disease
PTB Preterm birth
PPROM Preterm premature rupture of membranes
PROM Premature rupture of membranes
PTL Preterm labor
RCT Randomized controlled study
RDS Respiratory distress syndrome
ROM Rupture of membranes
SPTB Spontaneous preterm birth
STI Sexually-transmitted infections
TVU Transvaginal ultrasound
WHO World Health Organization

Preface

'As long as your kids do well, that's all that really matters'

As a father, I believe the health of our youngsters is of paramount importance. Almost 13 million babies every year worldwide are born preterm. Over 85% of preterm births occur in Asia and Africa. Over a million babies every year die of prematurity. So, every minute 2 babies die of preterm birth. This is shorter than the time it will take you to read this introduction. Since these deaths occur in infants supposed to live for 70–80 years, preterm birth represents one of the most important, if not the most important, cause of years-of-life lost. For the most part these are normal babies. I see them as innocent fetuses, then sick or dead neonates. We have to decrease this plague. I've dedicated my professional life to it.

When Wiley asked me to edit this book, I had to say yes. I want to thank some of the world's experts for writing wonderful chapters. I am honored to have collaborated with such esteemed and talented mentors and educators. We made sure that all randomized controlled trials and meta-analyses of such trials pertinent to prevention of preterm birth are included. So this is truly an evidence-based publication. My goal was to review for you all pertinent level 1 data, and present the data in summary for easy use in clinical practice, with ample use of tables, and algorithms. Key points at the beginning of every chapter should be helpful for a quick review. I wanted to keep it brief, clinician oriented, reasonably priced, and widely available.

Many authorities state that not much works for preventing preterm birth. I happen to see it differently. This book will prove to you that there are dozens of interventions that have been shown to significantly prevent preterm birth, and therefore save babies and improve their quality of life. I wanted to present them to you with the ultimate goal to see them used appropriately. We already know a lot, but often do not implement these often easy interventions. As physicians, we have to apply the many known interventions that we know work.

The chapters first review the impact, then the pathophysiology of preterm birth. In the remaining others, the emphasis is on prevention. First, primary prevention for all women is presented. Then chapters are organized by risk factors. This is because several interventions may be good in some clinical scenarios, and detrimental in others. So it is important first to review history and all possible risk factors before offering specific interventions. Many should be applied to reproductive age women before they get pregnant, in preconception counseling.

For the first time in decades the preterm birth incidence recently decreased in the United States. My hope is that this is the beginning of a new era. Prevention of preterm birth is a global health priority.

Vincenzo Berghella
Philadelphia, USA
January 2010

CHAPTER 1

The Global Impact of Preterm Birth

Jennifer Harris Requejo[1,2] *& Mario Merialdi*[3]

[1]Partnership for Maternal, Newborn, and Child Health and Department of Reproductive Health and Research, World Health Organization, Geneva, Switzerland; [2]Institute for International Programs, Johns Hopkins Bloomberg School of Public Health, Maryland, USA and [3]Improving Maternal and Perinatal Health, Department of Reproductive Health and Research, World Health Organization, Geneva, Switzerland

Key points

- An estimated 28% of the 4 million annual neonatal deaths worldwide are directly attributable to preterm birth (PTB).
- Approximately 12.9 million babies are born too early worldwide every year, representing an incidence of PTB of 9.6%. The global distribution of these births is uneven, with 85% of all PTBs occurring in Africa and Asia.
- The highest rates of PTB are in Africa and North America where 11.9% and 10.6% of all births are preterm, respectively.
- Available trend data on PTB rates show a dramatic increase over the past 20 years, particularly in indicated and 'near term' PTBs. Contributing factors to this upward trend include but are not limited to greater usage of assisted reproduction techniques, increasing rates of multiple births, increases in the proportion of births to women over 35 years of age, changes in clinical practice and more obstetric intervention.
- The enormous medical, educational, psychological, and social costs of PTB and the significant numbers of neonatal deaths associated with PTB indicate the urgent need for greater international attention on this issue. The overwhelming burden of PTBs in Africa and Asia suggest that strategies for improving access to effective obstetric and neonatal care and the development of appropriate diagnostic measures for use in these contexts must be a priority, particularly if the world is to achieve Millenium Development Goal 4.

Introduction

Preterm birth (PTB) is usually defined as delivery prior to 37 completed weeks or 259 days. For international comparisons, the World Health Organization (WHO) currently still recommends using 28 weeks completed gestation as a cut-off point for viability while acknowledging that viability varies at the local level depending upon the availability of medical resources [1]. **In this book, PTB is defined as a birth between 20 0/7 and 36 6/7 weeks.**

PTB is a major challenge for maternal and perinatal care and a leading cause of neonatal morbidity and mortality [1]. Globally, an estimated 28% of the 4 million annual neonatal deaths are directly attributable to PTB [2]. The percentage of neonatal deaths due to PTB varies between countries, correlating with the degree of neonatal mortality. In countries characterized by a very high neonatal mortality rate (NMR > 45 per 1000 live births), PTB represents around 20% of all neonatal deaths with most neonates dying from the largely preventable causes of infection and birth asphyxia. At low neonatal mortality levels (NMR < 15 per 1000 live births), the percentage of deaths attributable to PTB reaches nearly 40% and a substantially smaller proportion of neonates die from sepsis/pneumonia or asphyxia [2]. These pronounced differences in the cause distribution of neonatal deaths are a stark measure of health care inequities between low and high resource settings. Although the proportion of neonatal deaths linked to PTB is less in developing versus developed countries, 99% of all neonatal mortality occurs in the developing country context [1]. Thus, **the global burden of neonatal mortality due to prematurity is disproportionately shouldered by the developing world**.

Approximately **12.9 million babies worldwide are born too early every year, representing an incidence of PTB of 9.6%** [3]. The global distribution of these births is uneven, with **85% of all PTBs occurring in Africa and Asia** where almost 11 million births are estimated as preterm per year. In contrast, 0.9 million babies are born premature in Latin America and the Caribbean, and about 500 000 PTBs occur in both Europe and North America on an annual basis [3]. **The high absolute number of PTBs in Africa and Asia is associated with the substantially greater number of deliveries and fertility levels in these two contexts in comparison with other parts of the world.**

The rates of PTB which appear to be increasing worldwide show a slightly different picture, with broad discrepancies across regions and countries. The highest rates of PTB are in Africa and North America where 11.9% and 10.6% of all births are preterm, respectively [3]. In the United States, PTB has increased from 9.5% in 1981 to 12.7% in 2007. The range of PTB in other developed countries is 5–9% [4]. These aggregate figures mask **significant racial and ethnic disparities in PTB rates within countries**. In the United States, for example, non-Hispanic black infants are over two times more likely to be born preterm than non-Hispanic white infants, and this disparity in PTB accounts for a large proportion of the gap in black–white infant mortality levels [5, 6].

The growing concentration of child mortality in the neonatal period (38% of all deaths in children under 5 years of age were neonatal in 2000),

the high percentage of global neonatal deaths related to PTB (28%), and the increasing rates of PTB are all indications that achieving Millenium Development Goal 4 (MDG 4) will require focused attention on PTB [2]. MDG 4 calls for the two-thirds reduction of 1990 child mortality levels by 2015. The concentration of PTB in Africa and Asia — the two regions of the world characterized by the highest burden of newborn mortality — and the marked disparities in PTB along racial/ethnic lines in developed countries also indicate that **addressing PTB is critical for reducing the pronounced inequities in neonatal health**.

Following the call-to-action presented in the 2005 *Lancet* neonatal series, neonatal health in general and PTB in particular has received much overdue international attention. The continuum of care approach [1] has become widely adopted in public health; neonatal health is now a recommended part of Integrated Management of Childhood Illness programs, and greater political and donor commitment to maternal and newborn survival has been realized [7]. A special *Lancet* series dedicated to PTB was launched in early 2008, and a major international conference on prematurity and stillbirth to facilitate the development of a global plan of action to address data gaps in these two areas was held in May 2009 (Global Alliance to Prevent Prematurity and Stillbirths — GAPPS). In addition, WHO and March of Dimes jointly launched a white paper on preterm birth in the fall of 2009 and will launch the Preterm Birth Global Report in 2010. These are all encouraging signs that our knowledge base of PTB and ability to prevent and treat PTB will improve in the near future.

The **translation of the evidence into clinical practice** remains a challenge in many developing countries and is linked to resource constraints and shortfalls in capacity. The administration of corticosteroids to the mother during preterm labor and before the baby is born, for example, is a cost-effective intervention that helps develop the baby's lungs and reduce complications from respiratory distress syndrome — the primary cause of early neonatal mortality and disability in preterm infants [8] (Chapter 20). Studies show, however, that only 5–10% of appropriate candidates receive the intervention in low and middle income countries [9, 10]. These low coverage figures are in stark contrast to the approximate 80% maximum rate of use of the intervention in preterm babies below 34 weeks of age [10], and are indicative of the need for greater training opportunities and other innovative strategies to increase the implementation of this and other proven interventions in resource constrained settings.

The remaining paragraphs outline what is currently known about the main causes of PTB, how these causes vary in different parts of the world, and the health, social, and economic consequences of PTB.

Causes of preterm birth

The etiology of PTB is not completely understood and it is considered a syndrome initiated by multiple mechanisms (Chapter 2). It is unclear whether PTB results from the interaction of several pathways or the independent effect of each pathway. Causal factors linked to PTB include biological and genetic determinants, present pregnancy characteristics, pregnancy history, maternal demographic characteristics (e.g. age, socioeconomic status, education level), maternal nutritional and psychological status, fetal characteristics, environmental factors, and adverse behaviors [4, 11] (Chapter 4). A definitive explanation for racial disparities in PTB has not been proposed, although there is evidence of a possible role of gene–gene and gene–environmental interactions [12]. Importantly, while there is growing evidence of the biological basis of racial disparities in PTB, the promotion of **universal access to health care services** is widely accepted as a strategy for their reduction. It is important to note that the complex mechanisms leading to PTB differ between low and high resource settings. **Women living in low-resource settings are more likely to experience PTB because of the interplay of factors rooted in poverty including nutritional deprivation, lack of access to health services, and infections such as malaria.** In contrast, women in high-resource settings are more prone to deliver preterm because of the usage of assisted reproductive technologies and later maternal age. These differences are consequential for targeting populations with appropriate preventive and treatment strategies, and highlight the dire reproductive implications of the unacceptable global inequities in women's health.

PTB is categorized as either indicated or spontaneous [4] (Chapter 4). PTB can also be stratified by gestation age [4, 11] (see Definitions, page xi). Accurate classification of PTB by type and gestational age is essential for monitoring trends and for determining health service needs. Available trend data on PTB rates show **a dramatic increase over the past 20 years, particularly in indicated and 'near term' PTBs**. Contributing factors to this upward trend include but are not limited to greater usage of assisted reproduction techniques, increasing rates of multiple births, increases in the proportion of births to women over 35 years of age, changes in clinical practice and more obstetric intervention [3, 13]. Physicians, for example, are now more willing to perform elective Cesarean sections. The replacement of the usage of the last menstrual period with ultrasonography to estimate gestational age may have resulted in larger numbers of births being classified as preterm [11]. Inconsistent and changing classifications of spontaneous abortion, fetal loss, stillbirth, and early neonatal deaths have also likely contributed to the alarming increases in

PTB rates recorded in many developed countries in the previous two decades [4] (Chapter 4).

Health, social and economic consequences of preterm birth

PTBs account for 75% of perinatal mortality and make up more than 50% of long-term morbidity associated with poor perinatal outcomes [4]. While the survival rates of preterm infants have greatly improved over the past 20–30 years, the survival chances of a preterm infant are vastly different in developed and developing countries and are a reflection of **global gaps in the availability of quality obstetrical and neonatal care services. In many developing countries, infants weighing less than 2000 g (corresponding to about 32 weeks of gestation in the absence of intrauterine growth retardation) have little chance of survival**. In contrast, the survival rate of infants born at 32 weeks in developed countries where neonatal intensive care units are accessible nears the rate of full-term infants, and infants born at 25 weeks have a survival rate of around 50%. This discrepancy suggests that identifying innovative ways of delivering affordable neonatal care services in developing country settings where most PTBs occur needs to be a top priority [11].

While the survival chances of preterm infants have increased, studies show that infants born preterm have diminished long-term survival, and are particularly at risk for neurological impairments and respiratory disorders [14, 15] (Chapter 22). The severity of these risks is inversely related to gestational age at birth. Children born preterm have higher rates of cerebral palsy, hydrocephalus, learning disabilities, sensory deficits and respiratory illnesses. The risks of medical and psycho-social problems often extend into adolescence and adulthood, negatively impacting affected individuals, their families, health care services and societies [14, 15]. The estimated costs of PTB are staggering and affect multiple sectors of the economy including the health care and educational systems. In 2005, for example, more than US$26.2 billion was spent in the United States alone on the educational and medical expenses and lost productivity associated with PTB [3].

Concluding remarks

PTB is a devastating perinatal health problem impacting populations across the globe. The enormous medical, educational, psychological and social costs of PTB and the significant numbers of neonatal deaths associated with PTB indicate the **urgent need for greater international attention on this issue**. Additional research that defines the multiple causal pathways resulting in PTB is essential for developing effective preventive and treatment strategies with universal application. Research focused on modifying the neurological and other impairments associated with PTB, and prospective research on the long-term effects of PTB into middle-age are also crucial for the design of treatment modalities and for determining health service needs. The overwhelming burden of PTBs in Africa and Asia importantly suggest that strategies for improving access to effective obstetric and neonatal care and the development of appropriate diagnostic measures for use in these contexts must be a priority, particularly if the world is to achieve MDG 4.

References

1 WHO. *World Health Report: Making Every Mother and Child Count.* Geneva: World Health Organization, 2005.

2 Lawn JE, Cousens S, Zupan J, for the Neonatal Survival Steering Team. Four million neonatal deaths: when? where? why? Lancet 2005; 365: 891–900.

3 Beck S, Wojdyla D, Say L, *et al.* WHO systematic review on maternal mortality and morbidity: the global burden of preterm birth. Bull World Health Org 2009 available online, September 25, 2009.

4 Goldberg RL, Culhane JF, Iams JD, Romero R. Epidemiology and causes of preterm birth. Lancet 2008; 371: 75–84.

5 Ahern J, Picket KE, Selvin S, Abrams B. Preterm birth among African American and white women: a multi-level analysis of socioeconomic characteristics and cigarette smoking. J Epidemiol Community Health 2003; 57: 606–11.

6 Anachebe N, Sutton M. Racial disparities in reproductive health outcomes. Am J Obstet Gynecol 2003; 188: S37–42.

7 Lawn JE, Cousens SN, Darmstadt G, *et al.* for The Lancet Neonatal Survival Series Steering Team. One year after The Lancet Neonatal Survival Series — was the call for action heard? Lancet 2006; 367: 1541–7.

8 Dalziel RD. Antenatal corticosteroids for acceleration of fetal lung maturation for women at risk of preterm birth. Cochrane Systematic Reviews 2009, Issue 2. http://www.cochrane.org/reviews/en/ab004454.html

9 Jones G, Steketee R, Black RE, and the Bellagio Child Survival Study Group. How many child deaths can we prevent this year? Lancet 2003; 362: 65–71.

10 Darmstadt GL, Bhutta ZA, Cousens S, Adam T, Walker N, de Bernis L, for the Lancet Neonatal Survival Steering Team. Neonatal survival 2: evidence-based, cost-effective interventions: how many newborn babies can we save? Lancet 2005; 365: 977–88.

11 Tucker J, McGuire W. Epidemiology of preterm birth. BMJ 2004; 329: 675–8.

12 Menon R. Spontaneous preterm birth, a clinical dilemma: etiologic, pathophysiologic and genetic heterogeneities and racial disparity. Acta Obstet Gynecol Scand 2008; 87: 590–600.

13 Iams JD, Romero R, Culhane JF, Goldenberg RL. Primary, secondary, and tertiary interventions to reduce the morbidity and mortality of preterm birth. Lancet 2008; 371: 164–75.

14 Swamy GK, Ostbye T, Skjaerven R. Association of preterm birth with long-term survival, reproduction, and next-generation preterm birth. JAMA 2008; 299: 1429–36.

15 Saigal S, Doyle LW. An overview of mortality and sequelae of preterm birth from infancy to adulthood. Lancet 2008; 371: 261–9.

CHAPTER 2

Preterm Birth: A Complex Disease

Eric J. Hodgson & Charles J. Lockwood
Department of Obstetrics, Gynecology and Reproductive Sciences, Yale University School of Medicine, Connecticut, USA

Key points

- The rate of preterm birth (PTB) has gradually increased since 1990 to approximately 13% of all United States deliveries in 2007.
- PTB usually represents the final common pathway of four different inciting causes: maternal and/or fetal stress, inflammation, abruption (decidual bleeding), and pathological mechanical stretching of the uterus.
- Although arising from different causes, all spontaneous PTBs utilize a final common biochemical pathway that includes increased genital tract prostaglandin (PG) and protease production coupled with functional progesterone withdrawal.
- Disparities in PTB rates between racial groups may reflect both environmental stressors and differing genetic predispositions.

Introduction

Preterm birth (PTB) is a birth at or after 20 weeks but before 37 completed week's gestation. In 2007, the PTB rate in the United States was 12.7%. This represents an increase of approximately 21% since 1990. Although non-Hispanic white women saw the highest relative increase in PTB rates, non-Hispanic black women maintain an approximately 1.5-fold higher PTB rate and a 2.5-fold higher rate of very PTB (<32 weeks) [1]. The two principal drivers of the recent increase in PTBs among non-Hispanic white women have been the epidemic of multifetal gestations resulting from the increased availability of assisted reproductive technologies (ART) and PTBs indicated by deteriorating maternal or fetal health (Chapter 4).

Etiology and pathogenesis of spontaneous PTB: four paths converge

Spontaneous PTBs account for 70% of PTBs, while medically indicated and iatrogenic PTBs comprise the remainder. Despite distinct genetic

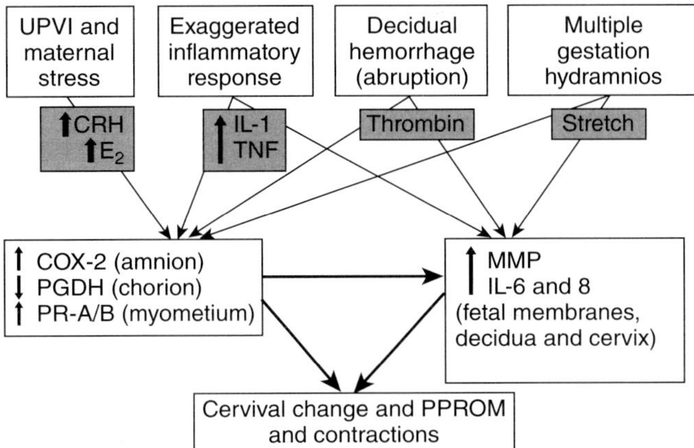

Figure 2.1 A schematic of the discrete pathogenic processes leading to prematurity and their final common biochemical pathway. UPVI, uteroplacental vascular insufficiency. CRH, corticotrophin-releasing hormone. IL, interleukin. TNF, tumor necrosis factor. COX-2, cyclooxygenase-2. MMP, matrix metalloproteinase. PGDH, prostaglandin dehydrogenase. PR, progesterone receptor. PPROM, preterm premature rupture of the membranes.

and/or epidemiological associations and biochemical triggers (Figure 2.1), **all spontaneous PTBs utilize a final common biochemical pathway that includes: (a) increased genital tract prostaglandin (PG) and protease production coupled with (b) functional progesterone withdrawal secondary to reductions in progesterone receptor (PR) isoform expression in the cervix, decidua and myometrium**.

The first path: maternal and/or fetal stress: premature activation of the placental–fetal hypothalamic–pituitary–adrenal (HPA) axis

Both **maternal and fetal stress** is associated with PTB. Maternal stress in the periconception period —including mood disorders such as anxiety and depression are associated with modest (twofold) increased rates of spontaneous PTB [2]. Pathological changes in the placenta due to fetal stress are three to seven times more common in patients with spontaneous PTB compared with term controls [3]. **Corticotropin-releasing hormone (CRH)** appears to be the mediator of stress-associated PTBs [4]. Rising CRH levels may also act as the trigger for term parturition, since placental-derived maternal plasma free CRH concentrations rise during the second half of pregnancy and peak during term labor [5]. This 41-amino-acid peptide hormone, initially discovered in the hypothalamus, is also expressed by placental, chorionic, amnionic and decidual cells. In the hypothalamus, glucocorticoids inhibit CRH release; however, cortisol enhances placental and reproductive tract production of CRH. Thus, rising maternal and cortisol levels enhance reproductive tract CRH expression while rising fetal cortisol levels enhance placental-derived CRH. The latter stimulate increasing release of fetal pituitary adrenocorticotropin (ACTH) to drive further fetal adrenal cortisol production which in turn, stimulates greater placental CRH release. Both maternal and fetal stress is associated with elevated maternal and/or fetal cortisol levels [6].

Elevated CRH levels stimulate the production and output of PGs whose pro-parturition effects are mediated by binding to uterotonic receptors in the uterine fundus and corpus. In amnionic, chorionic, decidual and placental cell culture, $PGF_{2\alpha}$ and/or estradiol (E_2) are induced by CRH, which in turn promotes calcium flux and expression of oxytocin receptor, connexin 43 (gap junctions), and cyclooxygenase-2 (COX-2) which triggers effective contractions, facilitates their transmission, and generates additional PGs, respectively [7].

Increased cortisol levels may directly **augment fetal membrane PGs output** by increasing amnionic COX-2 expression and inhibiting the chorionic PG metabolizing enzyme, prostaglandin dehydrogenase (PGDH) [8]. In addition, PGs promote cervical change and preterm premature membrane rupture (PROM) by enhancing fetal membrane and cervical matrix metalloproteinase (MMP) expression [9]. Moreover, PGs increase cervical expression of interleukin-8 (IL-8), which recruits and activates neutrophils, releasing additional MMPs and elastases. Finally, recent studies suggest PGs reduce reproductive tract PR expression [10].

With development of the fetal zone of the adrenal gland after 28–32 weeks gestation, stress-associated activation of the placental–fetal HPA axis increases ACTH-mediated production of dehydroepiandrosterone sulfate (DHEAS). Placental sulfatases cleave the conjugates of DHEAS and its 16-hydroxy hepatic derivative allowing their conversion to estradiol (E_2) and estrone (E_1), as well as estriol (E_3), respectively. Since reductions in PR-B expression lead to increases in the active form of the estrogen receptor (ER-α), estrogens are free to bind to ER-α and activate transcription factors (c-jun/fos) driving transcription of genes coding for contraction-associated proteins (CAPs) (oxytocin receptor and connexin 43) [11].

In summary, increased levels of maternal or fetal stress result in elevated levels of CRH, that increase production of cortisol promoting a positive feedback loop inducing higher levels of cortisol. Cortisol, in turn, induces production of PGs that mediate their effects by increasing gap junctions between uterine cells, enhancing myometrial oxytocin receptors formation, genital tract MMP release, and inhibition of myometrial PR expression [12]. Concurrently, elevated cortisol increases production of estrogens that increase the levels of myometrial CAPs.

The second path: decidual–amnion–chorion inflammation

Inflammation, both systemic and localized to the reproductive tract, has been associated with PTB; systemic inflammation due to **periodontal disease, pneumonia, sepsis, pancreatitis, acute cholecystitis, pyelonephritis and asymptomatic bacteriuria** as well as genital tract inflammatory states such **deciduitis, chorioamnionitis and intra-amniotic infections** are all associated with PTB [13]. Genital tract inflammation is the most common progenitor of very early PTBs, accounting for more than half of cases [14]. In particular, **bacterial vaginosis** (BV) has been associated with spontaneous PTB in multiple prospective cohort studies, especially when detected at less than 16 weeks (Chapter 14). The overgrowth of the bacteria that characterizes the BV milieu, *Gardnerella vaginalis*, and mycoplasma species creates an environment that promotes the 'overgrowth' of other bacterial species in the upper genital tract [15]. Gram negative bacteria such as *Escherichia coli* are more likely to colonize the vagina and urinary tract in the setting of BV. Importantly, asymptomatic bacteriuria and vaginal *E. coli* colonization are linked to a twofold increase in PTB [16].

The link between BV and bacteriuria with over-growth of lower and upper genital bacteria and PTB reflects the pivotal role of the innate immune response. In fact, the increased rates of PTB in certain ethnic groups may reflect a genetically determined, exaggerated inflammatory response by the maternal/fetal immune system. The most common microorganisms identified in the fetal membranes and amniotic fluid of patients with inflammation-associated PTB — *Ureaplasma Urealyticum, Mycoplasma hominis, Gardnerella vaginalis* and *bacteroides* species — are generally considered to have low virulence. Hence, **the maternal/fetal inflammatory response rather than the presence of specific microorganism is the causative factor for PTB** [17] (Chapter 7).

An exaggerated innate immune response ultimately leads to **functional progesterone withdrawal by PR down-regulation and promotes production of elastases and MMPs leading to PTB** [18]. Specifically, Gram-negative bacterial endotoxins bind to cervical and fetal membrane toll-like receptor (TLR)-4 and Gram-positive bacterial exotoxins bind to TLR-2 on decidual cells and leukocytes to elicit production of tumor necrosis factor-α (TNFα) and interleukin-1β (IL-1β) [19]. In turn, TNα, IL-1β and/or endotoxins such as lipopolysaccharide (LPS) induce expression of the transcription factor, NFkB, which enhances MMP-1, 3, and 9, and COX-2 expression and inhibits PGDH and PR-B gene expression in myometrium, decidua, fetal membranes and/or cervix while promoting programed cell death (apoptosis) in amnionic epithelial cells [20]. Moreover, TNFα, IL-1β and LPS also stimulated IL-6 production in amniochorion and decidua which further augments amnionic and decidual PG production.

Finally, IL-1β and TNFα induce IL-8 production in the fetal membranes, decidua and cervix, effects that are potentiated by rising IL-6 levels [21]. Given that IL-8 causes recruitment and activation of neutrophils that release additional MMPs and elastases, it further exacerbates the PTB-enhancing effects of genital tract inflammation.

The **genetic predisposition to inflammation-associated PTB** is suggested by the 15% recurrence risk of PTB, its high concordance in twin studies, and its aggregation in certain families. Specific polymorphisms of particular genes may also play a role in PTB. The T2 allele of the TNFα gene causes increased expression of TNFα and confers an increased risk of preterm PROM in African-American women. Moreover, African-American mothers harboring both this polymorphism and BV are at even greater risk of PTB [22]. An association between the IL-6 -174 promoter polymorphism and a decreased risk of PTB among women of European extraction has been shown. An increased frequency of PTB has been found among white infants carrying two polymorphisms for TLR-4 (Asp299Gly and Thr399Ile), the major endotoxin-signaling receptor. These findings may help account for disparate ethnic and racial patterns in PTB rates.

Fetal genotypes may also play a role in the genesis of PTB. The presence of fetal mutations in MMP-1 and MMP-9 has also been found to increase the risk of PROM when present in African-American fetuses, suggesting genetic influences on fetal membrane structural integrity contribute to preterm PROM [23]. Finally, **gene–environmental interactions** may also be important in inflammation-associated PTB. Polymorphisms in drug metabolizing genes, *CYP1A1 Hinc*II RFLP and *GSTT1* shorten gestation among Chinese women exposed to benzene and United States women exposed to cigarette smoke [24].

In summary, inflammation — both localized and systemic — is associated with PTB due to an exaggerated response by the innate immune system that increases production of inflammatory cytokines and induces functional progesterone withdrawal and increase in elastases and MMPs. Genetic differences in response to inflammation — both fetal and maternal — are implicated in PTB.

The third path: abruption-associated PTB

The third major progenitor of PTB is **abruption — placental or decidual hemorrhage**. Such hemorrhage originates in damaged spiral arteries or arterioles and presents clinically as vaginal bleeding, if the hemorrhage occurs at the placenta periphery near the internal os, or either a retroplacental or retrochorionic hematoma formation if the hemorrhage occurs remote from the os. When vaginal bleeding occurs in more than one trimester it is associated with a nearly 50% risk of preterm PROM [25]. Decidual hemosiderin deposition and retro-chorionic hematoma formation is present in 38% of patients with PTB between 22 and 32 weeks gestation due to preterm PROM and 36% of patients experiencing PTB after preterm labor compared with only 0.8% following term delivery. Utero-placental vascular lesions associated with abruption include spiral artery vascular thrombosis and failed physiological transformation of uteroplacental vessels. These vasculopathies may be associated with inherited and acquired thrombophilias and hypertension as well as environmental stimuli including heavy cigarette smoking, cocaine and trauma [26]. Abruption-associated PTBs are more common in older, married, parous, college-educated patients presenting a demographic profile distinct from that associated with patients with stress-induced PTBs (nulliparous, anxious or depressed patients) or inflammation-associated PTBs (African-American).

The decidua is a rich source of tissue factor, the primary initiator of clotting through the generation of thrombin [27]. Thus, decidual hemorrhage results in intense local thrombin production. Thrombin binding to its proteinase-activated receptor significantly enhances decidual cell expression of MMP-1 and 3 protein and mRNA [28]. Decidual neutrophils co-localized with areas of thrombin-induced fibrin deposition and thrombin/PAR-1 enhances decidual IL-8 mRNA and protein expression [29]. Neutrophils are a rich source of elastase and MMP-9 that contribute to PROM and cervical effacement [29].

The fourth path: mechanical stretching of the uterus

Mechanical stretch of the uterus has been associated with increased risk for PTB as illustrated by the decrease in the gestational age at delivery with increasing numbers of fetuses from 35.3 weeks with twins to 29.9 weeks with quadruplets. Mechanical dilation of the cervix promotes cervical ripening through the induction of endogenous PG and increased MMP-1 expression. Polyhydramnios and multifetal gestation-induced mechanical stretch increases amnion COX-2 expression and related PG production. Myometrial stretch also induces oxytocin receptor, COX-2, IL-8 and connexin 43 expression [30].

Final common pathway of PTB

As elucidated above, each of the four progenitors of PTB — stress, inflammation, decidual hemorrhage and myometrial stretch — induce preterm PROM and/or preterm labor through a final common pathway. **Ultimately, the generation of PGs and proteases occurs prior to all spontaneous labor whether occurring preterm or at term**. Concomitant with rising PG levels is the **up-regulation of myometrial PG receptors** prior to the onset of labor. As noted, PGs induce functional progesterone withdrawal, enhance sensitivity to estrogens, and increase MMP and IL-8 expression to mediate cervical change and fetal membrane rupture (see Figure 2.1). Prior to 20 weeks of gestation, the myometrium is quiescent due to high PR-B, low ERα, low circulating estrogen levels, and inhibition of CAP gene expression. Therefore, inflammation, abruption and excess stretch occurring prior to 24 weeks may present as 'incompetent cervix' with or without subsequent preterm PROM and not PTL.

References

1 Hamilton BE, Martin JA, Ventura SJ. Preliminary Births for 2006: Infant and Maternal Health. National Vital Statistics Reports, Volume 56, Number 7: National Center for Health Statistics. Released December 5, 2007.

2 Copper RL, Goldenberg RL, Das A, *et al.* The preterm prediction study: maternal stress is associated with spontaneous preterm birth at less than thirty-five weeks' gestation. National Institute of Child Health and Human Development Maternal-Fetal Medicine Units Network. Am J Obstet Gynecol 1996; 175: 1286–92.

3 Germain AM, Carvajal J, Sanchez M, Valenzuela GJ, Tsunekawa H, Chuaqui B. Preterm labor: placental pathology and clinical correlation. Obstet Gynecol 1999; 94: 284–9.

4 Challis JR, Lye SJ, Gibb W, Whittle W, Patel F, Alfaidy N. Understanding preterm labor. Ann NY Acad Sci 2001; 943: 225–34.

5 McLean M, Bisits A, Davies J, Woods R, Lowry P, Smith R. A placental clock controlling the length of human pregnancy. Nat Med 1995; 1: 460–3.

6 Lockwood CJ, Radunovic N, Nastic D, Petkovic S, Aigner S, Berkowitz GS. Corticotropin-releasing hormone and related pituitary-adrenal axis hormones in fetal and maternal blood during the second half of pregnancy. J Perinat Med 1996; 24: 243–51.

7 Olson DM. The role of prostaglandins in the initiation of parturition. Best Pract Res Clin Obstet Gynaecol 2003; 17: 717–30.

8 Zakar T, Hirst JJ, Mijovic JE, Olson DM. Glucocorticoids stimulate the expression of prostaglandin endoperoxide H synthase-2 in amnion cells. Endocrinology 1995; 136: 1610–9.

9 Yoshida M, Sagawa N, *et al.* Prostaglandin F(2alpha), cytokines and cyclic mechanical stretch augment matrix metalloproteinase-1 secretion from cultured human uterine cervical fibroblast cells. Mol Hum Reprod 2002; 8: 681–7.

10 Madsen G, Zakar T, Ku CY, Sanborn BM, Smith R, Mesiano S. Prostaglandins differentially modulate progesterone receptor-A and -B expression in human myometrial cells: evidence for prostaglandin-induced functional progesterone withdrawal. J Clin Endocrinol Metab 2004; 89:1010–3.

11 Di WL, Lachelin GC, McGarrigle HH, Thomas NS, Becker DL. Oestriol and oestradiol increase cell to cell communication and connexin43 protein expression in human myometrium. Mol Hum Reprod 2001; 7: 671–9.

12 Mesiano S, Chan EC, Fitter JT, Kwek K, Yeo G, Smith R. Progesterone withdrawal and estrogen activation in human parturition are coordinated by progesterone receptor A expression in the myometrium. J Clin Endocrinol Metab 2002; 87: 2924–30.

13 Locksmith G, Duff P. Infection, antibiotics, and preterm delivery. Semin Perinatol 2001; 25: 295–309.
14 Andrews WW, Hauth JC, Goldenberg RL, Gomez R, Romero R, Cassell GH. Amniotic fluid interleukin-6: correlation with upper genital tract microbial colonization and gestational age in women delivered after spontaneous labor versus indicated delivery. Am J Obstet Gynecol 1995; 173: 606–12.
15 Meis PJ, Goldenberg RL, Mercer B, *et al.* The preterm prediction study: significance of vaginal infections. National Institute of Child Health and Human Development Maternal-Fetal Medicine Units Network. Am J Obstet Gynecol 1995; 173: 1231–5.
16 Romero R, Oyarzun E, Mazor M, Sirtori M, Hobbins JC, Bracken M. Meta-analysis of the relationship between asymptomatic bacteriuria and preterm delivery/low birth weight. Obstet Gynecol 1989; 73: 576–8.
17 Clausson B, Lichtenstein P, Cnattingius S. Genetic influence on birthweight and gestational length determined by studies in offspring of twins. Br J Obstet Gynaecol 2000; 107: 375–81.
18 Oner C, Schatz F, Kizilay G, Murk W, Buchwalder LF, Kayisli UA, Arici A, Lockwood CJ. Progestin-inflammatory cytokine interactions affect matrix metalloproteinase-1 and -3 expression in term decidual cells: implications for treatment of chorioamnionitis-induced preterm delivery. J Clin Endocrinol Metab 2008; 93: 252–9.
19 Kim YM, Romero R, Chaiworapongsa T, *et al.* Toll-like receptor-2 and -4 in the chorioamniotic membranes in spontaneous labor at term and in preterm parturition that are associated with chorioamnionitis. Am J Obstet Gynecol 2004; 191: 1346–55.
20 Arechavaleta-Velasco F, Ogando D, Parry S, Vadillo-Ortega F. Production of matrix metalloproteinase-9 in lipopolysaccharide-stimulated human amnion occurs through an autocrine and paracrine proinflammatory cytokine-dependent system. Biol Reprod 2002; 67: 1952–8.
21 Lockwood CJ, Arcuri F, *et al.* Tumor necrosis factor-alpha and interleukin-1beta regulate interleukin-8 expression in third trimester decidual cells: implications for the genesis of chorioamnionitis. Am J Pathol 2006; 169: 1294–302.
22 Macones GA, Parry S, Elkousy M, Clothier B, Ural S, Strauss III JF. A polymorphism in the promoter region of TNF and bacterial vaginosis: preliminary evidence of gene-environment interaction in the etiology of spontaneous preterm birth. Am J Obstet Gynecol 2004; 190: 1504–8.
23 Fujimoto T, Parry S, Urbanek M, *et al.* A single nucleotide polymorphism in the matrix metalloproteinase-1 (MMP-1) promoter influences amnion cell MMP-1 expression and risk for preterm premature rupture of the fetal membranes. J Biol Chem 2002; 277: 6296–302. Epub 2001 Dec 11.
24 Wang X, Zuckerman B, Pearson C, *et al.* Maternal cigarette smoking, metabolic gene polymorphism, and infant birth weight. J Am Med Assoc 2002; 287: 195–202.
25 Harger JH, Hsing AW, Tuomala RE, *et al.* Risk factors for preterm premature rupture of fetal membranes: a multicenter case-control study. Am J Obstet Gynecol 1990; 163: 130–7.
26 Roque H, Paidas MJ, Funai EF, Kuczynski E, Lockwood CJ. Maternal thrombophilias are not associated with early pregnancy loss. Thromb Haemost 2004; 91: 290–5.
27 Lockwood C, Krikun G, Schatz F. The decidua regulates hemostasis in the human endometrium. Sem Reprod Endocrinol 1999; 17: 45–51.
28 Rosen T, Schatz F, Kuczynski E, Lam H, Koo AB, Lockwood CJ. Thrombin-enhanced matrix metalloproteinase-1 expression: a mechanism linking placental abruption with premature rupture of the membranes. J Matern Fetal Neonatal Med 2002; 11: 11–7.

29 Lockwood CJ, Toti P, Arcuri F, *et al.* Mechanisms of abruption-induced premature rupture of the fetal membranes: thrombin-enhanced interleukin-8 expression in term decidua. Am J Pathol 2005; 167: 1443–9.

30 Loudon JA, Sooranna SR, Bennett PR, Johnson MR. Mechanical stretch of human uterine smooth muscle cells increases IL-8 mRNA expression and peptide synthesis. Mol Hum Reprod 2004; 10: 895–9.

CHAPTER 3
Why Prevention?

Jason K. Baxter

Division of Maternal-Fetal Medicine, Department of Obstetrics and Gynecology, Thomas Jefferson University, Philadelphia, USA

Key points

- Primary, secondary, and tertiary preventions refer to universal, selective, and indicated interventions for the general population, those with risk factors, and those with the disease, respectively.
- Primary prevention of both spontaneous and iatrogenic preterm birth (PTB) encompasses interventions aimed at all women with a potential to be pregnant.
- Secondary or selective prevention involves screening for a risk factor in an asymptomatic or 'well' population, and either avoiding it or treating it.
- Tertiary or indicated prevention involves therapy to prevent PTB for women who already have symptoms of PTB.
- Tertiary prevention of PTB strategies have involved the most research, have been the most clinically applied, and have been the most expensive. They have been the most disappointing because they are applied too late in the preterm parturition process.
- The greatest medical improvements related to PTB have involved ameliorating treatments that don't actually decrease the rate of PTB.
- Primary and secondary prevention of PTB have been shown to be more efficacious and are probably more cost-effective than tertiary prevention.

Why prevention?

This book is designed based upon the thought process of a clinician or patient trying to prevent preterm birth (PTB). The chapters are titled mainly based upon clinical scenarios and risk factors that a woman might have for PTB. They are organized based upon problems that will then lead toward solutions with the idea that 'every problem is an opportunity in disguise'. This is in contrast to many textbooks about the prevention of PTB that focus on a growing armamentarium of 'therapies' for the prevention of PTB, some of which have subsequently been shown to not only not be helpful, but to actually cause harm. It has been said that 'when the only tool you own is a hammer, every problem begins to resemble a nail'. Our hope is that readers of this book will treat their patients appropriately

Preterm Birth. Edited by Vincenzo Berghella. © 2010 Blackwell Publishing

Table 3.1 Examples of strategies aimed at primary prevention of preterm birth in the general population.

Raise awareness of scope and significance of PTB
Standardized preconception care for everyone
Nutrition, diet, exercise and ideal BMI (19–25 kg/m^2) before and during pregnancy
Adequate folate (supplementation) for all reproductive aged women
Up-to-date vaccinations
Decrease unplanned pregnancy
Improved availability and utilization of reliable, acceptable contraception
Avoid pregnancy at extremes of age
Minimize uterine instrumentation (decrease abortions)
Inter-pregnancy interval of 18–24 months
Health policies minimizing prolonged standing, long work hours, and night shift work
Avoid substance abuse (tobacco, alcohol and illicit drugs)
Minimize stress (allostatic load)
Prevent sexually transmitted infections
Limit number of embryos transferred during IVF, minimizing multiple gestations
Prevent birth defects
Decrease preeclampsia and IUGR

based upon risk factors for PTB, rather than looking for appropriate patients upon which to use potential therapies. Even better, PTB may be prevented in the future via universally applied primary prevention strategies. Ultimately, our goal is not the prevention of PTB for its own sake, but rather to improve perinatal outcomes. Sometimes outcomes are improved by prematurely removing the fetus from a hostile environment. Preterm birth may be nature's way of telling us that it is better for the mother and baby for the baby to be outside the womb.

Primary, secondary, and tertiary preventions refer to universal, selective, and indicated interventions applied to the general population, those with risk factors, and those with the disease, respectively.

Primary or universal prevention is directed toward the general population. **Primary prevention of both spontaneous and iatrogenic PTB encompasses interventions aimed at all women with a potential to be pregnant**, regardless of any identifiable risk factors, and has been shown to be **more efficacious** than secondary or tertiary prevention. A wide variety of interventions fall under primary prevention (Table 3.1) and are described in detail in Chapter 9. Primary prevention of PTB may focus on a narrow group of women as do professional policies or laws that restrict in-vitro fertilization to single embryo transfer. Primary prevention of PTB may include prepubertal girls, optimizing their health, social conditions and education prior to menarche. It may include postmenopausal women, as they may be the best influences or educators for younger

Table 3.2 Criteria for screening tests for preterm birth.

Preterm birth causes significant harm
A pre-symptomatic stage of preterm birth exists
Screening test reliably predicts preterm birth
Screening test is acceptable to patients
Outcomes are better when diagnosis and intervention precede symptomatic disease
Benefit of diagnosis and intervention outweighs potential harm of false-positive tests
Cost is acceptable

women destined to have a PTB. Prevention of PTB even includes men: they may partner in responsible sexual activity, prevent transmission of sexually transmitted infections, stop abusive relationships, and provide nutritional, social, emotional and financial support.

Secondary or selective prevention involves screening for a risk factor in an asymptomatic or 'well' population, and either avoiding it or treating it. Criteria for good screening strategies are listed in Table 3.2. Asymptomatic cervical change (detected by ultrasound or physical exam) has been used as a screening test for PTB, but questions remain unanswered: how wide a screening net should be cast?; how should a positive screen be defined?; what intervention is appropriate in those women who screen positive? Shifting the focus from the classic 'PTB spectrum' (with painless cervical change versus preterm contractions as the ends of the spectrum) toward various risk factors or 'windows into the preterm parturition process' may be helpful. Examples of risk factors to screen for are listed in Table 3.3 and elaborated on in Chapters 10–17. Several management strategies aimed at preventing PTB identify an at-risk population and apply interventions. Two of the most commonly studied 'high-risk' populations are women with a prior PTB (Chapter 11) and those with multiple gestations (Chapter 16).

Tertiary or indicated prevention involves treatment to prevent PTB for women who already have symptoms of PTB. The apparent misnomer of tertiary prevention of PTB (i.e. treating PTB once it has actually occurred) is clarified when one considers the classic symptomatic precursors for PTB as preterm labor (PTL; Chapter 18) and preterm premature rupture of membranes (PPROM; Chapter 19). Strategies to prevent imminent PTB in these symptomatic women (Table 3.4) have taught us that prediction of PTB can be improved, and that the tertiary therapies to prevent PTB are not very effective. While much of Western medicine has focused on the expensive, hospital-based, intensive care of tertiary prevention, it is the least efficacious to prevent PTB as it is often 'too little, too late'. For PTB prevention, many consider 'the cat already out of the bag' when addressing true PTL, PPROM, preeclampsia or intrauterine growth restriction (IUGR).

Table 3.3 Examples of secondary prevention screening strategies and interventions for women in whom screening reveals them to be at higher risk for preterm birth.

Screen for:	Intervention:
Prior preterm birth	17-OH Progesterone caproate or history-indicated cerclage
Multiple gestation with first trimester ultrasound	Chapter 16
Uterine anomalies	Surgical correction
Prior or current risk for preeclampsia, IUGR	Low dose aspirin, as indicated (Chapter 9)
Birth defects	Fetal therapy, where indicated
Short cervical length or asymptomatic cervical changes	Ultrasound-indicated cerclage or progesterone
Medical diseases (e.g. diabetes, hypertension, asthma)	Optimize medical condition
	Optimize drug therapy (minimizing teratogenicity)
Asymptomatic bacteriuria	Treat with antibiotics, confirm test of cure
Sexually transmitted infections	Treat with antibiotics, confirm test of cure
Bacterial vaginosis (especially with prior PPROM)	Treat with antibiotics, confirm test of cure
Domestic violence	Ensure woman's safety, direct toward social support
Substance abuse: tobacco, alcohol, drug use	Encourage, assist with reduction and cessation
Abnormal BMI (<19 or >25)	Optimize nutrition and exercise
Fetal fibronectin	Chapter 13
IVF with multiple embryos transferred	Neonatal ICU tour and MFM consultation
High order multiples	Selective reduction to two or less

Table 3.4 Examples of strategies aimed at tertiary prevention through commonly used interventions in hopes of preventing 'imminent' preterm birth in symptomatic women.

Tocolysis, acute and maintenance
Prolonged hospitalization
Antibiotics for PPROM
Bedrest, pelvic rest
Fluids (oral or intravenous hydration)
Exam-indicated cerclage
Pessary

The **greatest medical improvements for PTB** in the last half century have involved **ameliorating treatments** that don't decrease the actual rate of PTB (Table 3.5). Focusing on the women thought to be at highest risk for PTB, these interventions have played a crucial role in lowering the United States infant mortality rate from 26 per 1000 in 1960 to about 6 per 1000 today. As PTB screening tests are not ideal, women who are over-diagnosed (false positives) may receive unnecessary, costly and potentially harmful interventions. It may be better to err on the side of

Table 3.5 Examples of ameliorating therapies to improve outcomes with preterm birth.

Transport of mother to tertiary center with neonatal ICU and specialized OB care
Glucocorticosteroids for fetal lung maturity
Antibiotics for GBS prophylaxis
Neonatal ICU care

over-diagnosis and over-treatment rather than risking PTBs without these ameliorating interventions. Minimizing the number of PTBs that do not receive timely ameliorating interventions will require screening broader populations or more primary prevention.

If 'an ounce of prevention is worth a pound of cure', **why is more emphasis placed upon tertiary care** in Western medicine? PTB tertiary prevention care may be **easier to provide** than primary prevention. It is easier to think of trying to prevent PTB at the bedside of a contracting preterm woman with a progressively dilating cervix than the consistent effort needed to lower the national (and local) PTB rate when seeing healthy women without risk factors. Providers want to do something with immediate, tangible results. **Success is much easier to identify** with tertiary or secondary prevention than it is with primary prevention. Labor and delivery staff will congratulate themselves when a woman presents with contractions, receives tocolysis, and doesn't deliver immediately. Doctors will take credit after progesterone, cerclage, or prophylactic bedrest recommendations 'lead to' a term delivery. New parents don't credit primary prevention when they have their expected healthy term delivery. The **effectiveness of PTB primary prevention strategies is difficult to evaluate**, requiring large, expensive, difficult-to-perform population studies. There is more literature on tertiary prevention than on the primary prevention of PTB. Primary prevention involves more time (years) and variables before a potential PTB than the shorter time (hours to weeks) and less variables affecting a woman with PTL or PPROM (or preeclampsia or IUGR), in the process of preterm parturition. Finally, the United States health care system provides perverse incentives making **tertiary care more profitable** than primary prevention. More money is made by the healthcare industry on tests, procedures, and drugs for PTB than is made on primary prevention of PTB enacted by policy makers, communities, schools, and leaders.

Few would argue against primary prevention of PTB. Improving population health and health education is a daunting goal. Primary prevention of PTB requires more of a 'global will' to implement. We need to place more emphasis on the study and provision of primary prevention of PTB.

CHAPTER 4

The Epidemiology of Preterm Birth

Robert L. Goldenberg[1] *& Elizabeth M. McClure*[2]

[1] Department of Obstetrics and Gynecology, Drexel University College of Medicine, Philadelphia, USA, [2] Department of Epidemiology, University of North Carolina School of Public Health, and Department of Statistics and Epidemiology, Research Triangle Institute, North Carolina, USA

Key points

- The United States preterm birth (PTB) rate is one of the highest in the developed world.
- The PTB rate is rising in most developed countries.
- PTBs can be categorized as following spontaneous labor, preterm membrane rupture or a decision that the delivery is indicated.
- The rise in PTBs in the United States is mostly due to an increase in indicated PTBs and an increasing number of preterm multiple births.
- The increase in indicated PTBs is mostly occurring in late PTBs and may be due to the use of less stringent criteria for delivery at these gestational ages.
- Black women have twice as many PTBs and three to four times more early PTBs than women of other ethnic groups.
- A number of genital and systemic infections are associated with PTB.
- Chorioamnionitis is strongly associated with early PTB.

Introduction

Preterm birth (PTB) is associated with over 75% of all perinatal mortality and more than 50% of perinatal and long-term morbidity [1]. Although the vast majority of preterm newborns survive, even late PTBs have a significantly greater risk of mortality than infants born at term. In addition, studies of short- and long-term outcomes find significantly higher rates of neurodevelopmental morbidity, sensorineural impairments, and other disabilities (e.g. cerebral palsy, and visual, auditory and intellectual impairments), and higher rates of complications of the respiratory, gastrointestinal and renal systems [2] (Chapter 22). Also, recent epidemiologic evidence suggests that PTB is significantly and

Preterm Birth. Edited by Vincenzo Berghella.

independently associated with increased risk of several chronic degenerative diseases in adulthood (the so-called 'fetal programing of adult disease' proposition), including coronary heart disease, stroke, hypertension, and type II diabetes mellitus [3]. PTB is also a major economic burden. In the United States, it is estimated that about 40% ($6–10 billion per year) of all the expenditures on infant health care is related to prematurity [4, 5] even though only about 12–13% of all infants are born preterm [6].

Definitions

PTBs are those that occur at <37 weeks' gestational age [7]. However, the lower gestational age cutoff, or that used to distinguish a PTB from spontaneous abortion, varies by location. In some geographic areas including the United States, **20 weeks is used as the lower gestational age limit**, while in other areas, especially lower and middle income countries, 28 weeks (or even 1000g birth weight) is often used as the lower limit. A precise description of the lower gestational age cutoff is necessary if comparisons between PTB rates are to be made from one time period to another in the same geographic area, or between different geographic areas. In this chapter and in this book, PTB is defined as occurring between 20 0/7 and 36 6/7 weeks.

Preterm labor (PTL) is usually defined as regular contractions accompanied by cervical change at 20–36 6/7 weeks (Chapter 18). Preterm premature rupture of membranes (PPROM) is defined as spontaneous membrane rupture at 20–36 6/7 weeks at least one hour prior to onset of contractions (Chapter 19). Many women (50–70%) with apparent PTL stop contracting and go on to deliver at term. Most women with PPROM begin labor spontaneously within several days of membrane rupture, but a small proportion remains undelivered for weeks or months. The earlier the gestational age at PPROM, the more likely there will be an extended latency period to delivery. Risk factors for PPROM are generally similar to those for spontaneous PTL with intact membranes and will not be discussed separately [8].

In the United States, the PTB rate is 12–13%, whereas in Europe and other high income countries, PTB rates often vary between 5% and 9% [9]. The PTB rate has recently risen in most industrialized countries, with the United States rate increasing from 9.5% in 1981 to 12.7% in 2007 [9, 10] (Figure 4.1). This increase occurred despite advancing knowledge of risk factors and mechanisms related to PTL, and the introduction of numerous public health and medical interventions designed to reduce PTB [10].

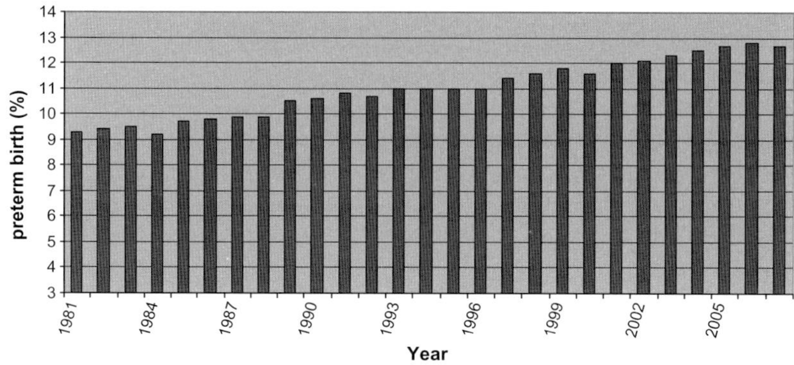

Figure 4.1 Incidence of preterm birth in the United States 1981–2007 (Data from Martin *et al.* [9]).

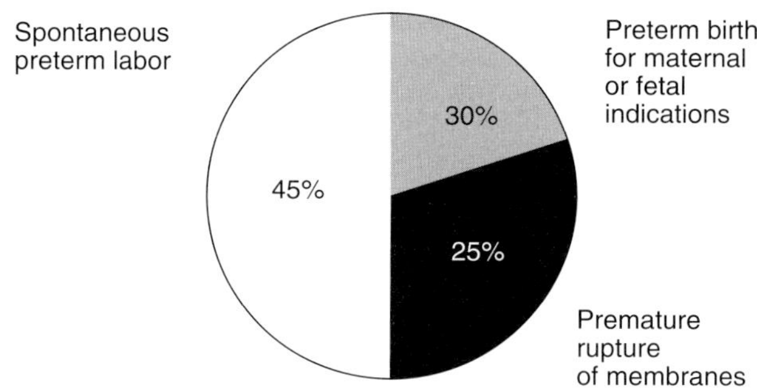

Figure 4.2 Obstetric precursors of preterm birth.

Types of preterm birth

The obstetric precursors leading to PTB include: (1) **spontaneous PTL with intact membranes**; (2) **PPROM regardless of whether delivery is vaginal or by Cesarean delivery**; and (3) **delivery for maternal or fetal indications** where labor is either induced or the infant delivered by pre-labor Cesarean delivery [11] (Figure 4.2). Common reasons for the decisions to undertake an indicated delivery include non-reassuring fetal testing, severe growth restriction and maternal preeclampsia and placental abruption. Those births following spontaneous PTL and PPROM together are often designated spontaneous PTBs. The relative contribution of these etiologies may differ by ethnic group. Preterm labor more commonly leads to PTB in white women, whereas PPROM is more common in black women [12].

PTBs can also be subdivided according to **gestational age**. About 5% occur at <28 weeks, about 12% at 28–31 weeks, about 13% at 32–33 weeks,

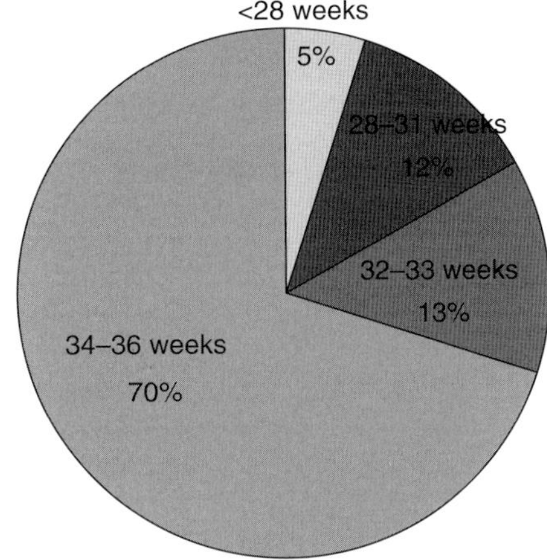

Figure 4.3 Gestational age distribution of all singleton preterm births in the United States.

and **about 70% at 34–36 weeks** [6, 7] (Figure 4.3). Differences in these numbers also are found in various ethnic groups. For example, black women appear to have a greater percentage of earlier gestational age PTBs.

Reasons for rate changes in preterm birth

In an analysis using United States vital statistics data, a large part of the increase in PTBs in singletons is explained by an increase in **indicated PTBs** [13] (Figure 4.4). Another reason is the considerable increase in PTBs associated with **multiple births** that occurs following the use of various **assisted reproductive techniques** [14]. Although the data are mixed, singleton infants conceived after in-vitro fertilization are also at greater risk for PTB [15]. Thus, PTBs coded as indicated and multiple births secondary to assisted reproductive technologies account for the vast majority of the increase in PTBs in the United States. In fact, **the increase in PTBs coded as indicated may be masking a smaller but important decrease in spontaneous PTBs, especially in black women** [13].

While in previous years most of the research and prevention efforts have been focused on the 20% of all preterm infants born at <32 weeks, more recently the **increasing number of late PTBs** — with their excess adverse outcomes compared with term births — has received more attention [16–19]. Why this increase is occurring is not clear, but there appears to be a trend toward delivering women early who have less severe complications that in previous years would not have led to an early delivery [19]. For example, a woman at 36 weeks with a blood pressure of 140/90, but no other signs of preeclampsia or non-reassuring fetal testing may be induced and signed out as an indicated PTB. As another example of the

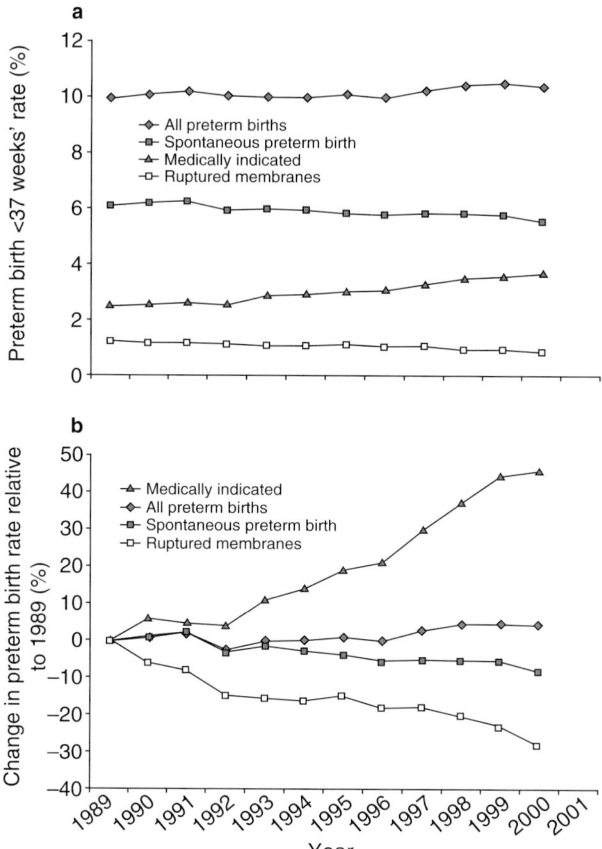

Figure 4.4 Temporal changes in preterm birth and those resulting from ruptured membranes, medically indicated and spontaneous PTB: United States, 1989–2000 (Reproduced from Ananth *et al.* [13] with permission from Lippincott Williams & Wilkins.).

difficulty in classifying deliveries as spontaneous or induced, a woman enters the hospital at 36 weeks with a history of contractions and a dilatation of 2 cm but is not contracting on admission. Oxytocin is started. She is signed out as spontaneous labor with augmentation. More than likely she would have delivered spontaneously at term if not 'augmented' electively at 36 weeks. The line dividing spontaneous PTBs from indicated PTB is not always clear; and indications for PTB are not uniform over time or across geographic areas [20]. In any case, evidence suggests that with the improved survival associated with newborn intensive care, both scenarios have become more common [19]. Thus, there are **many potential sources of bias in studies attempting to distinguish the obstetric origins of PTB**, especially those using administrative data bases as compared with chart review.

The etiology of preterm labor and PPROM

Both preterm labor and PPROM are now considered a syndrome initiated by multiple mechanisms including infection/inflammation, uteroplacental ischemia/hemorrhage, uterine overdistension, stress, and other immunologically mediated processes (see Figure 2.1) [21]. However, **a precise mechanism cannot be established in most cases**. Therefore, factors associated with PTB but not obviously in the causal pathway have been sought to explain PTL. It is postulated that, as occurs with other '**multifactorial**' disorders such as heart disease, an increasing number of risk factors interact to cause a transition from uterine quiescence toward PTL or PPROM [22].

Risk factors for preterm birth

Defining risk factors for prediction of PTB is a reasonable goal for several reasons. First, **identifying women at risk allows initiation of risk-specific treatment** [23]. Second, it may **define a population useful for studying particular interventions.** Finally, identifying risk factors may provide important **insights into mechanisms** leading to PTB. There are many maternal/fetal characteristics that have been associated with PTB, including maternal demographic characteristics, nutritional status, previous pregnancy history, current pregnancy characteristics, psychological characteristics, adverse behaviors, and infection [23] (Table 4.1). The most important examples of these factors are discussed below.

Previous pregnancy and gynecological history

The recurrence risk in women with a **prior PTB** ranges from 15% to more than 50%, depending on the number and gestational age of prior deliveries [24, 25]. Women with prior PTB have a 2.5-fold increased risk of PTB in their next pregnancy [24]. The earlier the gestational age, the greater the risk. Women with early spontaneous PTB are far more likely to have subsequent spontaneous PTBs, while women with indicated PTBs tend to repeat indicated PTBs [25]. Persistent or recurrent intrauterine infection likely explains many repetitive spontaneous PTBs [25]. The underlying condition causing an indicated PTB such as diabetes, hypertension or obesity, often persists between pregnancies. History of **cervical surgery** such as cone biopsy and LEEP procedures, multiple dilatation and evacuation (**D&Es**) procedures (for therapeutic or spontaneous terminations), diethylstilbestrol (**DES**) exposure, and various **anomalies of the uterus** are associated with PTB [26].

Table 4.1 Risk factors for preterm birth (PTB).

Prior obstetric/gynecologic history

- Prior PTB
- Cervical surgery (e.g. cone biopsy, LEEP, etc.)
- Multiple dilatations and evacuations
- Uterine anomalies

Maternal demographics

- <17, >35 years of age
- Less education (e.g. <12 grades)
- Single marital status
- Lower socioeconomic status
- Short inter-pregnancy interval (e.g. <6 months)
- Other social factors (e.g. poor access to care, physical abuse, acculturation)

Nutritional status/physical activity

- BMI < 19, or pre-pregnancy weight <50 kg (<120 lb)
- Poor nutritional status
- Long working hours (e.g. >80/week)
- Hard physical labor (e.g. shift work, standing >8 hours)

Current pregnancy characteristics

- Assisted reproductive techniques (e.g. IVF)
- Multiple gestations
- Fetal disease (e.g. chromosome anomaly, structural abnormality, growth restriction, death, etc.)
- Vaginal bleeding (e.g. first and second trimester, placenta previa, abruption)
- Poly- or oligohydramnios
- Maternal medical conditions (e.g. hypertension, diabetes, thyroid disease, asthma, etc.)
- Maternal abdominal surgery
- Psychological (e.g. stress, depression)
- Adverse behaviors
  - Smoking (e.g. tobacco)
  - Heavy alcohol consumption
  - Cocaine
  - Heroin
- Infection
  - Bacterial vaginosis
  - Trichomoniasis
  - Chlamydia
  - Gonorrhea
  - Syphylis
  - Urinary tract infection (e.g. asymptomatic bacteriuria, pyelonephritis)
  - Severe viral infections
  - Intrauterine infections
- Short cervical length between 14 and 28 weeks
- Positive fFN between 22 and 34 weeks
- Uterine contractions

Maternal demographic characteristics

In the United States and Great Britain, women classified as **black**, African-American and Afro-Caribbean are consistently found to be at higher risk for PTB. PTB rates in the range of 16–18% are often reported compared with 5–9% for white women. Black women are also three to four times more likely to have a very early PTB than are women from other racial or ethnic groups, with at least part of this discrepancy explained by higher rates of vaginal and intrauterine infections [27–30] (Figure 4.5). Also, the distribution of early black PTBs across metropolitan areas does not overlap those of white or Hispanic women [31] (Figure 4.6). Part of the discrepancy in PTB rates between the United States and other countries is likely explained by the high rate of PTB in the United States black population. Over time, the disparity in PTB between black and white women has remained largely unchanged and unexplained [32]. East Asian and Hispanic women typically have lower PTB rates. Women from south Asia including the Indian subcontinent have very high rates of low-birth weight mostly due to decreased fetal growth, but it is not clear if PTB is substantially increased (see also Chapter 1). Women **younger than 17 or older than 35** also are at higher risk of PTB. **Less education, single marital status and lower socioeconomic status** are also risk factors, although they probably are not independent of one other [33, 34].

Whether the differences in demographic or social or economic risks explain the high PTB rates in the United States relative to other developed nations or whether the frequent lack of health insurance and the absence of a strong supportive economic and social safety net contribute to this disparity is unknown (Table 4.2). It is also not clear if lower gestational age cutoffs for defining PTB used in the United States explain part of the

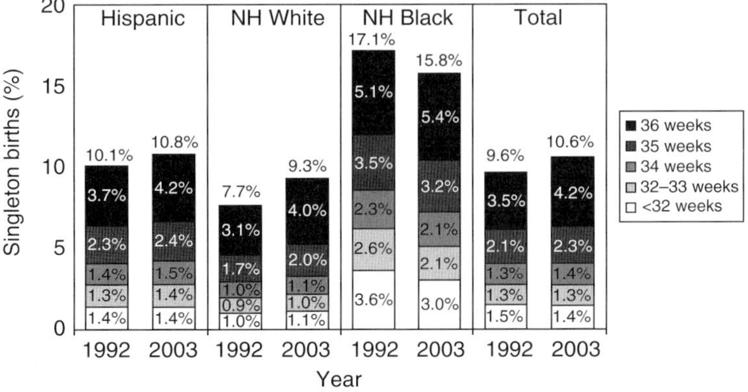

Figure 4.5 Comparison of singleton preterm birthrates by gestational age and ethnicity, 1992 and 2003 (Source [7]). NH, non-Hispanic.

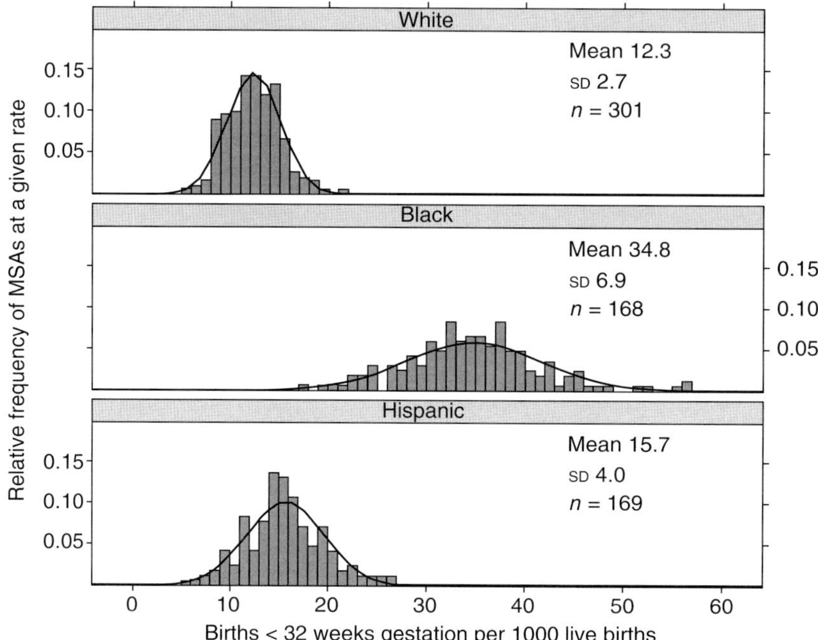

Figure 4.6 Rates of very preterm birth in United States metropolitan statistical areas (MSA) by race, 2002–2004 (source: National Center for Health Statistics Natality Files, 2002–2004; Singleton live births).

Table 4.2 Possible reasons for high incidence of preterm birth (PTB) in the United States.

- Lower gestational age criteria (in some areas, any fetus with movement, respirations or a heartbeat, regardless of gestational age is designated a PTB)
- High number of indicated PTBs
- Multiple births resulting from high incidence of assisted reproductive technology and the high numbers of embryos transferred in IVF
- High incidence of PTB in black women
- Wide disparities in socioeconomic status
- Relatively low levels of government economic and other support for pregnant women

difference. What does seem reasonably clear, however, is that among many United States immigrant groups, the greater the length of time living in the United States, the higher the PTB rate (acculturation effect) [35].

Pregnancies occurring within close temporal proximity to a previous delivery have an increased risk for PTB [36, 37]. An **inter-pregnancy interval less than 6 months** confers more than a twofold increased risk

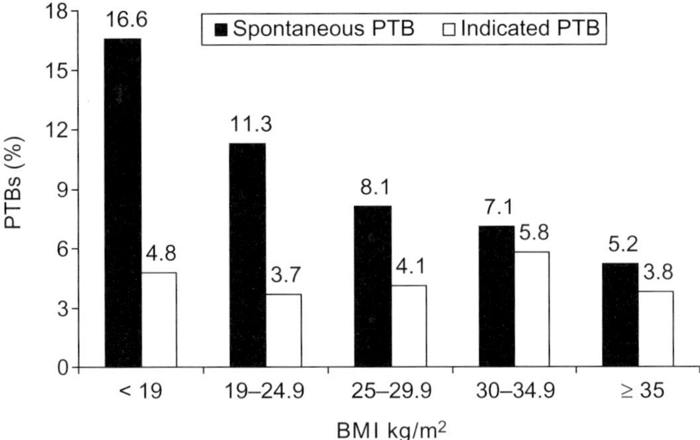

Figure 4.7 Spontaneous and indicated PTB by maternal body mass index (BMI) (Adapted from Hendler *et al.* [38]).

of PTB after adjusting for confounding variables [37]. While the mechanism is not clear, one potential explanation is that the uterus takes time to return to its normal state, including resolution of the 'inflammatory status' associated with the previous pregnancy. 'Maternal depletion' may be another cause since pregnancy consumes maternal stores of essential vitamins (such as folic acid), minerals and amino acids. A short interval decreases the opportunity to replenish these nutrients.

Nutritional status and physical activity

Nutritional status during pregnancy can be described by indicators of body size such as body mass index (BMI), nutritional intake and serum assessments for various analytes [38–42]. For example, a **low pre-pregnancy BMI** is associated with higher risks of spontaneous PTB, while obesity may be protective [38] (Figure 4.7). Women with low serum iron, folate or zinc levels have more PTBs than those with measurements in the normal range [39]. There are several mechanisms by which nutritional status may be related to PTB. For example, maternal thinness is associated with decreased blood volume and less uterine blood flow, with spontaneous PTB occurring via this mechanism [40]. Thin women also consume less vitamins and minerals, low levels of which are associated with decreased blood flow as well as increased maternal infections [41]. Obese women are more likely to have infants with congenital anomalies such as neural tube defects; these infants are more likely to be delivered preterm [42]. They are also more likely to develop preeclampsia and diabetes and have indicated PTBs associated with these conditions.

Observational studies involving **type of work and physical activity** have produced conflicting results related to PTB [43–45]. Evaluation of work-related risk is made difficult by confounding factors such as race and socioeconomic status. However, even after accounting for population differences, it appears that working long hours and performing hard physical labor under stressful conditions are likely to be associated with an increase in PTB risk. The level of physical activity, on the other hand, is not consistently related to the risk of PTB. In fact, moderate exercise is usually associated with lower risks of PTB compared with no exercise.

Current pregnancy characteristics

Multiple gestations carry a substantial risk of PTB [46]. Accounting for only 2–3% of infants, they are responsible for 15–20% of all PTBs. Nearly 60% of twins are born preterm. Approximately 40% of twins will have spontaneous labor or PPROM prior to 37 weeks, with others having an indicated PTB because of preeclampsia or other maternal or fetal conditions. Nearly all higher order multiple gestations deliver preterm.

Vaginal bleeding caused by placental abruption or previa is associated with a very high risk for PTB, but first and second-trimester bleeding not associated with either condition are also significantly associated with subsequent PTB [47]. Extremes in the **volume of amniotic fluid** — polyhydramnios or oligohydramnios — are associated with PTL and PPROM. **Maternal medical conditions** including thyroid disease, asthma, diabetes and hypertension, as well as maternal abdominal surgery, are associated with higher rates of PTB, many of which are indicated due to maternal complications.

Psychological characteristics

Mothers experiencing high levels of psychological or social **stress** are at increased risk for PTB (generally < twofold) even after adjusting for the effects of sociodemographic, medical, and behavioral risk factors [48–59]. Furthermore, exposure to objectively stressful conditions such as housing instability and severe material hardship has also been associated with PTB [50]. Clinical depression during pregnancy has been reported in up to 16% of women with up to 35% having some depressive symptoms [51]. There is an association (risks generally increased < twofold) between depression and PTB [52, 53]. Depression is associated with an increase in smoking, drug and alcohol use, and the relationship between depression and PTB may be mediated by these behaviors [54]. Nevertheless, in some studies that adjusted for these behaviors, the association between depression and PTB persisted, suggesting that this relationship may be due to more than confounding.

Adverse behaviors

In the United States, approximately 20–25% of pregnant women smoke and of these, 12–15% continue throughout pregnancy [55, 56]. **Tobacco**

use increases risk for PTB (<2.0 fold) after adjustment for other factors [56]. While heavy alcohol consumption has been associated with PTB, mild or moderate **alcohol** use is not generally considered a risk factor for PTB. **Cocaine and heroin** use have been associated with PTB in a number of studies.

Infection

Bacterial vaginosis (BV) is associated with PTB, and covered in detail in Chapter 14.

Whether other genital infections are causally associated with PTB is not always clear [57, 58] (Chapter 15). For many infections, a range of associations has been reported, varying from none to strong. Women with these infections commonly have other risk factors and many studies have not considered confounding variables. Nevertheless, **trichomoniasis** seems to be associated with PTB with a relative risk of about 1.3 [59]. **Chlamydia** is likely associated with PTB only in the presence of a maternal immune response, and most likely with a relative risk of about 2 [60]. **Syphilis** and **gonorrhea** are likely associated with PTB with a relative risk of about 2 [61]. Vaginal Group B *Streptococcus, Ureaplasma urealyticum* and *Mycoplasma hominis* colonizations are not associated with increased risk for PTB [57, 58].

Several **non-genital tract infections** such as pyelonephritis and asymptomatic bacteriuria, pneumonia and appendicitis are associated with and probably causal for PTB [57, 58, 62]. Recently, periodontal disease has received extensive scrutiny with some case-control studies suggesting increased risk independent of other factors [63–65].

In comparison with bacterial infections, the evidence that maternal **viral infections** are causal for PTB is sparse. However, when the mother is severely ill, such as with varicella pneumonia or severe acute respiratory syndrome (SARS), a PTB may occur [66]. In several studies where asymptomatic women undergoing genetic amniocentesis were evaluated for intra-amniotic viral infection using PCR techniques, a number of viral DNAs were identified in the amniotic fluid, but they were generally unrelated to subsequent PTB [67]. Therefore, it seems unlikely that maternal viral infection plays an important role in PTB, but controversy persists [68].

Intrauterine infection is a frequent and important mechanism leading to PTB [69]. Microbiologic studies suggest that intrauterine infection may account for 25–40% of PTB [69]. However, this may be a minimal estimate because intrauterine infection is difficult to detect with conventional culture techniques and using molecular microbiologic techniques, several investigators have demonstrated additional microbial footprints in the amniotic cavity [70, 71]. Furthermore, since the rate of microbial colonization of the chorioamnion is twice that observed in the amniotic cavity, basing rates of intrauterine infection only on amniotic fluid cultures substantially underestimates the level of association [72]. Importantly, the earlier the gestational age at which women present with PTL, the higher the frequency of intrauterine infection/inflammation [69, 73, 74]. At 21–24 weeks, most spontaneous births are associated with histologic chorioamnionitis compared with about 10% at 35–36 weeks [73]. Bacteria in the membranes and an associated inflammatory response in the amniotic fluid have been demonstrated in more than 80% of women in early preterm labor with intact membranes delivered by Cesarean section; thus this infection is likely causal for PTB [69].

Conclusion

PTB is a common pregnancy outcome associated with much of the pregnancy-related mortality and short and long-term morbidity in infants and children. PTB is far more common in black women than other racial/ethnic groups. Other important risk factors include multiple pregnancy, prior PTB, and maternal thinness. Maternal infection/inflammation, especially of the chorioamnion, is associated with the majority of early spontaneous PTBs. **The list of risk factors for PTB in Table 4.1 should be reviewed with each woman of reproductive age, and each pregnant woman**. As will be seen in subsequent chapters, only by identifying risk factors can appropriate risk-specific interventions be applied. Additional research that defines the mechanisms by which risk factors are related to PTB is crucial. Better understanding of these mechanisms should allow clinicians to design appropriate interventions so that the incidence of PTB and related fetal and neonatal morbidity and mortality will be reduced.

References

1 McCormick MC. The contribution of low birth weight to infant mortality and childhood morbidity. N Engl J Med 1985; 312: 82–90.
2 Saigal S, Doyle LW. An overview of mortality and sequelae of preterm birth from infancy to adulthood. Lancet 2008; 371: 261–9.
3 Barker DJ. The fetal and infant origin of disease. Eur J Clin Invest 1995; 25: 457–63.
4 Russell RB, Green NS, Steiner CA, *et al.* Cost of hospitalization for preterm and low birth weight infants in the United States. Pediatrics 2007; 120; e1–e9
5 St John EB, Nelson KG, Cliver SP, *et al.* Cost of neonatal care according to gestational age at birth and survival status. Am J Obstet Gynecol 2000; 182: 170–5.
6 Goldenberg RL, Culhane JF, Iams JD, Romero R. Epidemiology and causes of preterm birth. Lancet 2008; 371: 75–84.

7 Raju TNK. Epidemiology of late (near-term) preterm births. Clin Perinatol 2006; 33: 751–63.
8 Guinn DA, Goldenberg RL, Hauth JC, *et al.* Risk factors for the development of preterm premature rupture of the membranes after arrest of preterm labor. Am J Obstet Gynecol 1995; 173: 1310–5.
9 Martin JA, Kochanek KD, Strobino DM, *et al.* Annual summary of vital statistics–2003. Pediatrics 2005; 115: 619–34.
10 Goldenberg RL, Rouse DJ. The prevention of premature birth. N Engl J Med 1998; 339: 313–20.
11 Tucker JM, Goldenberg RL, Davis RO, *et al.* Etiologies of preterm birth in an indigent population: is prevention a logical expectation? Obstet Gynecol 1991; 77: 343–7.
12 Ananth CV, Vintzileos AM. Epidemiology of preterm birth and its clinical subtypes. J Matern Fetal Neonatal Med 2006; 19: 773–82.
13 Ananth CV, Joseph KS, Oyelese Y, *et al.* Trends in preterm birth and perinatal mortality among singletons: United States, 1989 through 2000. Obstet Gynecol 2005; 105: 1084–91.
14 Kuehn BM. Groups take aim at US preterm birth rate. J Am Med Assoc 2006; 296: 2907–8.
15 Jackson RA, Gibson KA, Wu YW, Croughan MS. Perinatal outcomes in singletons following in vitro fertilization: a meta-analysis. Obstet Gynecol 2004; 103: 551–63.
16 Fuchs K, Gyamfi C. The influence of obstetric practices on late prematurity. Clin Perinatol 2008; 35: 343–60.
17 Bastek JA, Sammel MD, Pare E, *et al.* Adverse neonatal outcomes: examining the risks between preterm, late preterm, and term infants. Am J Obstet Gynecol 2008; 1999: 367: e1–18.
18 Khashu M, Narayanan M, Bhargava S, Osiovich H. Perinatal outcomes associated with preterm birth at 33 to 36 weeks' gestation: a population based cohort study. Pediatrics 2009;123: 109–13.
19 Fuchs K, Wapner R. Elective Cesarean section and induction and their impact on late preterm births. Clin Perinatol 2006; 33: 793–801.
20 Klebanoff MA. Conceptualizing categories of preterm. Prenatal Neonatal Med 1998; 3: 13–15.
21 Romero R, Espinoza J, Kusanovic J, *et al.* The preterm parturition syndrome. Br J Obstet Gynaecol 2006; 113: 17–42.
22 Iams J, Romero R, Culhane JF, Goldenberg RL. The prevention of preterm birth. Lancet 2008; 371: 164–75.
23 Goldenberg RL, Goepfert AR, Ramsey PS. Biochemical markers for the prediction of preterm birth. Am J Obstet Gynecol 2005; 192: S36–46.
24 Mercer BM, Goldenberg RL, Moawad AH, *et al.* The preterm prediction study: effect of gestational age and cause of preterm birth on subsequent obstetric outcome. National Institute of Child Health and Human Development Maternal-Fetal Medicine Units Network. Am J Obstet Gynecol 1999; 181: 1216–21.
25 Goldenberg RL, Andrews WW, Faye-Petersen O, *et al.* The Alabama Preterm Birth Project: placental histology in recurrent spontaneous and indicated preterm birth. Am J Obstet Gynecol 2006; 195: 792–6.
26 Jakobsson M, Gissler M, Sainio S, *et al.* Preterm delivery after surgical treatment for cervical intraepithelial neoplasia. Obstet Gynecol 2007; 109: 309–13.
27 Fiscella, K. Race, perinatal outcome, and amniotic infection. Obstet Gynecol Surv 1996; 51: 60–6.
28 Fiscella K. Racial disparities in preterm births. The role of urogenital infections. Public Health Rep 1996; 111: 104–13.

29 Goldenberg RL, Cliver SP, Mulvihill FX, *et al.* Medical, psychosocial, and behavioral risk factors do not explain the increased risk for low birth weight among black women. Am J Obstet Gynecol 1996; 175: 1317–24.
30 Goldenberg RL, Klebanoff MA, Nugent R, *et al.* Bacterial colonization of the vagina during pregnancy in four ethnic groups. Am J Obstet Gynecol 1996; 175: 1317–24.
31 Kramer MR, Hogue C. Place matters: variation in the black/white very preterm birth rate across US Metropolitan Areas, 2002–2004. Public Health Reports 2008; 123: 576–85.
32 Collins JW, Jr, Hawkes EK. Racial differences in post-neonatal mortality in Chicago: what risk factors explain the black infant's disadvantage? Ethn Health 1997; 2: 117–25.
33 Smith LK, Draper ES, Manktelow BN, *et al.* Socioeconomic inequalities in very preterm birth rates. Arch Dis Child Fetal Neonatal Ed 2007; 92: F11–4.
34 Thompson JM, Irgens LM, Rasmussen S, Daltveit AK. Secular trends in socio-economic status and the implications for preterm birth. Paediatr Perinat Epidemiol 2006; 20: 182–7.
35 Wingate MS, Alexander GR. The healthy migrant theory: variations in pregnancy outcomes among US-born migrants. Soc Sci Med 2006; 62: 491–8.
36 Conde-Agudelo A, Rosas-Bermudez A, Kafury-Goeta AC. Birth spacing and risk of adverse perinatal outcomes: a meta-analysis. JAMA 2006; 295: 1809–23.
37 Smith GC, Pell JP, Dobbie R. Interpregnancy interval and risk of preterm birth and neonatal death: retrospective cohort study. BMJ 2003; 327: 313–18.
38 Hendler I, Goldenberg RL, Mercer BM, *et al.* The Preterm Prediction Study: association between maternal body mass index (BMI) and spontaneous preterm birth. Am J Obstet Gynecol 2005; 192: 882–6.
39 Tamura T, Goldenberg RL, Freeberg LE, *et al.* Maternal serum folate and zinc concentrations and their relationship to pregnancy outcome. Am J Clin Nutr 1992; 56: 365–70.
40 Neggers Y, Goldenberg RL. Some thoughts on body mass index, micronutrient intakes and pregnancy outcome. J Nutr 2003; 133: 1737S–40S.
41 Goldenberg RL. The plausibility of micronutrient deficiency in relationship to perinatal infection. J Nutr 2003; 133: 1645S–8S.
42 Goldenberg RL, Tamura T. Prepregnancy weight and pregnancy outcome. JAMA 1996; 275: 1127–8.
43 Saurel-Cubizolles MJ, Zeitlin J, Lelong N, *et al.* for the Europop Group. Employment, working conditions, and preterm birth: results from the Europop case-control survey. J Epidemiol Community Health 2004; 58: 395–401.
44 Pompeii LA, Savitz DA, Evenson KR, *et al.* Physicial exertion at work and the risk of preterm delivery and small-for-gestational-age birth. Obstet Gynecol 2005; 106: 1279–88.
45 Newman RB, Goldenberg RL, Moawad AH, *et al.* Occupational fatigue and preterm premature rupture of membranes. Am J Obstet Gynecol 2001; 184: 438–46.
46 Lee YM, Cleary-Goldman J, D'Alton ME. The impact of multiple gestations on late preterm (near-term) births. Clin Perinatol 2006; 33: 777–92
47 Krupa, FG, Faltin D, Cecatti JG, *et al.* Predictors of preterm birth. Int J Gynaecol Obstet 2006; 94: 5–11.
48 Copper RL, Goldenberg RL, Das A, *et al.* The preterm prediction study: maternal stress is associated with spontaneous preterm birth at less than thirty-five weeks gestation. National Institute of Child Health and Human Development Maternal-Fetal Medicine Units Network. Am J Obstet Gynecol 1996; 175: 1286–92.

49 Lobel M, Dunkerl-Schetter C, Scrimshaw SC. Prenatal maternal stress and prematurity: a prospective study of socioeconomically disadvantaged women. Health Psychology 1992; 11: 32–40.

50 Farley TA, Mason K, Rice J, *et al.* The relationship between the neighbourhood environment and adverse birth outcomes. Paediatr Perinat Epidemiol 2006; 20: 188–200.

51 Orr ST, Miller CA. Maternal depressive symptoms and the risk of poor pregnancy outcome: review of the literature and preliminary findings. Epidemiol Rev 1995; 17: 165–71.

52 Dayan J, Creveuil C, Marks MN, *et al.* Prenatal depression, prenatal anxiety, and spontaneous preterm birth: a prospective cohort study among women with early and regular care. Psychosom Med 2006; 68: 938–46.

53 Orr ST, James SA, Prince CB. Maternal prenatal depressive symptoms and spontaneous preterm births among African-American women in Baltimore, Maryland. Am J Epidemiol 2002; 156: 797–802.

54 Zuckerman B, Amaro H, Bauchner H, Cabral H. Depressive symptoms during pregnancy: relationship to poor health behaviors. Am J Obstet Gynecol 1989; 160: 1107–11.

55 Ebrahim SH, Floyd RL, Merritt RK, *et al.* Trends in pregnancy related smoking rates in the United States, 1987–1996. JAMA 2000; 283: 361–6.

56 Cnattingius S. The epidemiology of smoking during pregnancy: smoking prevalence, maternal characteristics, and pregnancy outcomes. Nicotine Tob Res 2004; 6: S125–40.

57 Goldenberg RL, Culhane JF, Johnson DC. Maternal infection and adverse fetal and neonatal outcomes. Clin Perinatol 2005; 32: 523–59.

58 Goldenberg RL, Andrews WW, Yuan AC, *et al.* Sexually transmitted diseases and adverse outcomes of pregnancy. Clin Perinatol 1997; 24: 23–41.

59 Cotch MF, Pastorek JG 2nd, Nugent RP, *et al.* Trichomonas vaginalis associated with low birth weight and preterm delivery. Sex Transm Dis 1997; 24: 353–60.

60 Sweet RL, Landers DL, Walker C, *et al.* Chlamydia trachomatis infection and pregnancy outcome. Am J Obstet Gynecol 1987; 156: 824–33.

61 Donders GG, Desmyter J, De Wet DH, *et al.* The association of gonorrhea and syphilis with premature birth and low birth weight. Genitourin Med 1993; 69: 98–101.

62 Romero R, Oyarzun E, Mazor M, *et al.* Meta-analysis of the relationship between asymptomatic bacteriuria and preterm delivery/low birth weight. Obstet Gynecol 1989; 73: 576–82.

63 Offenbacher S, Katz V, Fertik G, *et al.* Periodontal infection as a possible risk factor for preterm low birth weight. J Periodontol 1996; 67: 1103–13.

64 Jeffcoat MK, Geurs NC, Reddy MS, *et al.* Periodontal infection and preterm birth: results of a prospective study. J Am Dent Assoc 2001; 132: 875–80.

65 Goepfert AR, Jeffcoat M, Andrews WW, *et al.* Periodontal disease and upper genital tract inflammation in early spontaneous preterm birth. Am J Obstet Gynecol 2004; 104: 777–83.

66 Hardy JMB, Azarowicz EN, Mannini A, *et al.* The effect of Asian influenza on the outcome of pregnancy. Baltimore 1957–1958. Am J Public Health 1961; 51: 1182–8.

67 Wenstrom KD, Andrews WW, Bowles NE, *et al.* Intrauterine viral infection at the time of second trimester genetic amniocentesis. Obstet Gynecol 1998; 92: 420–4.

68 Srinivas SK, Ma Y, Sammel MD, *et al.* Placental inflammation and viral infection are implicated in second trimester pregnancy loss. Am J Obstet Gynecol 2006; 195: 797–802.

69 Goldenberg RL, Hauth JC, Andrews WW. Intrauterine infection and preterm delivery. N Engl J Med 2000; 342: 1500–7.
70 Jalava J, Mantymaa ML, Ekblad U, *et al.* Bacterial 16S rDNA polymerase chain reaction in the detection of intra-amniotic infection. Br J Obstet Gynaecol 1996; 103: 664–9.
71 Gardella C, Riley DE, Hitti J, *et al.* Identification and sequencing of bacterial rDNAs in culture-negative amniotic fluid from women in premature labor. Am J Perinatol 2004; 21: 319–23.
72 Cassell G, Andrews W, Hauth J, *et al.* Isolation of microorganisms from the chorioamnion is twice that from amniotic fluid at Cesarean delivery in women with intact membranes. Am J Obstet Gynecol 1993; 168: 424.
73 Russell P. Inflammatory lesions of the human placenta. I. Clinical significance of acute chorioamnionitis. Diagn Gynecol Obstet 1979; 1: 127–37.
74 Watts DH, Krohn MA, Hillier SL, *et al.* The association of occult amniotic fluid infection with gestational age and neonatal outcome among women in preterm labor. Obstet Gynecol 1992; 79: 351–7.

CHAPTER 5

Genetics of Preterm Birth

Heidi L. Thorson & Hyagriv N. Simhan
Division of Maternal-Fetal Medicine, Department of Obstetrics, Gynecology and Reproductive Sciences, University of Pittsburgh, Pittsburgh School of Medicine, USA

Key points

- Familial correlations in gestational length may be associated with fetal genes, of either maternal or paternal origin, as well as maternal genetic factors.
- Consistency in birth timing suggests that some factors remain stable from one pregnancy to the next. These factors may be both genetic and/or environmental.
- Correlations between siblings indicate that fetal genetic factors explain 11% of the variation in gestational age at delivery and maternal genetic factors explain 14% of the variation.
- Racial disparities in preterm birth cannot be fully explained by difference in socioeconomic status or maternal habits.
- Genetic variation in inflammatory response can affect birth timing.
- Gene expression can be modified by environmental factors.

Introduction

Preterm birth (PTB) is a complex disease characterized by multiple pathways (Figure 2.1), likely resulting from **multigene interactions, both maternal and fetal, as well as gene–environment interactions**. Recently, genetic research has shifted from single-gene disorders to multigene diseases, like PTB, resulting from complex polygenic inheritance. The complexity of PTB is the result of human genetic variation dictated by individual differences in our DNA.

Genetic contributions to PTB — epidemiologic evidence

PTB — complex phenotypic trait

When studying complex diseases it is important to **use a precise and standardized definition of the phenotype**; PTB — delivery between

Preterm Birth. Edited by Vincenzo Berghella.

16 weeks and 36 6/7 weeks gestation. PTB is often broadly thought of in three main categories: (1) preterm labor (PTL) leading to PTB (idiopathic); (2) preterm premature rupture of membranes (PPROM); and (3) medically indicated (iatrogenic) PTB (Figure 4.1) The focus of this chapter is on the first two categories of PTB, commonly referred to, collectively, as spontaneous PTB (SPTB).

In discussing genetic diseases it is impossible to ignore the simple Mendelian Laws of inheritance. Ehlers-Danlos syndrome (EDS) is one example of a group of Mendelian disorders that affects connective tissue and is linked to PTB secondary to PPROM [1]. It is mostly inherited in an autosomal dominant fashion although autosomal recessive patterns also exist. As an autosomal dominant disease it is unclear whether it is maternal or fetal factors influencing the risk for PPROM. Although EDS follows Mendelian inheritance, customarily, we **conceptualize PTB as a complex disease that does not follow Mendelian inheritance**.

Recurrence of PTB

The genetic heterogeneity of SPTB, like that of many complex diseases, makes it difficult to interpret and identify genetic influences. The first step is to identify the epidemiologic evidence suggestive of a genetic predisposition to PTB. One of the strongest risk factors for PTB is a prior PTB. Women with a prior SPTB carry a 2.5-fold increased risk of a subsequent spontaneous preterm delivery (95% CI, 1.9–3.2) [2]. The risk of PTB <37 weeks in the current pregnancy increases with decreasing gestational age of the earliest PTB. The risk of PTB also seems to increase with the number of prior consecutive PTBs [3]. Forty-nine percent of women with recurrent PTB deliver within one week of the previous PTB and 70% deliver within in two weeks [4]. **The consistency in birth timing suggests that some factors remain constant across pregnancies that may influence the timing of delivery. Factors that remain stable over time could be both genetic and environmental**.

Familiality of PTB

Familiality of PTB has been explored in intergenerational studies and studies of offspring in twins. Epidemiologists are able to use recurrence patterns of PTB in families across generations to assess genetic contributions. **Familial correlations in gestational length may be associated with fetal genes, of either maternal or paternal origin, as well as maternal genetic factors** [5]. Population-based twin and birth registries in Sweden provide insight into genetic effects of gestational length. **PTB concordance rates among twins were 0.22 for monozygotic twins** and 0.11 for dizygotic twins [5]. As one would expect the **higher concord-**

ance rate for monozygotic twins suggests a genetic component. When PTB was examined as a dichotomous variable, the heritability index is estimated at 36% and when examined as a continuous variable the heritability index was 31% [5]. An additional study supports this finding that heritable factors accounts for 27% of any PTB, and 17% if the PTB occurs in the first pregnancy [6].

Parent–offspring data was obtained from the Medical Birth Registry of Norway for the analysis of gestational age. Correlations between full siblings and half siblings indicate that **fetal genetic factors explain 11% of the variation in gestational age at delivery and maternal genetic factors explain 14% of the variation** [7]. In the Swedish birth registry, women whose sisters gave birth prematurely were at increased risk of delivering prematurely themselves (OR = 1.94; 95% CI 1.26–2.99) [8]. Using the Missouri Department of Health's maternally linked birth certificate database, the infant was identified as the proband and the risk to siblings delivering preterm investigated. The analysis was used to estimate the sibling risk ratio, λ_s, and sib-sib OR. Individuals whose older siblings were delivered preterm were at significantly greater risk for PTB than those whose older siblings were unaffected, λ_s was 4.3 (95% CI 4.0–4.6) and sib-sib adjusted OR 4.2 (95% CI 3.9–4.5) for all races [9]. The magnitude of λ_s reflects the mode of genetic etiology; for complex disorders, values range from 1.3 to 75. In contrast, Mendelian disorders show values of the magnitude greater than 500, indicating a more pure single gene influence. These comparisons between full and half siblings use the degree of genetic relatedness to estimate the relative importance of genetic versus environmental factors. However, familial aggregation is not enough to suggest a genetic influence as families share both genes and environments. The utility of these measures lies in establishing the family aggregation of disorders.

Maternal factors and PTB

A mother's gestational age at birth has an impact on the timing of her deliveries. A large Utah cohort comprised of parental birth records and offspring birth records were examined. In this cohort, 29 247 white women gave birth to 100 335 offspring. The distribution of gestational ages of the offspring born to women who themselves were born preterm earlier than that of women who were born at term. The frequency of preterm offspring compared with term offspring was 9.3% versus 4.4%; $P = 0.025$ at 36 completed weeks. As mothers' gestational age decreased at birth, the OR for PTB of her own offspring significantly increased, indicating an inverse relationship. They found that for women whom themselves were born preterm their risk of delivering preterm increased by nearly 20% [10]. Additional studies had similar findings that mothers born preterm had a relative risk of PTB of 1.54 (95% CI 1.42–1.67) and this association increased if the mother was born earlier <35 weeks (RR = 1.85, 95% CI: 1.52–2.27) [11].

Paternal factors and PTB

Evidence for paternal impact on PTB is conflicting. The genetic influences on PTB may include fetal genes paternally imprinted which control placental and membrane growth. Since the function of the placenta and fetal membranes can influence pregnancy outcome, fetal genes controlling these tissues may play a role in PTB. However, imprinted genes are relatively rare [12]. In a cohort from Norway, there was no significant contribution of paternal family history to risk of PTB [11], although previous studies have shown changing partners between pregnancies may reduce the risk for PTB [13, 14]. There were similar findings in a Danish population, where the change in female partner decreased the risk of PTB, suggesting a minimal impact of paternal genes on PTB [15]. In addition, unlike the correlation of maternal gestational age at delivery with PTB, paternal gestational age at birth does not significantly correlate with risk of PTB for his offspring [11].

Genetic basis for racial disparity in PTB

There is a predisposition for PTB among African-Americans when compared with Caucasians. This predisposition has often been confounded by **socioeconomic status**. However, **even when adjusting for these factors, an increased risk of PTB persisted among African-Americans** in an Alabama population [16]. Overall, African-Americans have a 3.5 times increased risk for PTB when compared with Caucasians, which cannot be fully explained by differences in socioeconomic status or maternal habits [16–19]. In addition, African-Americans have a higher rate of recurrent PTB than Caucasians [20]. Maternal and paternal ethnicity also plays a role in PTB. An increased risk of PTB <35 weeks (OR = 1.28, 95% CI 1.13–1.46) has been reported when the mother was Caucasian and the father African-American [21] and is confirmed in a cohort of more than 2.8 million singleton births [22].

Genetic contributions in pathways leading to PTB

Genetic variation in inflammatory response

Inflammatory response in both maternal and fetal tissues has been intensely studied as a pathway to PTB (Chapter 7). This response, mediated through the production of various pro- and anti-inflammatory cytokines, has been the primary interest in many recent studies. Single nucleotide polymorphisms (SNPs) are often found in the regulatory portion of genes therefore increasing or decreasing the production of these cytokines. Tumor necrosis factor-alpha has been the most widely studied gene and studies have shown conflicting results. The polymorphism at position −308 in the promoter region was initially associated with an increased risk of SPTB [23, 24] (Table 5.1) but a recent meta-analysis reviewing seven studies of this polymorphism found additional negative evidence [25]. Another study found that although the −308 promoter polymorphism was not significantly associated with idiopathic PTB it was associated with PPROM OR 3.18 (1.33–7.83) which leads to preterm delivery [26] (Table 5.1). Conflicting results may be the result of different patient populations. However, this information about various haplotypes of multiple polymorphisms may be more informative than individual polymorphisms. Studies into the TNF receptors 1 and 2 may also provide insight into PTB [27].

Interleukin 6 (IL-6) is a pro-inflammatory cytokine that has been implicated in the pathophysiology of infection- and inflammation-related PTB. Significant differences were found between AA (African Americans) and EA (Caucasians) in allele and genotype frequencies in the IL-6 and IL-6R for maternal and fetal samples [28]. Further investigation examined 30 polymorphisms in the IL-6 and IL-6R for association of IL-6 in the amniotic fluid, and for IL-6 and IL-6R SNPs for association with PTB [29] (Table 5.1). There was substantial evidence for linkage disequilibrium in IL-6 of Caucasians but little evidence for LD in African-Americans. Several statistically significant haplotypes were identified in both Caucasians and African-Americans that influence the risk of PTB. Polymorphisms may also be protective. In a cohort of Caucasian women, the polymorphism at −174 in the promoter region of IL-6 gene was associated with a decreased risk of PTB [30] (Table 5.1). In the same study this polymorphism was not identified in any of the African-American women with PTB, suggesting that this 'loss of function' polymorphism in Caucasians may be protective.

Further studies have also investigated the association of the polymorphisms in the β2-adrenergic receptor gene. Studies have demonstrated an increased risk of PTB associated with the polymorphism Arg16Gly (G allele at nucleotide 46) [31, 32]. However, other investigators have not found this same association in different populations [33].

Matrix metalloproteinases (MMP) degrade and digest collagen and have been identified as important molecules in the pathophysiology of PTB. MMP activity in the fetal membrane increases at the time of parturition and increases are associated with PPROM. MMP1 -1607, a polymorphism in the promoter region of the MMP1 gene, was found to be associated with PPROM in African-Americans. Identification of 1G/2G heterozygotes and 2G/2G homozygotes were higher in cases of PPROM than controls

Table 5.1 Genetic contributions in inflammatory pathways leading to preterm birth.

Polymorphism	Race/ethnicity	Sample	Preterm birth risk	PPROM risk	Reference
TNFα-308A	Mixed	Maternal	OR 2.2 (1.0–5.0) *P* = 0.026		24
TNFα-308A	Mixed	Maternal	OR 2.7 (1.7–4.5)		23
TNFα-308A	AA	Maternal	OR 2.5 (1.4–4.5)		23
TNFα-308A	Caucasian	Maternal	OR 1.6 (0.5–5.2)		23
TNFα-308A	AA	Maternal		OR 3.18 (1.33–7.83)	26
IL-6 haplotype (CAGC)	Caucasian	Maternal	OR 0.97 (0.66–1.42)		29
IL-6 haplotype (GGGG)	Caucasian	Maternal	OR 0.65 (0.33–1.29)		29
IL-6 haplotype (CGCG)	Caucasian	Maternal	OR 1.57 (0.77–3.22)		29
IL-6 haplotype (GAGC)	Caucasian	Maternal	OR 2.42 (0.92–6.85)		29
IL-6 haplotype (CTG)	Caucasian	Fetal	OR 1.01 (0.69–1.48)		29
IL-6 haplotype (CGG)	Caucasian	Fetal	OR 0.86 (0.56–1.38)		29
IL-6 haplotype (CTA)	Caucasian	Fetal	OR 1.19 (0.58–2.43)		29
IL-6 haplotype (GG)	AA	Maternal	OR 0.67 (0.37–1.17)		29
IL-6 haplotype (CC)	AA	Maternal	OR 1.01 (0.45–2.17)		29
IL-6 haplotype (CG)	AA	Fetal	OR 1.15 (0.51–2.46)		29
IL-6 haplotype (AG)	AA	Fetal	OR 0.32 (0.12–0.73)		29
IL-6 haplotype (AC)	AA	Fetal	OR 1.24 (0.48–3.03)		29
IL-6 (-174) C/C	Mixed	Maternal	OR 0.17 (0.04–0.74)		30
IL-6 (-174) C/C	White	Maternal	OR 0.14 (0.03–0.64)		30
IL-6 (-174) C/C	AA	Maternal	C/C variant not identified		30
MMP1-1607 1G/2G & 2G/2G	AA	Neonates		OR 2.29 (1.09–4.82)	34
MMP9 promoter	AA	Neonates		OR 3.06 (1.77–5.27)	35
Fetal IFN-γ (+874T)	Mixed	Fetal	OR 2.3 (1.2–4.4) p = 0.009 per T allele		42
Maternal IFN-γ (+874T)	Mixed	Maternal	OR 0.5 (0.3–0.98) p = 0.043 per T allele		42
IFN-γ (+874T) & IL-10 (-819) T/C or T/T	Mixed	Neonates	OR 7.2 (2.1–25.3)		42
IFN-γ (+874T) & IL-10 (-819) C/C	Mixed	Neonates	Not significant		42

OR 2.29 (1.09–4.82) [34] (Table 5.1). Similar associations have been found in the promoter region in MMP9 [35] (Table 5.1).

Thrombosis and PTB

Decidual hemorrhage is found in up to 45% of PTBs. Maternal data suggest that the strongest association with PTB lies in the complement-coagulation pathway. In a study examining SNPs in six genes, three were identified as significantly associated with PTB. These included factor V, factor VII and tissue plasminogen activator (tPA). The strongest effect was observed with tPA in allelic and genotypic association with PTB, OR 2.8 (1.77–4.44) for a recessive model. Multilocus analysis in the complement and coagulation pathway found a potentially significant interaction between factor V and factor VII ($P < 0.001$) [36]. Other studies have found that Factor V Leiden and prothrombin G20210A mutations are not significantly associated with PTB [37, 38]. However, there may be an association between the prothrombin G20210A mutation in white women with PTB [37].

Gene–gene and gene–environment interaction

PTB is a complex phenotype with both epidemiologic and pathophysiologic heterogeneity involving multiple pathways [25, 39]. **It is unlikely that a single gene locus can be the cause of PTB**. It is more likely that there is epistasis, literally 'to stand above'. The phenomenon of epistasis is essentially synonymous with **gene–gene interaction**. The influence of a SNP, haplotype or sequence variant on a phenotype depends upon another SNP, haplotype or sequence variant. Previous studies have shown that gene expression can be modified by environmental factors, such as smoking [40]. Recent documentation found that infants with homozygous polymorphism in the glutathione S-transferase TI gene are at increased risk of preterm delivery when exposed to cigarette smoke during pregnancy [41]. A gene–environmental interaction between TNF-α and bacterial vaginosis (BV) leads to increased risk of preterm delivery compared with women with either the TNF-α-308 polymorphism or BV alone [23]. Investigations in this regard are few in the published literature, but several large studies are ongoing and hold great promise for filling this gap in our knowledge.

Maternal–fetal interactions

Studies focusing on both maternal and fetal genes and their interactions also exist. Genotype and haplotype frequencies have been compared in maternal and fetal DNA for IFN-γ [42]. After adjusting for maternal genotypes for IFN-γ alleles they found that the fetal IFN-γ allele (+847T) was associated with increased risk of PTB. Whereas adjusting for the fetal genotype for IFN-γ, the maternal IFN-γ allele (+847T) was protective against PTB. They also found significant interactions between the maternal and fetal IFN-γ genotypes and the risk of PTB. Multi-locus interactions were identified between the IL-10 (-819) and IFN-γ allele (+847T) loci for the increased risk of PTB in both additive and dominant models [42] (Table 5.1).

Conclusions

At the time of this writing, **genetic testing to define risk of PTB is not clinically indicated**. Understanding the genetics of PTB provides a major opportunity in several ways. First, **identifying gene sequence variants that predispose to PTB could allow us to identify a group of women worthy of inclusion in interventional trials to prevent PTB**. Furthermore, **understanding the genetic contributors to PTB will also give us insight into pathways of causation of PTB so that diagnostic and therapeutic strategies may be tailored in biologically-plausible, mechanistically-appropriate fashion**. As a corollary, ongoing work in this field is likely to reveal that 'risk' genotypes differ depending upon critical environmental contexts. Understanding this interaction will help us disentangle the relation between particular environmental exposures (e.g. smoking, BV) and PTB.

Glossary

Allele — one of several alternative forms of a gene occupying a given locus on a chromosome

Homozygous — the presence of two identical alleles at a specified locus

Heterozygous — the presence of two different alleles at a specified locus

Heritability index — (variance from genetic factors)/(variance from genetic factors + variance from environmental factors)

Single nucleotide polymorphisms (SNP) — the occurrence in a population of different nucleotides at particular sites in the genome, not disease causing

Haplotype — a set of closely linked alleles on a single chromosome that tend to be inherited *en bloc*

Linkage disequilibrium — probability of the occurrence of particular DNA variants at two sites physically close to one another is significantly greater than expected from the product of the observed allelic frequencies at each site independently

Epistasis — the interaction between genes

Epigenetic — any heritable influence on chromosome or gene function not accompanied by a change in DNA sequence

References

1 Volkov N, Nisenblat V, Ohel G, Gonen R. Ehlers-Danlos syndrome: insights on obstetric aspects. Obstet Gynecol Survey 2007; 62: 51–7.
2 Mercer BM, Goldenberg RL, Moawad AH, *et al.* The preterm prediction study: effect of gestational age and cause of preterm birth on subsequent obstetric outcome. Am J Obstet Gynecol 1999; 181: 1216–21.
3 Iams JD, Goldenberg RL, Mercer BM, *et al.* The preterm prediction study: recurrence risk of spontaneous preterm birth. Am J Obstet Gynecol 1998; 178: 1035–40.
4 Bloom S, Yost N, McIntire D, Leveno K. Recurrence of preterm birth in singleton and twin pregnancies. Obstet Gynecol 2001; 98: 379–85.
5 Clausson B, Lichtenstein P, Cnattingius S. Genetic influence on birthweight and gestational length determined by studies in offspring of twins. Br J Obstetrics Gynaecol 2000; 107: 375–81.
6 Treloar SA, Macones GA, Mitchell LE, Martin NG. Genetic influences on premature parturition in an Australian twin sample. Twin Res 2000; 3: 80–2.
7 Lunde A, Melve KK, Gjessing HK, Skjaerven R, Irgens LM. Genetic and environmental influences on birth weight, birth length, head circumference and gestational age by use of population-based parent-offspring data. Am J Epidemiol 2007; 165: 734–41.
8 Winkvist A, Morgren I, Hogbert U. Familial patterns in birth characteristics: impact on individual and population risks. Int J Epidemiol 1998; 27: 248–54.
9 Plunkett J, Borecki, Morgan T, Stamilio, Muglia L. Population-based estimate of sibling risk for preterm birth, preterm premature rupture of membranes, placental abruption and pre–eclampsia. BMC Genetics 2008; 9: 44.
10 Porter TF, Fraser AM, Hunter CY, Ward RH, Varner MW. The risk of preterm birth across generations. Obstet Gynecol 1997; 90: 63–67.
11 Wilcox AJ, Skjaerven R, Lie RT. Familial patterns of preterm delivery: maternal and fetal contributions. Am J Epidemiol 2008; 167: 474–9.
12 Morison IM, Ramsay JP, Spencer H. A census of mammalian imprinting. Trends Genet 2005; 21: 457–65.
13 Li KD. Changing paternity and the risk of preterm delivery in the subsequent pregnancy. Epidemiology 1999; 10: 148–52.
14 Vatten LJ, Skjaerven R. Effects on pregnancy outcome of changing partner between first two births: prospective population study. BMJ (clinical research edition) 2003; 327: 1138.
15 Basso O, Olsen J, Christensen K. Low birthweight and prematurity in relation to paternal factors: a study of recurrence. Int J Epidemiol 1999; 28: 695–700.
16 Goldenberg RL, Cliver SP, Mulvihill FX, *et al.* Medical psychosocial and behavior risk factors do not explain the increased risk for low birth weight among black women. Am J Obstet Gynecol 1996; 175: 1317–24.
17 Foster HW, Wu L, Bracken MB, Semenya K, Thomas J, Thomas J. Intergenerational effects of high socioeconomic status on low birthweight and preterm birth in African Americans. J Nat Med Assoc 2000; 92: 213–21.
18 Lu MC, Halfon N. Racial and ethnic disparities in birth outcomes: a life-course perspective. Maternal Child Health J 2003; 7: 13–20.
19 Zhang J, Savitz DA. Preterm birth subtypes among blacks and whites. Epidemiology 1992; 3: 428–33.
20 Adams MM, Elam-Evans LD, Wilson HG, Gilbertz DA. Rates of and factors associated with recurrence of preterm delivery. JAMA 2000; 283: 1591–6.

21 Palomar L, DeFranco EA, Lee KA, Allsworth JE, Muglia JL. Paternal race is a risk factor for preterm birth. Am J Obstet Gynecol 2007; 197: 152.e1–152.e7.

22 Simhan HN, Krohn MA. Paternal race and preterm birth. Am J Obstet Gynecol 2008; 198: 644.e1–644.e6.

23 Macones GA, Parry S, Elkousy M, Clothier B, Ural SH, Strauss III JF. A polymorphism in the promoter region of TNF and bacterial vaginosis: preliminary evidence of gene–environment interaction in the etiology of spontaneous preterm birth. Am J Obstet Gynecol 2004; 190: 1504–8.

24 Moore S, Ide M, Randhawa M, Walker JJ, Reid JG, Simpson NA. An investigation into the association among preterm birth, cytokine gene polymorphisms and periodontal disease. Br J Obstet Gynaecol 2004; 191: 125–32.

25 Menon R, Merialdi M, Betran AP, *et al.* Analysis of association between tumor necrosis factor-alpha promoter polymorphism (-308), TNF concentration, and preterm birth. Am J Obstet Gynecol 2006; 195: 1240–8.

26 Roberts AK, Monzon–Bordonaba F, Van Deerlin PG, *et al.* Association of polymorphism within the promoter of the tumor necrosis factor alpha gene with increased risk of preterm premature rupture of the fetal membranes. Am J Obstet Gynecol 1999; 180: 1297–302.

27 Menon R, Velez DR, Thorsen P, *et al.* Ethnic differences in key candidate genes for spontaneous preterm birth: TNF-alpha and its receptors. Hum Hered 2006; 62: 107–18.

28 Velez DR, Menon R, Thorsen P, *et al.* Ethnic difference in interleukin 6 (IL–6) and IL6 receptor genes in spontaneous preterm birth and effects on amniotic fluid protein levels. Annals Human Genet 2007; 71: 586–600.

29 Velez DR, Fortunato SJ, Williams SM, Menon R. Interleukin–6 (IL-6) and receptor (IL6-R) gene haplotypes associate with amniotic fluid protein concentrations in preterm birth. Human Mol Genet 2008; 17: 1619–30.

30 Simhan HN, Krohn MA, Roberts JM, Zeevi A, Caritis SN. Interleukin-6 promoter–174 polymorphism and spontaneous preterm birth. Am J Obstet Gynecol 2003; 189: 915–18.

31 Landau R, Xie H-G, Dishy V, *et al.* Beta2-adrenergic receptor genotype and preterm delivery. Am J Obstet Gynecol 2002; 187: 1294–8.

32 Don K, Sziller I, Vardhana S, *et al.* Beta2-adrenergic receptor gene polymorphisms and pregnancy outcome. J Perinat Med 2004; 32: 413–7.

33 Ozkur M, Dogulu F, Ozkur A, *et al.* Association of the Gln27Glu polymorphism of the beta-2-adrenergic receptor with preterm labor. Int J Gynaecol Obstet 2002; 77: 209–15.

34 Fujimoto T, Parry S, Urbanek M, *et al.* A single nucleotide polymorphism in the matrix metalloproteinases-1 (MMP–1) promoter influences amnion cell MMP–1 expression and risk for preterm premature rupture of the fetal membranes. J Biol Chem 2002; 277: 6296–302.

35 Ferrand PE, Parry S, Sammel M, *et al.* A polymorphism in the matrix metalloproteinases-9 promoter is associated with increased risk of preterm premature rupture of membranes in African Americans. Mol Hum Reprod 2002; 8: 494–501.

36 Velez DR, Fortunato SJ, Thorsen P, Lombardi SJ, Williams SM, Menon R. Preterm birth in Caucasians is associated with coagulation and inflammation pathway gene variants. PloS ONE 2008; 3: e3283.

37 Kocher O CC, Malynn E, Rowland C, *et al.* Obstetric complications in patients with hereditary thrombophilia identified using the LCx Microparticle Enzyme Immunoassay. Am J Clin Pathol 2007; 127: 68–75.

38 Hartel C, von Otte S, Koct J, *et al.* Blood coagulation, fibrinolysis and cellular haemostatis. Thromb Haemost 2005; 94: 88–92.

39 Menon R, Velez DV, Simhan H, *et al.* Multilocus interactions at maternal TNF-a, IL–6 genes predict spontaneous preterm labor in European-American women. Am J Obstet Gynecol 2006; 194: 1616–4.

40 Van Baal CGM, Bloomsma DI. Etiology of individual differences in birthweight of twins as a function of maternal smoking during pregnancy. Twin Res 1998; 1: 123–30.

41 Nukui T, Day RD, Sims CS, Ness RB, Romkes M. Maternal/newborn GSTT1 null genotype polymorphism, and infant birth weight. JAMA 2002; 287: 241–42.

42 Speer EM, Gentile DA, Zeevi A, Pillage G, Huo D, Skoner DP. Role of single nucleotide polymorphisms of cytokine genes in spontaneous preterm delivery. Human Immunology 2006; 67: 915–23.

CHAPTER 6

The Cervix

Vincenzo Berghella
Division of Maternal-Fetal Medicine, Thomas Jefferson University, Philadelphia, USA

Key points

- The cervix has to open to allow vaginal birth. Therefore the cervix has a central role in the etiology of preterm birth (PTB), as well as its potential prevention strategies.
- The cervix is 80–85% connective tissue, with collagen I making up 70% of all collagen.
- The process of parturition takes months of preparation, and early changes can be detected in humans.
- Gradual and slow cervical changes during pregnancy can be divided in four phases: (1) remodeling of the collagen fibrillar network; (2) increased synthesis of proteoglycans, hydrophilic glycosaminoglycans, and collagen; (3) leukocyte invasion and release (by them) of proteases and collagenases; (4) resolution of inflammation and edema.
- Cervical insufficiency should be defined as the presence of both: a prior PTB(s) and/or second trimester loss(es); *and* cervical shortening or dilatation before 24 weeks in the current pregnancy.
- Possible etiologies of cervical etiology of PTB include cervical surgery, inflammation/infection, multiple dilatations and evacuations, uterine anomaly, diethylstilbestrol exposure, Ehler-Danlos syndrome, and others.

Introduction

The cervix has to open to allow vaginal birth. Therefore the cervix has a central role in the etiology of preterm birth (PTB), as well as its potential prevention strategies.

Histology of the cervix

While the cervix was thought in the past to be just an 'appendage' of the uterus, we know now that its histology and properties are very different than the womb. While the uterus is smooth muscle, the cervix is made of

>80–85% connective tissue, 10–15% smooth muscle, and the rest elastin (about 1%) and other less common components [1, 2].

Collagen makes up about 50% of the dry weight of the cervix, and 80% of the protein component. The extracellular matrix is 75–80% water. **Collagen I** accounts for 70%, III for 30%, and IV for <1% of the total cervical collagen. The extracellular matrix contains cells and **proteoglycans**. Decorin is a small proteoglycan making up 85% of the non-pregnant dermatan sulfate (66% of the glycosaminoglycan of the cervix). Many other proteoglycans (e.g. fibromodulin, aggrecan, biglycan, versican, etc.), glycoproteins (e.g. fibronectin), and collagenases (e.g. metalloproteinanses [MMPs]) make up the matrix component of the cervix.

The minimal amount of muscle in the cervix can contract, but, being heavily interspersed with fibrous tissue, appears to have minimal sphincteric capabilities. **The percentage of smooth muscle decreases progressively in the cervix** from the internal (up to 29%) to the external os (6%) region. So there is a region where the lower uterine segment, made of >95% smooth muscle, changes to mostly cervical connective tissue. This change can occur abruptly or over a 5–10 cm region. This histologic internal os does not correspond always to the anatomic one, which may be 6–10 mm superior to this [1].

Cervical changes in pregnancy leading to birth

The process of parturition takes months of preparation, and early changes can be detected in humans (Figure 6.1). While PTB was often

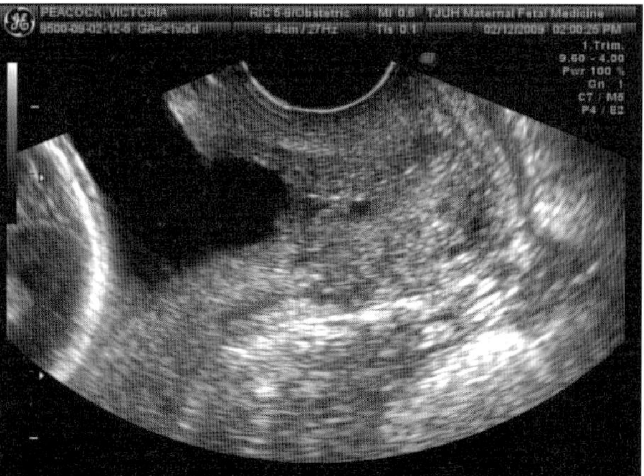

Figure 6.1 Short cervical length (24 mm) and funneling at 21 weeks. Please also note small amount of **sludge**.

characterized in the past as something happening suddenly and unexpectantly, the **changes are gradual and usually very slow**. In fact, in many high-risk women delivering preterm, the cervix starts to shorten a couple of months before preterm labor (PTL) or preterm premature rupture of membranes (PPROM) occurs (Chapter 12). For endocrine change, including estrogen, progesterone, and relaxin, see also Chapter 8.

Basic science studies have divided these cervical changes in **four phases** [3].

The **first** phase involves slow **remodeling of the collagen fibrillar network**. The cervix slowly 'softens'. Even from the first month of pregnancy, the cervical stroma has hypertrophy, the cervical glands both hypertrophy and hyperplasia, and the entire cervix increased vascularity and edema. Inflammatory cells are rare, while collagen bundles are dense and organized. Collagen synthesis is increased, maintaining the force of this softened cervix. Crossed-linked collagen (type I and III) fibers give the cervix its tensile strength. Therefore, the endocervical epithelial cells, scant in the non-pregnant cervix, proliferate to occupy up to 50% of cervical mass by the end of pregnancy. There are many ways in which these cells maintain the strength of the cervix. Expression of Toll-like receptors in these cells binds bacterial toxins. Cervical epithelial cells express enzymes that promote high tissue levels of progesterone [3].

Some of these changes can be detected even **on ultrasound**. For example, the absence of these cervical glands is associated with PTB [4]. Sonoelastometry and quantitative ultrasound of the cervix are two other techniques with potential for prediction of PTB.

The **second** phase, often called '**ripening**', is physiologically a third trimester phenomenon, but can happen earlier and lead to PTB. It involves **increased synthesis of proteoglycans, hydrophilic glycosaminoglycans, and collagen**. Total collagen content of the cervix increases in pregnancy. Nonetheless, cervical ripening at term is characterized by collagen bundles that get more dispersed. This decrease in tissue collagen and proteoglycans (e.g. decorin) concentrations is due to the more pronounced increase in hydrophilic glycosaminoglycans, non-collagenous proteins, and slight increase in water content. In late pregnancy, decreases in the glycoprotein decorin (which normally binds and immobilizes cervical bundles) and increases in hydrophilic hyaluronan, cause collagen dispersal. Much research is being conducted on the role of extracellular metalloproteases (MMPs) and cytokines in cervical ripening.

Prostaglandinds (PGs) can induce ripening of the cervix, causing changes similar to what we just described. But PGs may not be physiologic mediators of cervical ripening [3]. While progesterone levels do not decrease prior to parturition in humans, the function of progesterone receptors

Table 6.1 Possible etiologies for early (14–24 weeks) development of a short cervix (cervical length <25 mm) leading to preterm birth.

- Intrinsic weakness of the cervix, or cervical insufficiency (e.g. from cervical surgery, multiple dilatations and evacuations, repeated cervical dilatations, Ehlers-Danlos, DES exposure, etc.).
- Inflammatory or infectious processes (cause or effect?).
- Mullerian anomalies, multiple gestations, etc.
- Contractions (cause or effect?).

(PG) declines progressively during pregnancy. PG isoforms can be altered by PGs. Local progesterone metabolism and changes in PG isoforms may be what facilitates early ripening.

The clinically detectable manifestation of this second phase occurring too early, in the second trimester, is a **short cervical length** (CL) on transvaginal ultrasound (TVU) (Chapter 12). Early changes happen at the internal os (Figure 6.1). Ultrasound has now shown that this lower part of the uterus begins to show changes weeks before eventual birth. It is unclear how ultrasound changes and the sonographic internal os correlate with histology. Leading hypotheses regarding the etiology of short CL leading to PTB are listed in Table 6.1.

This phase usually precedes contractions. Cervical light-induced fluorescence detected by a collascope decreases progressively in pregnancy, and may be a useful tool for predicting PTB [5]. Uterine electromyographic signals can assess (before clinically apparent contractions) the contractile function of the uterus, just like the EKG is used for the heart.

In this phase, the cervix is more easily stretched if examined. In advanced stages, asymptomatic contractions can be detected on the monitor, making it difficult to understand if cervical changes are due to 'pressure' from the uterine contractions, or if cervical changes then lead to uterine stimulation. In any case, uterine contractions are a relatively late event in the continuum to parturition.

The **third** phase is the one we as clinicians see as it is associated with gross changes. Cervical dilation is associated with **leukocyte invasion and release (by them) of proteases and collagenases** into the extracellular matrix. The signal for recruitment of white blood cells is unknown. Collagen is lysed. Collagen bundles consequently become more dispersed. Macrophages invade the cervix, recruiting other inflammatory cells. The presence of these inflammatory cells invading the cervix and even the amniotic cavity is seen on ultrasounds as sludge (Figure 6.1). Loss of the protective cervical barrier, including cervical mucus, allows opportunistic microbial invasion of the uterus. Cervical glands are collapsed. Apoptosis may also play a role [6]. Clinically, we see contractions on monitoring, and palpable cervical dilation.

The **final** phase is remodeling after delivery. **Inflammation and edema resolve**, and dense connective tissue and normal non-pregnant structure is restored [3].

Cervical insufficiency

Cervical insufficiency (CI) was previously defined as recurrent painless dilatation leading to second trimester losses, and was called incompetence. Current understanding leads us to propose a new definition. Cervical insufficiency should be defined as the presence of both a **prior PTB(s) and/or second trimester loss(es) *and* cervical shortening or dilatation before 24 weeks in the current pregnancy.**

Histologically, the 'insufficient' or 'weak' cervix is characterized by decreased collagen (to only 67%) [1], decreased crosslinks between tropocollagen molecules of collagen I, and decreased elastin [7]. Genetic changes are an exiting area of research, recently reviewed [8]. The processes described above clearly show that **the path to PTB is a continuous progress, with CI being a most severe manifestation, while third trimester PPROM or PTL are less severe phenotypes.** Known risk factors for pathologic cervical function leading to CI and PTB are reviewed below (Table 6.1).

Cervical surgery

Pregnant women with a history of cervical cone biopsy by cold knife, loop electrosurgical excision procedure (LEEP), or laser are at increased risk for PTB. The risk is proportional to the amount of tissue removed. Maximum heights of <2.0 cm for cold knife cone, <1.5 cm for LEEP, and <1.0 cm for laser cone are usually not associated with an increase in PTB in subsequent pregnancies [9]. Laser vaporization, cryotherapy and most lacerations are also not associated with PTB, while trachelectomy is a huge risk factor for PTB.

Multiple terminations

Two or more prior dilatations and evacuations, especially from terminations (induced abortions) are associated with an increased risk of PTB [10]. Even one termination can slightly increase the risk of PTB [11].

Infection and the cervix

It is unclear if infection causes or is the consequence of the process leading to PTB. Probably both mechanisms are in play, mostly in different patients. The shorter the CL, the higher is the incidence of intra-amniotic infection.

Clearly, in many cases the shorter cervix allows ascending infection from the vagina, full of bacteria, to the sterile uterine cavity. Amniocentesis of women with singleton gestations, a poor obstetrical history and a TVU CL <25 mm in the second trimester has revealed that the incidence of intra-amniotic infection in these women is about 1–9%. Chorioamnionitis, endometritis, and higher IL-6 levels have all been associated with a shorter CL, the higher the earlier the short CL is detected.

The presence of **bacterial vaginosis** (Chapter 14) further increases the risk of PTB in women with a short cervix. There are as yet no studies on any association between other infections that contribute to PTB (e.g. Chlamydia, gonorrhea, etc.) and TVU CL.

Mullerian anomalies

Uterine anomalies are associated with PTB. TVU CL is predictive of PTB in these pregnancies, too [12]. The mechanisms leading to PTB in these pregnancies are unclear, but they might relate more to the abnormal uterine shape than to a pathology of the cervix.

Diethylstilbestrol exposure

Diethylstilbestrol (DES), taken by mothers until the early 1970s, can cause changes in the cervix and PTB in female offspring. Up to half of these women have second trimester cervical changes [13].

Ehlers-Danlos syndrome

This is a genetic disorder characterized by disorganization of collagen fibrils and PTB. The classic variety (EDS I) is autosomal dominant and due to mutations in type V collagen, but many types of this disorder, inheritance patterns, and different collagen mutations can lead to its phenotype.

Understanding where the problem starts

The cascade leading to PTB has probably many possible 'matches' that can start the 'fire'. Progress could be improved by better correlation between histologic, inflammatory, and genetic sampling obtained safely in pregnancy and other clinical information such as cervical ultrasound. Finding out early in the process leading to PTB which is the 'match', such as intrinsic weakness of the cervix, infection or inflammation, uterine overdistension, hormonal changes, or a combination of these and other factors (Chapters 2 and 4) could lead to much more effective use of interventions.

References

1 Danfort DN. The fibrous nature of the human cervix, and its relation to the isthmic segment in gravid and nongravid uteri. Am J Obstet Gynecol 1947; 53: 5410.

2 House M, Kaplan DL, Socrate S. Relationships between mechanical properties and extracellular matrix constituents of the cervical stroma during pregnancy. Sem Perinatol 2009; 33: 300–7.

3 Word RA, Li X-H, Hnat M, Carrick K. Dynamics of cervical remodeling during pregnancy and parturition: mechanisms and current concepts. Seminars Repro Med 2007; 25: 69–79.

4 Fukami T, Ishihara K, Sekira T, Araki T. Is transvaginal ultrasonography at midtrimester useful for predicting early spontaneous preterm birth? J Nippon Med Sch 2003; 70: 135–40.

5 Maul H, Olson G, Fittkow CT, Saade GR, Garfield RE. Cervical light-induced fluorescence in humans decreases throughout gestation and before delivery: preliminary observations. Am J Obstet Gynecol 2003; 188: 537–41.

6 Allaire AD, D'Andrea N, Truong P, McMahon MJ, Lessey BA. Cervical stroma apoptosis in pregnancy. Obstet Gynecol 2001; 97: 399–403.

7 Leppert PC, Yeh SY, Keller S, Cerreta J, Mandl I. Decreased elastic fibers and desmosine content in incompetent cervix. Am J Obstet Gynecol 187; 157: 1134–9.

8 Warren JE, Silver RM. Genetics of the cervix in relation to preterm birth. Sem Perinatol 2009; 33: 308–11.

9 Berghella V, Pereira L, Gariepy A, Simonazzi G. Prior cone biopsy: prediction of preterm birth by cervical ultrasound. Am J Obstet Gynecol 2004; 191: 1393–7.

10 Visintine J, Berghella V, Henning D, Baxter J. Cervical length for prediction of preterm birth in women with multiple prior induced abortion. Ultrasound Obstet Gynecol 2008; 31: 198–200.

11 Swingle HM, Colaizy TT, Zimmerman MB, Morriss FH. Abortion and the risk of subsequent preterm birth. J Reprod Med 2009; 54: 95–108.

12 Airoldi J, Berghella V, Sehdev H, Ludmir J. Transvaginal ultrasound of the cervix to predict preterm birth in women with uterine anomalies. Obstet Gynecol 2005; 106: 553–6.

13 Ludmir J, Landon MB, Gabbe SG, Samuels P, Mennuti MT. Management of the diestylbestrol-exposed pregnant patient: a prospective study. Am J Obstet Gynecol 1987; 157: 665–9.

CHAPTER 7

Inflammation and Infection

Roberto Romero[1,2,3], *Francesca Gotsch*[1], *Shali Mazaki-Tovi*[1,3] *&* *Juan Pedro Kusanovic*[1,3]

[1]Perinatology Research Branch, *Eunice Kennedy Shriver* National Institute to Child Health and Human Development, National Institutes of Health, Michigan, USA, [2]Center for Molecular Medicine and Genetics and [3]Department of Obstetrics and Gynecology, Wayne State University, Perinatology Research Branch, *Eunice Kennedy Shriver* National Institute of Child Health and Human Development, National Institutes of Health, Michigan, USA

Key points

- The amniotic cavity in a normal pregnancy is considered to be sterile for bacteria using standard cultivation techniques.
- The frequency of microbial invasion of the amniotic cavity varies according to the presence or absence of labor, gestational age at presentation, cervical dilation, and status of membrane rupture.
- Microbial invasion of the amniotic cavity is present in 25% of all preterm births, and it is largely subclinical in nature.
- The frequency of a positive amniotic fluid culture for microorganisms in women undergoing midtrimester amniocentesis for genetic indications is approximately 0.4%. These patients frequently have an adverse pregnancy outcome. Thus, subclinical infection in the midtrimester is often followed by spontaneous preterm labor and delivery.
- The prevalence of a positive amniotic fluid culture for microorganisms in women with preterm labor leading to preterm delivery is 12%; in patients with preterm premature rupture of membranes (PPROM) it is 32% at the time of presentation. However, 75% of patients with PPROM have a positive amniotic fluid culture at the time of the onset of labor. Thus, microbial invasion of the amniotic cavity increases during the latency period. As many as 50% of women with acute cervical insufficiency (cervix dilated ≥2 cm by digital exam between 14 and 24 weeks) have a positive amniotic fluid culture for microorganisms, and the placement of a cerclage in such infected patients is associated with adverse pregnancy outcome.
- The prevalence of a positive amniotic fluid culture for microorganisms among women with a sonographic short cervix (<25 mm) at 14–24 weeks of gestation is 9%. Some of these patients have been treated with antibiotics, with resolution of the infection and term delivery.
- The most frequent organisms isolated in the amniotic fluid are genital mycoplasmas (*Ureaplasma urealyticum* and *Mycoplasma hominis*). These microorganisms cannot be seen with a Gram stain of amniotic fluid.

(Continued)

- The molecular mechanisms involved in the onset of preterm parturition involve inflammatory mediators such as pattern-recognition receptors (e.g. Toll-like receptors), chemokines (e.g. interleukin (IL)-8, monocyte chemotactic protein-1, etc.), and proinflammatory cytokines such as IL-1β and tumor necrosis factor-α.
- The optimal method currently to diagnose intra-amniotic infection/inflammation is examination of amniotic fluid with a Gram stain, amniotic fluid white blood cell count, amniotic fluid glucose concentration and amniotic fluid culture for aerobic and anaerobic bacteria, as well as genital mycoplasmas. The most promising tests are the measurement of matrix metalloprotein-8 (MMP-8) and IL-6 in amniotic fluid. The use of molecular microbiologic techniques is expected to improve the speed of detection of microorganisms.

Introduction

Infection/inflammation is an important cause of spontaneous preterm labor (PTL) and delivery [1–8]. Moreover, intrauterine infection may lead to fetal invasion and the development of a fetal systemic inflammatory response, which may participate in signaling the onset of preterm labor and, when exaggerated, may lead to fetal injury (fetal inflammatory response syndrome, in which several organs are involved including the fetal lung and brain).

Prevalence of microbial invasion of the amniotic cavity

The amniotic cavity in normal pregnancies is considered to be sterile for bacteria, as **less than 1% of women not in labor at term have bacteria in the amniotic fluid (AF)** [9]. Therefore, the isolation of bacteria from the AF, which is defined as **'microbial invasion of the amniotic cavity' (MIAC)**, is a **pathologic finding**. Most of these infections are subclinical in nature and cannot be detected without AF analysis. The frequency of MIAC depends upon the clinical presentation and gestational age (Table 7.1). **In patients with preterm labor with intact membranes, the rate of positive AF cultures is 12.8%** [10]. However, among those who have PTL with intact membranes and deliver a preterm neonate, the frequency is 22%. Among women with **preterm prelabor rupture of membranes (PPROM), the overall rate of positive AF cultures at admission is 32.4%** [10], but at the time of the subsequent onset of labor, as many as 75% will have MIAC [11], suggesting that MIAC may also occur during the latency period. The frequency of MIAC among women with **cervical insufficiency is up to 51%** [12] and **9% in cases of sonographic short cervix** (cervical length <25 mm in the midtrimes-

Table 7.1 Prevalence of microbial invasion of the amniotic cavity according to gestational age and clinical presentation. TVU, transvaginal ultrasonography. PPROM, preterm prelabor rupture of the membranes. PROM, prelabor rupture of the membranes.

Pregnancy status	Prevalence of infection
Gestational age <37	
Midtrimester [25]	0.4% (9/2,461)
Short cervix (TVU <25 mm) [13]	9% (5/57)
PPROM without labor on admission [11]	25.6% (41/160)
PPROM with labor on admission [11]	39% (24/61)
Preterm labor with intact membranes [10]	12.8% (379/2,963)
Cervical insufficiency [12]	51.5% (17/33)
Twin gestation with preterm labor [14]	10.8% (5/46)
Gestational age ≥37	
Intact membranes, no labor [98]	1.4% (2/143)
Intact membranes, with labor [98]	18.8% (17/90)
PROM [99]	34.3% (11/32)

ter) [13]. Finally, the frequency of MIAC in **twin gestations is 10.8%** [14]. Of interest, in twin gestations in whom MIAC is detected, the presenting sac is nearly always involved, while the other amniotic cavity may not have MIAC [14]. Patients with a positive AF culture and PTL with intact membranes are more likely to have spontaneous preterm birth (PTB), rupture the membranes spontaneously, and develop clinical chorioamnionitis than patients with a negative AF culture for microorganisms.

Microbiology of intrauterine infection

The most common microorganisms found in the AF are genital Mycoplasmas, particularly *Ureaplasma urealyticum* [15]. **Other microorganisms include *Mycoplasma hominis, Streptococcus agalactiae, Escherichia coli, Fusobacterium* species, and *Gardnerella vaginalis.*** Interestingly, with the use of molecular microbiologic techniques, organisms normally found in the oral cavity have been detected in AF of women with PTL [16]. In general, microorganisms may gain access to the amniotic cavity and fetus using any of the following pathways: (1) ascending from the vagina and the cervix; (2) hematogenous dissemination through the placenta; (3) retrograde seeding from the peritoneal cavity through the fallopian tubes; and (4) accidental introduction at the time of invasive procedures such as amniocentesis, cordocentesis, chorionic villous sam-

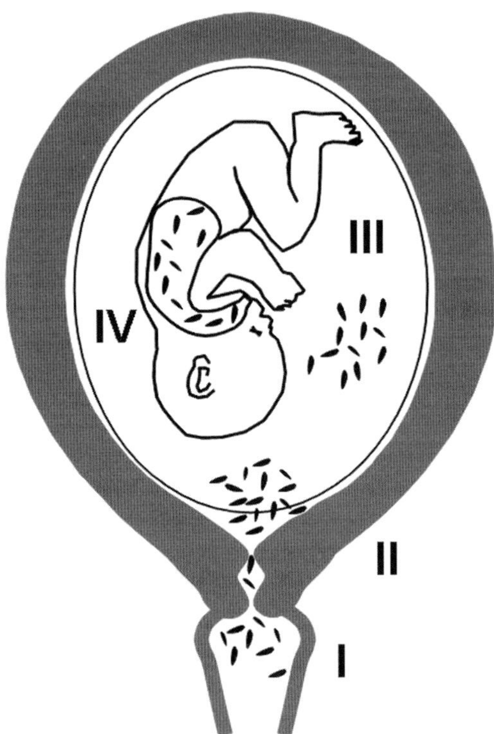

Figure 7.1 Stages of ascending intrauterine infection. Stage I: the first stage consists of an overgrowth of facultative organisms or the presence of the pathologic organisms in the vagina, cervix, or both. Stage II: the microorganisms gain access to the intrauterine cavity through a restricted cervical region. Stage III: the infection may invade the fetal vessels (choriovasculitis) or proceed through the amnion (amnionitis) into the amniotic fluid, leading to microbial invasion of the amniotic cavity. Stage IV: once in the amniotic cavity, the bacteria may gain access to the fetus by different ports of entry. Modified with permission from Kim MJ, Romero R, Gervas MT *et al.* *Lab Invest.* 2009; 89: 924–36.

pling, or shunting [3]. The most common pathway of intrauterine infection is the ascending route (Figure 7.1).

What is the significance of microbial invasion of the amniotic cavity detected only by molecular microbiology techniques?

The prevalence of MIAC described in the previous paragraphs is based on the results of standard microbiologic methods (cultivation techniques). However, a positive culture can only be obtained if the conditions in the laboratory are able to support the growth of a particular microorganism. Thus, **while a positive culture is indicative of MIAC, a negative culture does not necessarily rule out MIAC**. A negative culture indicates that the laboratory was not able to grow a particular bacterium from the specimen of AF, either because bacteria were absent or because the conditions used for cultivation did not support the growth of a specific microorganism. This is an important point since **only 1% of the microbial world can be detected by cultivation techniques** [17]. Consequently, the frequency of MIAC represents a minimum estimate, and it is likely to increase with the introduction of more sensitive methods for microbial recovery and identification [18–21].

The question of the clinical significance of MIAC detected only by molecular microbiology techniques, but which cannot be detected by cultivation techniques, has been answered. Patients with a positive polymerase chain reaction (PCR) for *Ureaplasma urealyticum*, but negative culture, have similar adverse outcomes as patients with a positive AF culture for this microorganism and worse than patients with sterile AF and negative PCR [22, 23]. Moreover, these patients also have the same degree of inflammation as those with a positive AF culture [23]. Collectively, this evidence suggests that **the presence of microbial footprints detected by PCR is associated with adverse outcome**. Similar observations have been made using conserved primers of the bacterial genome [21].

Microbial invasion of the amniotic cavity as a chronic process

Although chorioamnionitis is traditionally considered an acute process, a growing body of evidence suggests that **MIAC exists for an extended period of time**: (1) Cassell *et al.* [24] recovered genital Mycoplasmas from 6.6% of AF samples collected in mid-trimester amniocentesis. Women with *Mycoplasma hominis* delivered at 34 and 40 weeks without neonatal complications, while those with *Ureaplasma urealyticum* had PTB, neonatal sepsis and neonatal death at 24 and 29 weeks; (2) Gray *et al.* [25] reported a 0.37% prevalence of positive cultures for *Ureaplasma urealyticum* in AF samples obtained during genetic amniocentesis. All women with positive AF cultures had either a fetal loss or PTB within four weeks of amniocentesis, and all had histologic chorioamnionitis; (3) Horowitz *et al.* [26] detected *Ureaplasma urealyticum* in 2.8% of mid-trimester AF samples. The rate of adverse pregnancy outcome was significantly higher in women with a positive AF culture than in those with a negative culture (50% vs 12%); (4) Gerber *et al.* [27] identified *Ureaplasma urealyticum* using PCR in 11% of AF samples obtained between 15 and 17 weeks of gestation.

Patients with *Ureaplasma urealyticum* had a significantly higher rate of subsequent PTL (58% vs 4%) and PTB (24% vs 0.4%) than those with a negative result; (5) Markenson *et al.* [28] detected bacterial 16S ribosomal DNA in 18% of mid-trimester AF samples; (6) Nguyen *et al.* [29] identified *Mycoplasma hominis* in 6.4% of AF samples obtained between 15 and 17 weeks. The rate of PTL in women with a positive PCR for *Mycoplasma hominis* was significantly higher than in those with negative PCR (14% vs 3%); and (7) Perni *et al.* [30] detected *Mycoplasma hominis* and *Ureaplasma urealyticum* by PCR in 6.1% and 12.8% of mid-trimester amniocentesis, respectively. Preterm PROM or spontaneous PTB with intact membranes occurred in 2.8% of women. This compelling evidence suggests that **MIAC could be chronic in nature and sub-clinical in the midtrimester of pregnancy and that pregnancy loss or PTB due to infection may take weeks to occur**.

Evidence that infection is causally linked to preterm labor and delivery

Infection is a frequent and important mechanism of disease in premature labor and delivery [1, 10, 15, 31]. The evidence in support of this includes: (1) in pregnant animals intrauterine infection or systemic administration of microbial products to pregnant animals can result in PTL and PTB [31–36]; (2) extra-uterine maternal infections such as malaria [37], pyelonephritis [38, 39] pneumonia [40] and periodontal disease have been associated with PTB [41–43]; (3) subclinical intrauterine infections are associated with PTL and PTB [44]; and (4) treatment of asymptomatic bacteriuria prevents PTB [45, 46].

Fetal attack rate

MIAC is a risk factor for fetal invasion with microorganisms. This attack rate varies, but has been extensively studied in the case of genital mycoplasmas. It has been determined that **approximately 30% of fetuses of mothers who have MIAC have positive blood cultures for microorganisms** [47]. Moreover, in a recent study in which umbilical cord blood cultures for *Ureaplasma urealyticum* and *Mycoplasma hominis* were obtained from mothers who delivered between 23 and 32 weeks, the rate of bacteremia was 23% [48]. Thus, the infection does not remain confined to the amniotic cavity, but can extend into the human fetus. **The ports of entry are the airways, skin, gastrointestinal tract and ears**. Microbial products can elicit a systemic inflammatory response in the human fetus, which we have termed a **fetal inflammatory response syndrome (FIRS)** [5, 6]. This condition is operationally **defined by an elevation in umbilical cord concentration of IL-6**, and is associated with a high rate of perinatal morbidity and mortality as well as multi-systemic involvement. FIRS is a risk factor for the subsequent development of chronic lung disease and cerebral palsy [49, 50]. For more details about the involvement of the adrenal glands [51], the cardiac system [52] and the matrix-degrading enzymes [53], the reader is referred to the original studies.

Inflammation: the mechanism for the onset of preterm parturition in the context of infection

Inflammation is the fundamental mechanism to deal with insults, both of an infectious and non-infectious-related nature. However, inflammation has a broad spectrum, and could be physiologic or pathologic. **There is a common misconception that in the absence of systemic clinical signs of inflammation (e.g. fever, chills, leucocytosis, etc.), infection is unlikely. This is not the case in intrauterine infection**. Histologic chorioamnionitis, both at term and in preterm gestations, may be diagnosed in the absence of any maternal or fetal clinical signs or symptoms of inflammation/infection. Moreover, **inflammation also plays a central role in physiologic processes**, particularly in the reproductive tract: the rupture of an ovarian follicle, implantation, menstruation, and parturition are characterized by cellular and molecular events which are found in pathologic inflammation.

The first line of defense against infection is provided by the innate immune system, which provides immediate protection from microbial challenge by recognizing the presence of microorganisms, thus preventing tissue invasion and/or eliciting a host response to limit microbial proliferation. One of the mechanisms by which the innate immunity recognizes microorganisms is by using **pattern recognition receptors (PRRs)** that bind to repeating patterns of molecular structures present in the surfaces of microorganisms. PRRs are classified based on their function and subcellular localization into the following groups: (1) soluble PRRs, such as 'the acute phase proteins' Mannan Binding Lectin (MBL) and C-Reactive Protein (CRP), which act as opsonins to neutralize and clear pathogens through the complement and phagocytic systems; (2) transmembrane PRRs, including scavenger receptors, C-type lectins and the **Toll-like receptors (TLRs)**; and (3) intracellular PRRs, including Nod1 and Nod2, RIG-1 and MDA-5, which mediate recognition of intracellular pathogens (e.g. viruses) [54].

The genital tract and trophoblast have innate immune receptors

Ten different TLRs have been identified in humans. TLR-4 recognizes the presence of lypopolysaccharide (LPS; Gram-negative bacteria), TLR-2 recognizes peptidoglycans, lipoproteins, and zymosan (Gram-positive bacteria, mycoplasmas, and fungi), TLR-3 recognizes double-stranded RNA (viruses), and the ligand for TLR-5 is flagellin [55]. Toll-like receptors (TLR)-1, 2, 3, 5 and 6, have been identified in the epithelia from the vagina, ecto- and endocervix, endometrium, and uterine tubes [56]. Of note, TLR-4 has only been demonstrated in the endocervix, endometrium, and uterine tubes, but not in the vagina and ectocervix [56]. This has been interpreted as evidence that TLR-4 may participate in the modulation of immunological tolerance in the lower parts of the female reproductive tract and in host defense against infection [56]. Similarly, trophoblast cells are able to recognize and respond to pathogens through the expression of Toll-like receptors. We have demonstrated that trophoblast cells are able to recognize pathogens through the expression of TLR-2 and TLR-4. However, activation of different TLRs appears to generate distinct trophoblast cell responses. Indeed, TLR-4 ligation by LPS promotes cytokine production, while ligation of TLR-2 to peptidoglycan and lipoteichoic acid induces apoptosis in first trimester trophoblast cells [57]. These findings suggest that pathogens, through TLR-2, may directly promote trophoblast cell death [57] observed in a number of pregnancy complications including spontaneous abortion, intrauterine growth restriction and preeclampsia.

Since TLRs are crucial for the recognition of microorganisms, it is be anticipated that **defective signaling through this pattern recognition receptor may impair bacteria-induced PTL**. A strain of mice which has a spontaneous mutation for TLR-4 is less likely to deliver preterm after intrauterine inoculation of heat-killed bacteria or LPS (bacterial endotoxin) than wild type mice [58]. In pregnant women, TLR-2 and TLR-4 are expressed in the amniotic epithelium [59]. Moreover, spontaneous labor at term and PTB with histologic chorioamnionitis, regardless of the membrane status (intact or ruptured), are associated with an increased mRNA expression of TLR-2 and TLR-4 in the chorioamniotic membranes [59]. These observations suggest that the innate immune system plays a role in parturition, whether or not there is demonstrable intra-amniotic infection/inflammation.

The role of pro-inflammatory cytokines

A solid body of evidence indicates that cytokines play a central role in the mechanisms of inflammation/infection-induced preterm parturition. **IL-1** was the first cytokine [60] to be implicated in the onset of PTL associated with infection. IL-1 is produced by human decidua in response to bacterial products [61], can stimulate prostaglandin production by human amnion and decidua [62], and its concentration and bioactivity is increased in the AF of women with PTL and infection [63]. Additional cytokines such as **TNF-α** [31, 33, 64–68], **IL-6** [69–72], **IL-10** [73–75], **IL-16** [76], **IL-18** [77], **colony stimulating factors (CSFs)** [78, 79], **macrophage migration inhibitory factor (MIF)** [80], and **chemokines** including IL-8 [81, 82], monocyte chemotactic protein-1 (MCP-1) [83], epithelial cell-derived neutrophil-activating peptide (ENA)-78 [84]. Regulated on Activation Normal T cell Expressed and Secreted (RANTES) [85] have also been implicated in the mechanisms of disease in PTL and PTB. The redundancy of the cytokine network implicated in parturition is such that a blockade on a single factor is insufficient to prevent PTB in the context of infection. Indeed, PTL can occur in knockout mice for the IL-1 type I receptor after exposure to infection, suggesting that IL-1 is sufficient, but not necessary, for the onset of parturition in the context of intra-amniotic infection/inflammation [86].

The role of anti-inflammatory cytokines

IL-10 is thought to be a key cytokine for the maintenance of pregnancy. Indeed, IL-10 production is significantly reduced in the term no labor placenta compared with that from first- and second-trimester tissues, suggesting that down-regulation of IL-10 is a physiologic event that favors an inflammatory state around the time of onset of labor [87]. IL-10 has also been implicated in the control of preterm parturition associated with inflammation [74]. Indeed, IL-10 expression was reduced in placental tissues of pregnancies complicated by PTL and chorioamnionitis when compared with placental tissues from normal controls [74].

Tests for diagnosis of microbial invasion of the amniotic cavity

The **tests used for the rapid analysis** of AF include a Gram stain to detect the presence of microorganisms, the AF white blood cell (WBC) count, AF glucose concentration, and the concentration of inflammatory markers, such as IL-6 and matrix metalloproteinase-8 (MMP-8).

A **Gram stain** of AF is universally available in clinical centers. This test has a limited sensitivity in the detection of MIAC, genital mycoplasmas, which are the most frequent pathogens found in the AF, cannot be seen in a Gram stain because of their small size. However, a positive Gram stain has a specificity of 99%, in other words, a false-positive rate of only 1%. We recommend that Gram stain examinations be performed by

Table 7.2 Diagnostic indices of amniotic fluid white blood cell (WBC) count in detecting microbial invasion of the amniotic cavity in patients with preterm labor (PTL) and intact membranes and in those with prelabor premature rupture of the membranes (PPROM).

Reference	Year	Condition	*n*	WBC cutoff (cell/mm^3)	Sensitivity (%)	Specificity (%)	Predictive value	
							Positive (%)	Negative (%)
Romero *et al.* [100]	1991	PTL	195	≥100	66	92.9	58.6	95.2
Romero *et al.* [100]	1991	PTL	195	≥50	80	87.6	48.8	96.7
Romero *et al.* [88]	1993	PTL	120	≥50	63.6	94.5	53.8	96.3
Romero *et al.* [89]	1993	PPROM	110	≥30	57.1	77.9	61.5	74.6

experienced laboratory staff because artifacts and crystals of the reagents may be confused with bacteria by inexperienced individuals.

Neutrophils are not normally present in the AF. The presence of neutrophils is an indication that an inflammatory process is present, and the most frequent cause of inflammation is intra-amniotic infection. An AF WBC count can be performed easily in a hemocytometer chamber, which is also universally available in hospitals around the world. It is the same chamber used to determine a WBC count in blood. An **AF WBC count ≥50 cells/mm^3** had a sensitivity of 80% and a specificity of 87.6% in the detection of MIAC in patients in preterm labor with intact membranes (Table 7.2). Patients with an AF WBC count ≥50 cells/mm^3, but a negative AF culture, are at risk for PTB and frequently have infections caused by genital mycoplasmas [88]. We have proposed a different cutoff value of WBC count for the diagnosis of MIAC in patients with PPROM (≥30 cells/mm^3) [89].

Glucose is a normal constituent of AF, and the concentration of glucose decreases with advancing gestational age. In the presence of intra-amniotic inflammation/infection, the concentration of glucose in the AF decreases. This has been attributed to the consumption of glucose by microorganisms or the consumption of glucose by activated neutrophils engaged in the process of microbial killing. A glucose concentration of **<14 mg/dl** in patients with **PTL** and intact membranes has a high sensitivity and specificity for the detection of intra-amniotic infection/inflammation. The cutoff used in patients who have PPROM is <10 mg/dl. It is important to inform the laboratory that a request for glucose determination of AF is being made because analyzers commonly available in hospitals are optimized for the determination of glucose concentration in blood, which is substantially higher than that of AF. However, AF glucose determination is similar to the glucose determination that is a standard test in the analysis of cerebrospinal fluid in the diagnosis of meningitis. This is a test that is universally available, and so should AF glucose determination for the diagnosis of intra-amniotic infection.

IL-6 has been studied as a rapid test for the detection of MIAC [88, 89]. Patients with MIAC have significantly higher AF IL-6 concentrations than patients with a negative culture. An AF IL-6 concentration of **≥2.6 ng/ml** identifies patients at risk for a positive AF culture for microorganisms and impending delivery. Moreover, patients with an elevated AF IL-6 concentration are also at increased risk for perinatal morbidity and mortality. Interestingly, the outcome of patients with spontaneous preterm labor with intra-amniotic inflammation and a negative AF culture is similar to that of patients with MIAC. Using an AF IL-6 concentration ≥2.6 ng/ml in patients with spontaneous preterm labor and intact membranes, Yoon *et al.* [8] demonstrated that intra-amniotic inflammation was more common than intra-amniotic infection. The rate of spontaneous preterm delivery <37 weeks and adverse pregnancy outcome was higher in patients with intra-amniotic inflammation than in those with a negative culture and without inflammation. Similar observations have been reported in patients with PPROM [90]. Thus, the detection of inflammation using IL-6 may be as important as the detection of a positive AF culture. The advantage of IL-6 is that the **results can be available in as little as 3 hours because the assay is an ELISA**. The importance of IL-6 determination needs to be conveyed to the laboratory because the management of premature labor cannot wait for results that take 24 hours or a week to determine.

MMP-8 plays an important role in MIAC, PPROM, and term and preterm labor. Spontaneous preterm labor and PPROM associated with infection have high concentrations of AF MMP-8 [90–92]. Indeed, among patients with spontaneous preterm labor, the median AF concentration of MMP-8 is more than 50-fold higher in patients with MIAC than in those without [92].

Comparison between amniotic fluid tests

The use of a Gram stain, AF WBC count, and AF glucose determination remain valuable tools for clinical decision making. The determinations of IL-6 and MMP-8 appear superior when they are clinically available. MMP-8 has demonstrated to be an excellent marker of intra-amniotic infection. A comparison between ROC curves demonstrated that the diagnostic performance of AF MMP-8 concentration is superior to that of IL-6 and AF WBC count for the prediction of a positive AF culture [92]. The diagnostic performance of AF IL-6, MMP-8 and glucose concentrations, WBC count, and Gram stain in patients with preterm labor and intact

Table 7.3 Diagnostic indices and predictive values of amniotic fluid tests for detection of positive amniotic fluid culture in patients with preterm labor and intact membranes. WBC, white blood cells. IL-6, interleukin 6.

Amniotic fluid tests	Sensitivity (%)	Specificity (%)	Predictive value	
			Positive (%)	Negative (%)
Gram stain	63.6	99.1	87.5	96.4
IL-6 ≥11.3 ng/ml	100	82.6	36.7	100
WBC ≥50/mm^3	63.6	94.5	53.8	96.3
Glucose ≤14 mg/dl	81.8	81.6	31.0	97.8
Gram stain + WBC count (≥50/mm^3)	90.9	93.6	58.8	99.0
Gram stain + glucose (≤14 mg/dl)	90.9	80.7	32.3	98.9
Gram stain + IL-6 (≥11.3 ng/ml)	100	81.6	35.5	100
Gram stain + glucose (≤14 mg/dl) + WBC count (≥50/mm^3)	90.9	78	29.4	98.8
Gram stain + WBC count (≥50/mm^3) + IL-6 (≥11.3 ng/ml)	100	79.8	33.3	100
Gram stain + glucose (≤14 mg/dl) + IL-6 (≥11.3 ng/ml)	100	71.6	26.2	100
Gram stain + WBC count (≥50/mm^3) + glucose (≤14 mg/dl) + IL-6 (≥11.3 ng/ml)	100	69.7	25	100

membranes and patients with PPROM are displayed in Tables 7.3 and 7.4, respectively.

Bedside rapid test for diagnosis of MIAC

Since the outcome of patients with intra-amniotic inflammation and a negative AF culture is similar to that of patients with MIAC, **our group has proposed that the management of patients with spontaneous preterm labor [8] or PPROM [90] should be based on the diagnosis of intra-amniotic inflammation rather than the diagnosis of MIAC**, because the results of the AF culture will not be available earlier than 48 hours. Recently, a bedside test has been developed to detect intra-amniotic inflammation based on the detection of an elevated concentration of AF MMP-8 [93]. The **MMP-8 PTD Check test** (SK Pharma Co. Ltd, Kyunggi-do, Korea) is similar to a rapid pregnancy test, it requires only 20 µl of AF and no laboratory equipment, and the results are available within 15 minutes. Among patients admitted with PTL and intact membranes [94], the efficiency of a positive MMP-8 rapid test result in the identification of MIAC and intra-amniotic inflammation was 94% and 97%, respectively (Table 7.5). Patients with a positive MMP-8 rapid test had a significantly

Table 7.4 Diagnostic indices and predictive values of amniotic fluid tests for detection of positive amniotic fluid culture in patients with preterm prelabor rupture of the membranes.

Amniotic fluid tests	Sensitivity (%)	Specificity (%)	Predictive value	
			Positive (%)	Negative (%)
Gram stain	23.8	98.5	90.9	67.8
IL-6 ≥7.9 ng/ml	80.9	75	66.7	86.4
MMP-8 >30 ng/ml	76.1	61.8	62.5	75.6
WBC count ≥30 cells/μl	57.1	77.9	61.5	74.6
WBC count ≥50 cells/μl	52.4	83.8	66.7	74
Glucose <10 mg/dl	57.1	73.5	57.1	73.5
Glucose ≤14 mg/dl	71.4	51.5	47.6	74.5
Gram stain + WBC count (≥30 cells/μl)	61.9	77.9	63.4	76.8
Gram stain + glucose (<10 mg/dl)	66.7	73.5	60.9	78.1
Gram stain + IL-6 (≥7.9 ng/ml)	80.9	75	66.7	86.4
Gram stain + MMP-8 (>30 ng/ml)	82.6	61.8	64.4	81
WBC count (≥30 cells/μl) + MMP-8 (>30 ng/ml)	80	60	62.1	78.6
Gram stain + WBC count (≥30 cells/μl) + glucose (<10 mg/dl)	76.2	60.3	61	80.4
Gram stain + WBC count (≥30 cells/μl) + IL-6 (≥7.9 ng/ml)	85.7	61.8	58.1	87.5
Gram stain + WBC count (≥30 cells/μl) + MMP-8 (>30 ng/ml)	84.4	60	63.3	82.5
Gram stain + glucose (<10 mg/dl) + IL-6 (≥7.9 ng/ml)	85.7	52.9	52.9	85.7
Gram stain + WBC count (≥30 cells/μl) + glucose (<10 mg/dl) + IL-6 (≥7.9 ng/ml)	92.9	52.9	52	91.4

Table 7.5 Diagnostic indices, predictive values and likelihood ratios of MMP-8 PTD Check™ for the detection of intra-amniotic infection and inflammation. CI, confidence interval. *A positive amniotic fluid culture for microorganisms. †Amniotic fluid interleukin 6 concentration ≥2.6 ng/ml. Reproduced with permission from Nien JK, Yoon BH, Espinoza J, *et al.* Am J Obstet Gynecol 2006; 195: 1025–30.

	Prevalence	Sensitivity	Specificity	Positive predictive value	Negative predictive value	Positive likelihood ratio (95% CI)	Negative likelihood ratio (95% CI)
Intra-amniotic infection*	7.3% (24/331)	83% (20/24)	95% (291/307)	56% (20/36)	99% (291/295)	15.9 (9.6–26.6)	0.2 (0.1–0.3)
Intra-amniotic inflammation†	11.5% (38/331)	84% (32/38)	99% (289/293)	89% (32/36)	98% (289/295)	61.7 (23.1–164.8)	0.2 (0.1–0.4)

Table 7.6 Diagnostic indices, predictive values and likelihood ratios of MMP-8 PTD Check™ for the identification of patients with spontaneous preterm delivery within 48 h, 7 days, 14 days and <32 and <34 weeks. CI, confidence interval. Reproduced with permission from Nien JK, Yoon BH, Espinoza J, *et al.* Am J Obstet Gynecol 2006; 195: 1025–30.

	Prevalence	Sensitivity	Specificity	Positive predictive value	Negative predictive value	Positive likelihood ratio (95% CI)	Negative likelihood ratio (95% CI)
Delivery within 48 hours	11.6% (38/327)	61% (23/38)	97% (279/289)	70% (23/33)	95% (279/294)	17.5 (9–33.9)	0.4 (0.2–0.8)
Delivery within 7 days	20.2% (66/327)	47% (31/66)	99% (259/261)	94% (31/33)	88% (259/294)	61.3 (15.1–250)	0.5 (0.1–2.2)
Delivery within 14 days	24.5% (80/327)	39% (31/80)	99% (245/247)	94% (31/33)	83% (245/294)	50 (12–196)	0.6 (0.2–2.5)
Delivery <32 weeks	21.1% (32/152)	56% (18/32)	98% (117/120)	86% (18/21)	89% (117/131)	22.5 (7.1–71.7)	0.5 (0.1–1.4)
Delivery <34 weeks	22.4% (61/272)	44% (27/61)	98% (207/211)	87% (27/31)	86% (207/241)	23.4 (8.5–64.2)	0.6 (0.2–1.6)

shorter amniocentesis-to-delivery interval than patients with a negative test. Interestingly, a patient with a positive MMP-8 rapid test is at a substantial risk for spontaneous PTB within 48 hours, 7 days, and 14 days (Table 7.6) [94]. These findings demonstrated that the MMP-8 PTD Check is a sensitive and specific test for the identification of both MIAC and intra-amniotic inflammation among patients with PTL and intact membranes.

The management of patients with intra-amniotic infection/inflammation

The detection of microorganisms or intra-amniotic inflammation is a poor prognostic sign. Patients with PTL with intact membranes and documented intra-amniotic infection/inflammation are unlikely to respond to tocolysis, and are at risk of developing pulmonary edema if attempts are made to delay delivery with tocolysis. Therefore, our approach is to **suspend the administration of tocolysis**. We continue to administer steroids because there is evidence that they cross the placenta and may down-regulate the fetal inflammatory response syndrome. In patients with PPROM, the management depends upon gestational age. The higher the gestational age (e.g.

>33 weeks), the better the outcome if the decision is to deliver the patient. On the other hand, at a gestational age of <32 weeks, treatment must be individualized. We have previously reported that **it is possible to eradicate intra-amniotic infection** in patients with PPROM [95, 96] as well as in patients with a short cervix with antibiotic treatment [13].

A particular challenge is the patient with proven intra-amniotic infection/inflammation around the time of viability. The reader is referred to our original sources to obtain information about antibiotic treatment and the planned amniocentesis to monitor the response to therapy [95, 96]. **It is likely that in the future, anti-inflammatory agents will be coupled with antibiotic treatment** because it is not only the infection, but the inflammatory response that may cause fetal injury and predispose to short and long-term complications, such as chronic lung disease and cerebral palsy. The use of antibiotics in women with PTL or PPROM is discussed in Chapters 18 and 19, respectively. It is important to note that in the context of PPROM, the administration of antibiotics can delay the onset of labor and reduce the rate of proven maternal and neonatal infection. However, the administration of antibiotics neither eradicates established intra-amniotic infection in all cases nor prevents subsequent subclinical microbial invasion of the amniotic cavity while the patient remains undelivered [97]. This observation has important implications for patients and clinicians.

Acknowledgment

This research was supported by the Perinatology Research Branch, Division of Intramural Research, Eunice Kennedy Shriver National Institute of Child Health and Human Development, NIH, DHHS.

References

1 Minkoff H. Prematurity: infection as an etiologic factor. Obstet Gynecol 1983; 62: 137–44.
2 Naeye RL, Ross SM. Amniotic fluid infection syndrome. Clin Obstet Gynaecol 1982; 9: 593–607.
3 Romero R, Mazor M. Infection and preterm labor. Clin Obstet Gynecol 1988; 31: 553–84.
4 Gibbs RS, Romero R, Hillier SL, Eschenbach DA, Sweet RL. A review of premature birth and subclinical infection. Am J Obstet Gynecol 1992; 166: 1515–28.
5 Romero R, Gomez R, Ghezzi F, *et al.* A fetal systemic inflammatory response is followed by the spontaneous onset of preterm parturition. Am J Obstet Gynecol 1998; 179: 186–93.

6 Gomez R, Romero R, Ghezzi F, Yoon BH, Mazor M, Berry SM. The fetal inflammatory response syndrome. Am J Obstet Gynecol 1998; 179: 194–202.

7 Goldenberg RL, Hauth JC, Andrews WW. Intrauterine infection and preterm delivery. N Engl J Med 2000; 342: 1500–7.

8 Yoon BH, Romero R, Moon JB, *et al.* Clinical significance of intra-amniotic inflammation in patients with preterm labor and intact membranes. Am J Obstet Gynecol 2001; 185: 1130–6.

9 Seong HS, Lee SE, Kang JH, Romero R, Yoon BH. The frequency of microbial invasion of the amniotic cavity and histologic chorioamnionitis in women at term with intact membranes in the presence or absence of labor. Am J Obstet Gynecol 2008; 199: 375.

10 Goncalves LF, Chaiworapongsa T, Romero R. Intrauterine infection and prematurity. Ment Retard Dev Disabil Res Rev 2002; 8: 3–13.

11 Romero R, Quintero R, Oyarzun E, *et al.* Intraamniotic infection and the onset of labor in preterm premature rupture of the membranes. Am J Obstet Gynecol 1988; 159: 661–6.

12 Romero R, Gonzalez R, Sepulveda W, *et al.* Infection and labor. VIII. Microbial invasion of the amniotic cavity in patients with suspected cervical incompetence: prevalence and clinical significance. Am J Obstet Gynecol 1992; 167: 1086–91.

13 Hassan S, Romero R, Hendler I, *et al.* A sonographic short cervix as the only clinical manifestation of intra-amniotic infection. J Perinat Med 2006; 34: 13–19.

14 Romero R, Shamma F, Avila C, *et al.* Infection and labor. VI. Prevalence, microbiology, and clinical significance of intraamniotic infection in twin gestations with preterm labor. Am J Obstet Gynecol 1990; 163: 757–61.

15 Romero R, Sirtori M, Oyarzun E, *et al.* Infection and labor. V. Prevalence, microbiology, and clinical significance of intraamniotic infection in women with preterm labor and intact membranes. Am J Obstet Gynecol 1989; 161: 817–24.

16 Bearfield C, Davenport ES, Sivapathasundaram V, Allaker RP. Possible association between amniotic fluid micro-organism infection and microflora in the mouth. Br J Obstet Gynaecol 2002; 109: 527–33.

17 Relman DA. The search for unrecognized pathogens. Science 1999; 284: 1308–10.

18 Jalava J, Mantymaa ML, Ekblad U, *et al.* Bacterial 16S rDNA polymerase chain reaction in the detection of intra-amniotic infection. Br J Obstet Gynaecol 1996; 103: 664–9.

19 Hitti J, Riley DE, Krohn MA, *et al.* Broad-spectrum bacterial rDNA polymerase chain reaction assay for detecting amniotic fluid infection among women in premature labor. Clin Infect Dis 1997; 24: 1228–32.

20 Gardella C, Riley DE, Hitti J, Agnew K, Krieger JN, Eschenbach D. Identification and sequencing of bacterial rDNAs in culture-negative amniotic fluid from women in premature labor. Am J Perinatol 2004; 21: 319–23.

21 DiGiulio DB, Romero R, Amogan HP, *et al.* Microbial prevalence, diversity and abundance in amniotic fluid during preterm labor: a molecular and culture-based investigation. PLoS ONE 2008; 3: e3056.

22 Yoon BH, Romero R, Kim M, *et al.* Clinical implications of detection of *Ureaplasma urealyticum* in the amniotic cavity with the polymerase chain reaction. Am J Obstet Gynecol 2000; 183: 1130–7.

23 Yoon BH, Romero R, Lim JH, *et al.* The clinical significance of detecting *Ureaplasma urealyticum* by the polymerase chain reaction in the amniotic fluid of patients with preterm labor. Am J Obstet Gynecol 2003; 189: 919–24.

24 Cassell GH, Davis RO, Waites KB, *et al.* Isolation of *Mycoplasma hominis* and *Ureaplasma urealyticum* from amniotic fluid at 16–20 weeks of gestation: potential effect on outcome of pregnancy. Sex Transm Dis 1983; 10: 294–302.
25 Gray DJ, Robinson HB, Malone J, Thomson RB, Jr. Adverse outcome in pregnancy following amniotic fluid isolation of *Ureaplasma urealyticum*. Prenat Diagn 1992; 12: 111–7.
26 Horowitz S, Mazor M, Romero R, Horowitz J, Glezerman M. Infection of the amniotic cavity with *Ureaplasma urealyticum* in the midtrimester of pregnancy. J Reprod Med 1995; 40: 375–9.
27 Gerber S, Vial Y, Hohlfeld P, Witkin SS. Detection of *Ureaplasma urealyticum* in second-trimester amniotic fluid by polymerase chain reaction correlates with subsequent preterm labor and delivery. J Infect Dis 2003; 187: 518–21.
28 Markenson GR, Adams LA, Hoffman DE, Reece MT. Prevalence of Mycoplasma bacteria in amniotic fluid at the time of genetic amniocentesis using the polymerase chain reaction. J Reprod Med 2003; 48: 775–9.
29 Nguyen DP, Gerber S, Hohlfeld P, Sandrine G, Witkin SS. Mycoplasma hominis in mid-trimester amniotic fluid: relation to pregnancy outcome. J Perinat Med 2004; 32: 323–6.
30 Perni SC, Vardhana S, Korneeva I, *et al. Mycoplasma hominis* and *Ureaplasma urealyticum* in midtrimester amniotic fluid: association with amniotic fluid cytokine levels and pregnancy outcome. Am J Obstet Gynecol 2004; 191: 1382–6.
31 Romero R, Mazor M, Wu YK, *et al.* Infection in the pathogenesis of preterm labor. Semin Perinatol 1988; 12: 262–79.
32 McDuffie RS, Jr, Sherman MP, Gibbs RS. Amniotic fluid tumor necrosis factor-alpha and interleukin-1 in a rabbit model of bacterially induced preterm pregnancy loss. Am J Obstet Gynecol 1992; 167: 1583–8.
33 Fidel PL, Jr, Romero R, Wolf N, *et al.* Systemic and local cytokine profiles in endotoxin-induced preterm parturition in mice. Am J Obstet Gynecol 1994; 170: 1467–75.
34 Gravett MG, Witkin SS, Haluska GJ, Edwards JL, Cook MJ, Novy MJ. An experimental model for intraamniotic infection and preterm labor in rhesus monkeys. Am J Obstet Gynecol 1994; 171: 1660–7.
35 Romero R, Munoz H, Gomez R, *et al.* Antibiotic therapy reduces the rate of infection-induced preterm delivery and perinatal mortality. Am J Obstet Gynecol 1994; 170: 390.
36 Elovitz MA, Mrinalini C. Animal models of preterm birth. Trends Endocrinol.Metab 2004; 15: 479–87.
37 Kalanda BF, Verhoeff FH, Chimsuku L, Harper G, Brabin BJ. Adverse birth outcomes in a malarious area. Epidemiol.Infect 2005; 28: 1–8.
38 Patrick MJ. Influence of maternal renal infection on the foetus and infant. Arch Dis Child 1967; 42: 208–13.
39 Wren BG. Subclinical renal infection and prematurity. Med J Aust 1969; 2: 596–600.
40 Benedetti TJ, Valle R, Ledger WJ. Antepartum pneumonia in pregnancy. Am J Obstet Gynecol 1982; 144: 413–17.
41 Goepfert AR, Jeffcoat MK, Andrews WW, *et al.* Periodontal disease and upper genital tract inflammation in early spontaneous preterm birth. Obstet Gynecol 2004; 104: 777–83.
42 Jarjoura K, Devine PC, Perez-Delboy A, Herrera-Abreu M, D'Alton M, Papapanou PN. Markers of periodontal infection and preterm birth. Am J Obstet Gynecol 2005; 192: 513–19.

43 Offenbacher S, Boggess KA, Murtha AP, *et al.* Progressive periodontal disease and risk of very preterm delivery. Obstet Gynecol 2006; 107: 29–36.

44 Gomez R, Ghezzi F, Romero R, Munoz H, Tolosa JE, Rojas I. Premature labor and intra-amniotic infection. Clinical aspects and role of the cytokines in diagnosis and pathophysiology. Clin Perinatol 1995; 22: 281–342.

45 Romero R, Oyarzun E, Mazor M, Sirtori M, Hobbins JC, Bracken M. Meta-analysis of the relationship between asymptomatic bacteriuria and preterm delivery/low birth weight. Obstet Gynecol 1989; 73: 576–82.

46 Smaill F. Antibiotics for asymptomatic bacteriuria in pregnancy. Cochrane Database Syst Rev 2001; CD000490.

47 Carroll SG, Papaioannou S, Ntumazah IL, Philpott-Howard J, Nicolaides KH. Lower genital tract swabs in the prediction of intrauterine infection in preterm prelabour rupture of the membranes. Br J Obstet Gynaecol 1996; 103: 54–9.

48 Goldenberg RL, Andrews WW, Goepfert AR, *et al.* The Alabama Preterm Birth Study: umbilical cord blood *Ureaplasma urealyticum* and *Mycoplasma hominis* cultures in very preterm newborn infants. Am J Obstet Gynecol 2008; 198: 43–5.

49 Yoon BH, Romero R, Kim KS, *et al.* A systemic fetal inflammatory response and the development of bronchopulmonary dysplasia. Am J Obstet Gynecol 1999; 181: 773–9.

50 Yoon BH, Romero R, Park JS, *et al.* Fetal exposure to an intra-amniotic inflammation and the development of cerebral palsy at the age of three years. Am J Obstet Gynecol 2000; 182: 675–81.

51 Yoon BH, Romero R, Jun JK, *et al.* An increase in fetal plasma cortisol but not dehydroepiandrosterone sulfate is followed by the onset of preterm labor in patients with preterm premature rupture of the membranes. Am J Obstet Gynecol 1998; 179: 1107–14.

52 Romero R, Espinoza J, Goncalves LF, *et al.* Fetal cardiac dysfunction in preterm premature rupture of membranes. J Matern Fetal Neonatal Med 2004; 16: 146–57.

53 Romero R, Athayde N, Gomez R, *et al.* The fetal inflammatory response syndrome is characterized by the outpouring of a potent extracellular matrix degrading enzyme into the fetal circulation. Am J Obstet Gynecol 1998; 178: S3.

54 Hargreaves DC, Medzhitov R. Innate sensors of microbial infection. J Clin Immunol 2005; 25: 503–10.

55 Pasare C, Medzhitov R. Toll-like receptors: linking innate and adaptive immunity. Microbes Infect 2004; 6: 1382–7.

56 Fazeli A, Bruce C, Anumba DO. Characterization of Toll-like receptors in the female reproductive tract in humans. Human Reprod 2005; 20: 1372–8.

57 Abrahams VM, Bole-Aldo P, Kim YM, *et al.* Divergent trophoblast responses to bacterial products mediated by TLRs. J Immunol 2004; 173: 4286–96.

58 Wang H, Hirsch E. Bacterially-induced preterm labor and regulation of prostaglandin-metabolizing enzyme expression in mice: the role of toll-like receptor 4. Biol Reprod 2003; 69: 1957–63.

59 Kim YM, Romero R, Chaiworapongsa T, *et al.* Toll-like receptor-2 and -4 in the chorioamniotic membranes in spontaneous labor at term and in preterm parturition that are associated with chorioamnionitis. Am J Obstet Gynecol 2004; 191: 1346–55.

60 Romero R, Durum S, Dinarello C, Hobbins JC, Mitchell M. Interleukin-1: A signal for the initiation of labor in chorioamnionitis. Society for Gynecologic Investigation (33rd Annual Meeting), 71. 1986. Abstract.

61 Romero R, Wu YK, Brody DT, Oyarzun E, Duff GW, Durum SK. Human decidua: a source of interleukin-1. Obstet Gynecol 1989; 73: 31–4.

62 Romero R, Durum S, Dinarello CA, Oyarzun E, Hobbins JC, Mitchell MD. Interleukin-1 stimulates prostaglandin biosynthesis by human amnion. Prostaglandins 1989; 37: 13–22.

63 Romero R, Brody DT, Oyarzun E, *et al.* Infection and labor. III. Interleukin-1: a signal for the onset of parturition. Am J Obstet Gynecol 1989; 160: 1117–23.

64 Romero R, Manogue KR, Mitchell MD, *et al.* Infection and labor. IV. Cachectin-tumor necrosis factor in the amniotic fluid of women with intraamniotic infection and preterm labor. Am J Obstet Gynecol 1989; 161: 336–41.

65 Casey ML, Cox SM, Beutler B, Milewich L, MacDonald PC. Cachectin/tumor necrosis factor-alpha formation in human decidua. Potential role of cytokines in infection-induced preterm labor. J Clin Invest 1989; 83: 430–6.

66 Romero R, Mazor M, Manogue K, Oyarzun E, Cerami A. Human decidua: a source of cachectin-tumor necrosis factor. Eur J Obstet Gynecol Reprod Biol 1991; 41: 123–7.

67 Chwalisz K, Benson M, Scholz P, Daum J, Beier HM, Hegele-Hartung C. Cervical ripening with the cytokines interleukin 8, interleukin 1[beta] and tumour necrosis factor [alpha] in guinea-pigs. Hum Reprod 1994; 9: 2173–81.

68 Watari M, Watari H, DiSanto ME, Chacko S, Shi GP, Strauss JF, III. Pro-inflammatory cytokines induce expression of matrix-metabolizing enzymes in human cervical smooth muscle cells. Am J Pathol 1999; 154: 1755–62.

69 Romero R, Avila C, Santhanam U, Sehgal PB. Amniotic fluid interleukin 6 in preterm labor. Association with infection. J Clin Invest 1990; 85: 1392–400.

70 Hillier SL, Witkin SS, Krohn MA, Watts DH, Kiviat NB, Eschenbach DA. The relationship of amniotic fluid cytokines and preterm delivery, amniotic fluid infection, histologic chorioamnionitis, and chorioamnion infection. Obstet Gynecol 1993; 81: 941–8.

71 Gomez R, Romero R, Galasso M, Behnke E, Insunza A, Cotton DB. The value of amniotic fluid interleukin-6, white blood cell count, and gram stain in the diagnosis of microbial invasion of the amniotic cavity in patients at term. Am J Reprod Immunol 1994; 32: 200–10.

72 Andrews WW, Hauth JC, Goldenberg RL, Gomez R, Romero R, Cassell GH. Amniotic fluid interleukin-6: correlation with upper genital tract microbial colonization and gestational age in women delivered after spontaneous labor versus indicated delivery. Am J Obstet Gynecol 1995; 173: 606–12.

73 Sadowsky DW, Novy MJ, Witkin SS, Gravett MG. Dexamethasone or interleukin-10 blocks interleukin-1beta-induced uterine contractions in pregnant rhesus monkeys. Am J Obstet Gynecol 2003; 188: 252–63.

74 Hanna N, Bonifacio L, Weinberger B, *et al.* Evidence for interleukin-10-mediated inhibition of cyclo- oxygenase-2 expression and prostaglandin production in preterm human placenta. Am J Reprod Immunol 2006; 55: 19–27.

75 Gotsch F, Romero R, Kusanovic JP, *et al.* The anti-inflammatory limb of the immune response in preterm labor, intra-amniotic infection/inflammation, and spontaneous parturition at term: a role for interleukin-10. J Matern Fetal Neonatal Med 2008; 21: 529–47.

76 Athayde N, Romero R, Maymon E, *et al.* Interleukin 16 in pregnancy, parturition, rupture of fetal membranes, and microbial invasion of the amniotic cavity. Am J Obstet Gynecol 2000; 182: 135–41.

77 Pacora P, Romero R, Maymon E, *et al.* Participation of the novel cytokine interleukin 18 in the host response to intra-amniotic infection. Am J Obstet Gynecol 2000; 183: 1138–43.

78 Saito S, Kato Y, Ishihara Y, Ichijo M. Amniotic fluid granulocyte colony-stimulating factor in preterm and term labor. Clin Chim Acta 1992; 208: 105–9.

79 Goldenberg RL, Andrews WW, Mercer BM, *et al.* The preterm prediction study: granulocyte colony-stimulating factor and spontaneous preterm birth. National Institute of Child Health and Human Development Maternal-Fetal Medicine Units Network. Am J Obstet Gynecol 2000; 182: 625–30.
80 Chaiworapongsa T, Romero R, Espinoza J, *et al.* Macrophage migration inhibitory factor in patients with preterm parturition and microbial invasion of the amniotic cavity. J Matern Fetal Neonatal Med 2005; 18: 405–16.
81 Romero R, Ceska M, Avila C, Mazor M, Behnke E, Lindley I. Neutrophil attractant/activating peptide-1/interleukin-8 in term and preterm parturition. Am J Obstet Gynecol 1991; 165: 813–20.
82 Saito S, Kasahara T, Kato Y, Ishihara Y, Ichijo M. Elevation of amniotic fluid interleukin 6 (IL-6), IL-8 and granulocyte colony stimulating factor (G-CSF) in term and preterm parturition. Cytokine 1993; 5: 81–8.
83 Esplin MS, Romero R, Chaiworapongsa T, *et al.* Monocyte chemotactic protein-1 is increased in the amniotic fluid of women who deliver preterm in the presence or absence of intra-amniotic infection. J Matern.Fetal Neonatal Med 2005; 17: 365–73.
84 Keelan JA, Yang J, Romero RJ, *et al.* Epithelial cell-derived neutrophil-activating peptide-78 is present in fetal membranes and amniotic fluid at increased concentrations with intra-amniotic infection and preterm delivery. Biol Reprod 2004; 70: 253–9.
85 Athayde N, Romero R, Maymon E, *et al.* A role for the novel cytokine RANTES in pregnancy and parturition. Am J Obstet Gynecol 1999; 181: 989–94.
86 Hirsch E, Muhle RA, Mussalli GM, Blanchard R. Bacterially induced preterm labor in the mouse does not require maternal interleukin-1 signaling. Am J Obstet Gynecol 2002; 186: 523–30.
87 Hanna N, Hanna I, Hleb M, *et al.* Gestational age-dependent expression of IL-10 and its receptor in human placental tissues and isolated cytotrophoblasts. J Immunol 2000; 164: 5721–8.
88 Romero R, Yoon BH, Mazor M, *et al.* The diagnostic and prognostic value of amniotic fluid white blood cell count, glucose, interleukin-6, and gram stain in patients with preterm labor and intact membranes. Am J Obstet Gynecol 1993; 169: 805–16.
89 Romero R, Yoon BH, Mazor M, *et al.* A comparative study of the diagnostic performance of amniotic fluid glucose, white blood cell count, interleukin-6, and gram stain in the detection of microbial invasion in patients with preterm premature rupture of membranes. Am J Obstet Gynecol 1993; 169: 839–51.
90 Shim SS, Romero R, Hong JS, *et al.* Clinical significance of intra-amniotic inflammation in patients with preterm premature rupture of membranes. Am J Obstet. Gynecol 2004; 191: 1339–45.
91 Maymon E, Romero R, Pacora P, *et al.* Human neutrophil collagenase (matrix metalloproteinase 8) in parturition, premature rupture of the membranes, and intrauterine infection. Am J Obstet.Gynecol 2000; 183: 94–9.
92 Maymon E, Romero R, Chaiworapongsa T, *et al.* Amniotic fluid matrix metalloproteinase-8 in preterm labor with intact membranes. Am J Obstet Gynecol 2001; 185: 1149–55.
93 Romero R, Gomez R, Nien JK, *et al.* Metabolomics in premature labor: a novel approach to identify patients at risk for preterm delivery. Am J Obstet Gynecol 2004; 191: S2.
94 Nien JK, Yoon BH, Espinoza J, *et al.* A rapid MMP-8 bedside test for the detection of intra-amniotic inflammation identifies patients at risk for imminent preterm delivery. Am J Obstet Gynecol 2006; 195: 1025–30.

95 Romero R, Scioscia AL, Edberg SC, Hobbins JC. Use of parenteral antibiotic therapy to eradicate bacterial colonization of amniotic fluid in premature rupture of membranes. Obstet Gynecol 1986; 67: 15S–17S.

96 Romero R, Hagay Z, Nores J, Sepulveda W, Mazor M. Eradication of Ureaplasma urealyticum from the amniotic fluid with transplacental antibiotic treatment. Am J Obstet Gynecol 1992; 166: 618–20.

97 Gomez R, Romero R, Nien JK, *et al.* Antibiotic administration to patients with preterm premature rupture of membranes does not eradicate intra-amniotic infection. J Matern Fetal Neonatal Med 2007; 20: 167–73.

98 Romero R, Nores J, Mazor M, *et al.* Microbial invasion of the amniotic cavity during term labor. Prevalence and clinical significance. J Reprod Med 1993; 38: 543–8.

99 Romero R, Mazor M, Morrotti R, *et al.* Infection and labor. VII. Microbial invasion of theamniotic cavity in spontaneous rupture of membranes at term. Am J Obstet Gynecol 1992; 166: 129–33.

100 Romero R, Quintero R, Nores J, *et al.* Amniotic fluid white blood cell count: a rapid and simple test to diagnose microbial invasion of the amniotic cavity and predict preterm delivery. Am J Obstet Gynecol 1991; 165: 821–30.

CHAPTER 8

The Endocrine Regulation of Human Labor

Roger Smith[1,2], *Julia I. Smith*[1] *& Andrew M. Bisits*[3]

[1] Mothers and Babies Research Centre and [2] Endocrine Unit, John Hunter Faculty of Health/School of Medicine and Public Health, University of Newcastle and [3] Division of Obstetrics and Gynaecology, John Hunter Hospital, NSW, Australia

Key points

- Placental corticotrophin releasing hormone (CRH) determines the length of pregnancy.
- CRH drives fetal adrenal production of dehydroepiandrosterone sulfate (DHEAS).
- DHEAS is converted into estriol in the placenta.
- Estriol and estradiol are competitive antagonists at equimolar concentrations but both are estrogen agonists at high concentrations.
- Labor is associated with an excess of estriol over estradiol.
- High levels of estriol lead to myometrial expression of connexin 43 and cyclo-oxygenase.
- Myometrial expression of connexin 43 and prostaglandins leads to synchronised myometrial contractions and the onset of labor.

Does the fetus start labor?

In some species, delivery is linked to maturation of the lungs; it is not clear if this plays a part in human labor. Survival of the fetus following delivery is dependent on the degree of maturity of several organ systems, notably the lungs. Recent work in rodents has linked the onset of labor to maturation of the lungs and their secretion of surfactant protein A (SPA) [1]. In the rodent the presence of fetal lung-derived SPA in the amniotic fluid activates fetal macrophages which then migrate into the myometrium, releasing inflammatory factors that promote uterine contraction. This mechanism links fetal maturation with the onset of labor. Several groups have tested for a similar system in women but have been unable to identify fetal macrophages in human myometrium at the time of labor [2, 3]. SPA has, however, been identified in the fetal membranes and **it remains possible that production of SPA from this site plays a role in the onset of labor to link lung maturation with delivery** [4].

Preterm Birth. Edited by Vincenzo Berghella.

In most mammals studied, however, **progress towards the onset of labor is associated with increasing concentrations of cortisol in the fetal circulation which promote fetal lung maturation**. This was first demonstrated by Liggins *et al.* [5] in the sheep leading to the introduction of glucocorticoid therapy for fetal lung maturation in women in preterm labor.

In the human, placental production of corticotrophin releasing hormone (**CRH**) is **linked to the onset of labor** [6, 7]. CRH is **able to stimulate fetal pituitary adrenocorticotropic hormone (ACTH) production and therefore fetal cortisol synthesis, potentially linking the onset of labor to fetal lung maturation**. CRH also has direct actions to promote lung maturation in the baboon [8], but it is not known if this occurs in humans.

Placental CRH

The onset of human labor is regulated by placental production of CRH, likely acting through placental production of progesterone and different estrogens [7, 9, 10]. Human pregnancy lasts approximately 38 weeks after conception, with minor variations among different racial groups [11]. In humans, the length of gestation is associated with development of the placenta and, in particular, expression of the *CRH* gene by the placenta [12]. In several large cohort studies, the length of gestation has been associated with levels of maternal plasma CRH, of placental origin [6, 13–15]. Maternal plasma CRH increases exponentially as pregnancy advances, peaking at the time of delivery. **In women destined to deliver preterm the exponential increase is more rapid**, whereas in women destined to deliver after the median date of delivery, the rise is slower (Figure 8.1). These findings suggest that a **placental clock** determines the length of gestation and the ultimate timing of delivery [6]. Unfortunately the presence of circulating binding proteins in peripheral maternal plasma interferes with CRH assay unless the sample is extracted to remove these interfering effects prior to assay [16]; additionally maternal plasma levels are very low in early pregnancy. Several negative reports have appeared in which samples were taken early in pregnancy or the assay was performed on unextracted plasma, and this has confused the literature in this area.

Production of CRH by the placenta is restricted to primates and even within the order of primates the pattern of production varies considerably. In New and Old World monkeys there is a pronounced peak in CRH production in mid-gestation [17, 18], but only in the great apes is there an exponential production similar to the rise in maternal CRH in humans

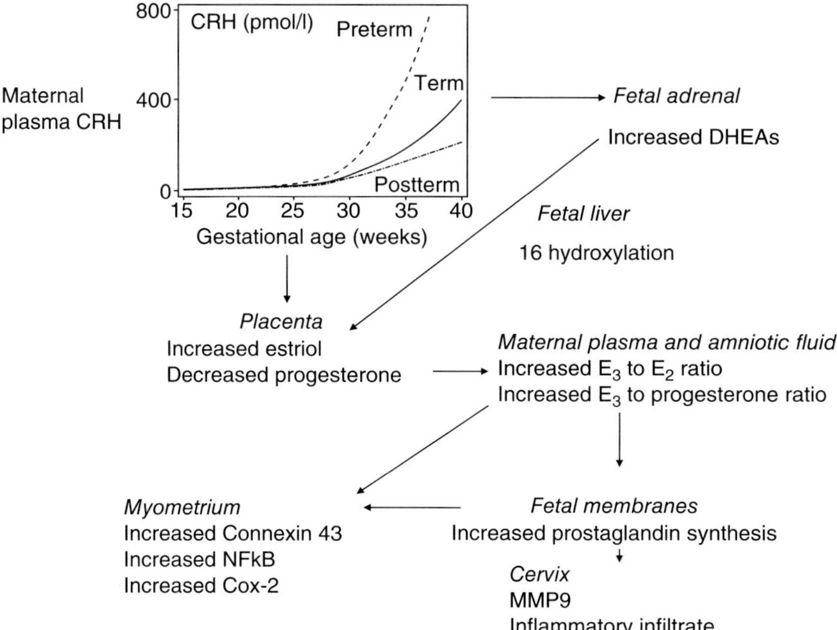

Figure 8.1 Relationships between placental production of corticotrophin releasing hormone (CRH) and the onset of labor. DHEAS, dehydroepiandrosterone sulfate.

[19]. Humans and great apes also produce **a circulating binding protein for CRH (CRHBP)** [20]. **At the end of pregnancy, CRHBP levels fall, thereby increasing the bioavailability of CRH** [21, 22].

Glucocorticoids stimulate expression of the *CRH* gene and production of CRH by the placenta [23–25]. **In turn, CRH stimulates ACTH production by the pituitary and this ACTH causes release of cortisol by the adrenal cortex. This arrangement permits a positive feed forward system** which has been shown by mathematical modelling to mimic the changes observed in human pregnancy [25]. Placental CRH production is also modified by estrogen, progesterone and nitric oxide, which is inhibitory, and by a range of neuropeptides which are stimulatory [26–29]. In each individual woman, levels of placental CRH in maternal blood follow an exponential function to produce a particular trajectory for that pregnancy. Small changes in the exponential function describing CRH production lead to large differences between different women later in pregnancy. Given the large variations between individuals, it is likely that **the rate of rise of maternal concentrations of CRH** is the biological trigger for physiological changes that lead to labor and is the most accurate predictor of outcome [7, 13, 30]. In assessing

CRH values it is also necessary to allow for **racial background**. African-Americans have lower maternal plasma CRH concentrations than other racial groups, although among African- American women, CRH concentrations continue to correlate with the length of gestation and the timing of birth [31].

The placenta predominantly secretes CRH into the maternal blood, but physiologically relevant amounts are also released into the fetal circulation [32]. CRH acts primarily through binding to the CRH type 1 receptor, a member of the 7 transmembrane, G-protein coupled receptor superfamily [33]. In the mother, CRH receptors are present in the pituitary, the myometrium, and probably the adrenal. In the fetus, there are CRH receptors on the pituitary, the adrenal gland, and perhaps the lung. Rising levels of CRH can therefore potentially act at multiple sites in mother and fetus to initiate the changes associated with parturition.

In the mother, **increased placental CRH drives the increase in maternal cortisol and ACTH as gestation advances**, although the effect is moderated by the circulating binding protein and desensitization of CRH receptors by continuous exposure to high concentrations of CRH [34, 35]. The increased levels of CRH and ACTH promote cortisol and dehydroepiandrosterone sulfate (**DHEAS**) production by the maternal adrenal, and this may stimulate further placental release of CRH (by cortisol) and provide substrate for placental estradiol synthesis (from DHEAS). There are several different forms of **CRH receptor** in the human myometrium [36]. Ligand binding to the most common form (CRHR1α) activates adenylate cyclase, stimulating the formation of cAMP which promotes relaxation of the myometrium. At term, CRH receptors change to a form that is less efficient at activating relaxation pathways in the myometrium. Instead, they activate the $G\alpha_q$ pathway that is linked to protein kinase C activation, and contractile pathways [37]. Nevertheless, the predominant action of CRH on the myometrium for the majority of pregnancy is probably to promote relaxation.

Placental CRH is also released into the **fetus**, and although circulating fetal CRH concentrations are lower than in the maternal circulation, they still rise with advancing gestation [38]. In the fetus, CRH receptors are present on the pituitary [39] and on the cells that form the fetal zone of the adrenal [40]. **Stimulation of the fetal pituitary by CRH increases ACTH production** and consequently the synthesis of cortisol by the fetal adrenal gland and maturation of the fetal lung. The rising fetal cortisol concentrations further stimulate placental CRH production and the cortisol-induced maturation of the fetal lung is associated with increased production of surfactant protein A and phospholipids. These have **pro-inflammatory actions and may stimulate myometrial contractility**

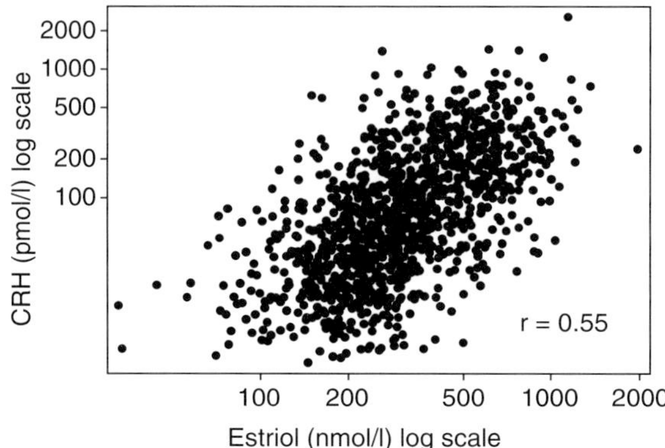

Figure 8.2 Relationship between maternal corticotrophin releasing hormone (CRH) and estriol concentrations in the third trimester. r, correlation coefficient.

through increased production of prostaglandins by fetal membranes and the myometrium itself. CRH may also directly stimulate fetal lung development and surfactant phospholipid synthesis [8].

CRH stimulation of the fetal adrenal zone cells, which lack 3β hydroxysteroid dehydrogenase, preferentially promotes the formation of **DHEAS** [40]. DHEAS is 16 hydroxylated in the fetal liver and then converted into estriol by aromatase and sulfatase in the placenta. The fetal zone of the adrenal involutes rapidly after placental delivery, consistent with the idea that placental factors, such as CRH, maintain the fetal zone. CRH therefore stimulates adrenal steroidogenesis and provides the substrate for increased placental production of estriol. In maternal plasma in the third trimester maternal plasma CRH concentrations are correlated with maternal plasma estriol concentrations supporting this schema for the endocrine regulation of estriol production (Figure 8.2).

In twin gestations the endocrinology of pregnancy is altered by the presence of multiple placentas in dichorionic twins. This is associated with levels of progesterone, estradiol, estriol and CRH that are considerably elevated relative to singleton pregnancies[7] (Figure 8.3).

Regulation of the onset of labor

As pregnancy advances, the production of estriol, derived from the fetal adrenal precursors, increases more rapidly than the production of estradiol, derived predominantly from maternal sources; this leads to a progressive rise in the ratio of estriol to estradiol [7]. This is relevant to the onset of parturition as these two estrogens are mutual antagonists at the estrogen receptor at roughly equimolar concentrations

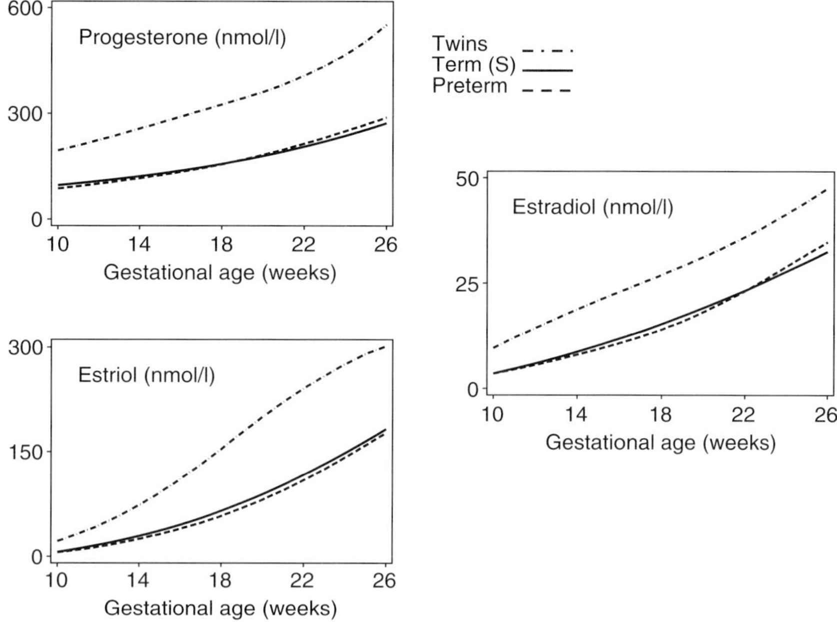

Figure 8.3 Gestational age-related changes in maternal estriol, estradiol and progesterone in singletons that deliver at term, twin gestations and singletons that deliver preterm.

but agonists when present in substantial molar excess [41]. **High ratios of estriol to estradiol in the maternal plasma and in the amniotic fluid at the end of pregnancy can therefore generate the estrogenic environment that promotes the expression of the contraction associated genes** such as connexin 43 required for the onset of labor [42, 43].

In many mammals **progesterone** has a dominant role in maintaining pregnancy and the onset of labor coincides with a fall in maternal progesterone concentrations. No such dramatic fall has been documented in humans. This has led to a search for alternative mechanisms of progesterone withdrawal that might participate in the regulation of the onset of human labor. **Several potential mechanisms have been identified including changes in the co-factors required for progesterone receptor action** [44], **increases in progesterone metabolising enzymes** [45], **antagonism by the transcription factor NFκB** [46] **and changes in progesterone receptor isoforms**. Two main forms of the **progesterone receptor** exist, progesterone receptor A and progesterone receptor B. Progesterone receptor B is the usual receptor mediating progesterone effects on target genes, while progesterone receptor A acts as a dominant negative that can block the action of progesterone. Mesiano

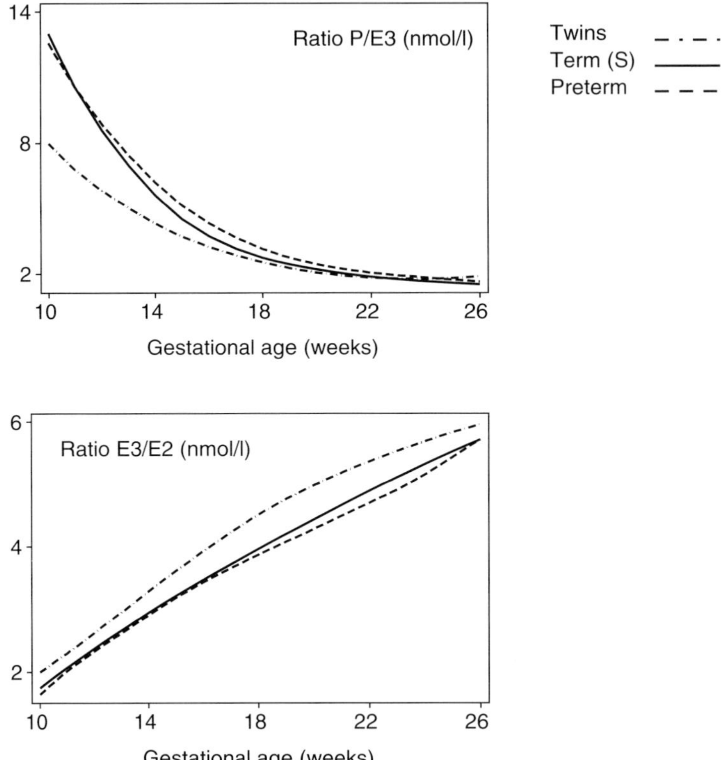

Figure 8.4 The changing ratios of estriol to estradiol and estriol to progesterone as pregnancy progresses. P, progesterone; E2, estradiol; E3, estriol.

et al. [47] have shown that as labor approaches the expression of the different isoforms of the progesterone receptor changes so that the ratio of progesterone receptor A to receptor B increases, potentially mediating a functional progesterone withdrawal in this critical target tissue. The importance of this changing ratio for the function of the myometrium is strengthened by the demonstration that the ratio correlates with the expression of the estrogen receptor alpha gene and the expression of the key contraction associated proteins connexin 43 and cyclooxygenase 2.

Recent data, however, also indicates that **the rate of rise of maternal plasma progesterone changes in late gestation**, flattening off considerably and in some women actually falling [7]. Further it has been shown *in vitro* that CRH can inhibit the placental synthesis of progesterone [9]. The combination of a decline in the rate of rise of progesterone and an increase in the rate of rise of estriol, both potentially driven by rising CRH concentrations, leads to a relative decline in circulating progesterone to estriol ratios as parturition unfolds. This occurs regardless of whether the pregnancy is a singleton term delivery, a twin gestation or a preterm labor

[7] (Figure 8.4). **As estriol shows a diurnal rhythm with peaks levels occurring at night this may explain the nocturnal onset of labor in many women.**

In summary, it appears that positive feed forward systems in the mother and fetus drive an exponential increase in placental CRH production as gestation advances. The increasing placental CRH production drives a change in fetal cortisol concentrations leading to fetal lung maturation. Concurrently, the increasing CRH inhibits placental progesterone synthesis and stimulates the formation of estriol; these events combine to change the progesterone dominated environment of pregnancy to the estrogen dominated environment of labor. The presence of multiple independent pathways, each capable of stimulating parturition, provides robustness to the system and helps to explain why the onset of labor in humans is an inevitable consequence of conception.

References

1 Condon JC, Jeyasuria P, Faust JM, Mendelson CR. Surfactant protein secreted by the maturing mouse fetal lung acts as a hormone that signals the initiation of parturition. Proc Natl Acad Sci USA, 2004; 101: 978–83.

2 Kim CJ, Kim J, Kim Y, *et al.* Fetal macrophages are not present in the myometrium of women with labor at term. Am J Obstet Gynecol 2006: 195: 829–33.

3 Leong AS, Norman JE, Smith R. Vascular and myometrial changes in the human uterus at term. Reprod Sci 2008; 15: 59–65.

4 Han YM, Romero R, Kim YM, *et al.* Surfactant protein-A mRNA expression by human fetal membranes is increased in histological chorioamnionitis but not in spontaneous labour at term. J Pathol 2007; 211: 489–96.

5 Liggins GC, Fairclough RJ, Grieves SA, Kendall JZ, Knox BS. The mechanism of initiation of parturition in the ewe. Rec Prog Horm Res 1973; 29: 111–59.

6 McLean M, Bisits A, Davies J, Woods R, Lowry P, Smith R. A placental clock controlling the length of human pregnancy [see comments]. Nat Med 1995; 1: 460–3.

7 Smith R, Smith JI, Shen X, *et al.* Patterns of plasma corticotrophin-releasing hormone, progesterone, estradiol and estriol change and the onset of human labor. J Clin Endocrinol Metab 2009; 94: 1886–9.

8 Emanuel RL, Torday JS, Asokananthan N, Sunday ME. Direct effects of corticotropin-releasing hormone and thyrotropin-releasing hormone on fetal lung explants. Peptides 2000; 21: 819–29.

9 Yang R, You X, Tang X, Gao X, Ni X. Corticotropin-releasing hormone inhibits progesterone production in cultured human placental trophoblasts. J Mol Endocrinol 2006; 37: 533–40.

10 You X, Yang R, Tang X, Gao L, Ni X. Corticotropin-releasing hormone stimulates estrogen biosynthesis in cultured human placental trophoblasts. Biol Reprod 2006; 74: 1067–72.

11 Patel RR, Steer P, Doyle P, Little MP, Elliott P. Does gestation vary by ethnic group? A London-based study of over 122,000 pregnancies with spontaneous onset of labour. Int J Epidemiol 2004; 33: 107–13.

12 Smith R. Parturition. N Engl J Med 2007; 356: 271–83.
13 Leung TN, Chung TK, Madsen G, Lam PK, Sahota D, Smith R. Rate of rise in maternal plasma corticotrophin-releasing hormone and its relation to gestational length. Br J Obstet Gynaecol 2001; 108: 527–32.
14 Ellis MJ, Livesey JH, Inder WJ, Prickett TC, Reid R. Plasma corticotropin-releasing hormone and unconjugated estriol in human pregnancy: gestational patterns and ability to predict preterm delivery. Am J Obstet Gynecol 2002; 186: 94–9.
15 Sandman CA, Glynn L, Schetter CD, *et al.* Elevated maternal cortisol early in pregnancy predicts third trimester levels of placental corticotropin releasing hormone (CRH): priming the placental clock. Peptides 2006; 27: 1457–63.
16 Ellis MJ, Livesey JH, Donald RA. Circulating plasma corticotrophin-releasing factor-like immunoreactivity. J Endocrinol 1988; 117: 299–307.
17 Goland RS, Wardlaw SL, Fortman JD, Stark RI. Plasma corticotropin-releasing factor concentrations in the baboon during pregnancy. Endocrinology 1992; 131: 1782–6.
18 Smith R, Chan EC, Bowman ME, Harewood WJ, Phippard AF. Corticotropin-releasing hormone in baboon pregnancy. J Clin Endocrinol Metab 1993; 76: 1063–8.
19 Smith R, Wickings EJ, Bowman ME, *et al.* Corticotropin-releasing hormone in chimpanzee and gorilla pregnancies. J Clin Endocrinol Metab 1999; 84: 2820–5.
20 Bowman ME, Lopata A, Jaffe RB, Golos TG, Wickings J, Smith R. Corticotropin-releasing hormone-binding protein in primates. Am J Primatol 2001; 53: 123–30.
21 Linton EA, Behan DP, Saphier PW, Lowry PJ. Corticotropin-releasing hormone (CRH)-binding protein: reduction in the adrenocorticotropin-releasing activity of placental but not hypothalamic CRH. J Clin Endocrinol Metab 1990; 70: 1574–80.
22 Linton EA, Perkins AV, Woods RJ, *et al.* Corticotropin releasing hormone-binding protein (CRH-BP): plasma levels decrease during the third trimester of normal human pregnancy. J Clin Endocrinol Metab 1993; 76: 260–2.
23 Robinson BG, Emanuel RL, Frim DM, Majzoub JA. Glucocorticoid stimulates expression of corticotropin-releasing hormone gene in human placenta. Proc Natl Acad Sci USA 1988; 85: 5244–8.
24 Korebrits C, Yu DH, Ramirez MM, Marinoni E, Bocking AD, Challis JR. Antenatal glucocorticoid administration increases corticotrophin-releasing hormone in maternal plasma. Br J Obstet Gynaecol 1998; 105: 556–61.
25 Emanuel RL, Robinson BG, Seely EW, *et al.* Corticotrophin releasing hormone levels in human plasma and amniotic fluid during gestation. Clin Endocrinol (Oxf) 1994; 40: 257–62.
26 Ni X, *et al.* Nitric oxide inhibits corticotropin-releasing hormone exocytosis but not synthesis by cultured human trophoblasts. J Clin Endocrinol Metab 1997; 82: 4171–5.
27 Ni X, Nicholson RC, King BR, Chan EC, Read MA, Smith R. Estrogen represses whereas the estrogen-antagonist ICI 182780 stimulates placental CRH gene expression. J Clin Endocrinol Metab 2002; 87: 3774–8.
28 Ni X, Hou Y, Yang R, Tang X, Smith R, Nicholson RC. Progesterone receptors A and B differentially modulate corticotropin-releasing hormone gene expression through a cAMP regulatory element. Cell Mol Life Sci 2004; 61: 1114–22.
29 Petraglia F, Sutton S, Vale W. Neurotransmitters and peptides modulate the release of immunoreactive corticotropin-releasing factor from cultured human placental cells. Am J Obstet Gynecol 1989; 160: 247–51.

30 McGrath S, McLean M, Smith D, Bisits A, Giles W, Smith R. Maternal plasma corticotropin-releasing hormone trajectories vary depending on the cause of preterm delivery. Am J Obstet Gynecol 2002; 186: 257–60.
31 Holzman C, Jetton J, Siler-Khodr T, Fisher R, Rip T. Second trimester corticotropin-releasing hormone levels in relation to preterm delivery and ethnicity. Obstet Gynecol 2001; 97: 657–63.
32 Goland RS, Jozak S, Warren WB, Conwell IM, Stark RI, Tropper PJ. Elevated levels of umbilical cord plasma corticotropin-releasing hormone in growth-retarded fetuses. J Clin Endocrinol Metab 1993; 77: 1174–9.
33 Hillhouse EW, Grammatopoulos D, Milton NG, Quartero HW. The identification of a human myometrial corticotropin-releasing hormone receptor that increases in affinity during pregnancy. J Clin Endocrinol Metab 1993; 76: 736–41.
34 Thomson M, Smith R. The action of hypothalamic and placental corticotropin releasing factor on the corticotrope. Mol Cell Endocrinol 1989; 62: 1–12.
35 Livesey JH, Evans MJ, Mulligan R, Donald RA. Interactions of CRH, AVP and cortisol in the secretion of ACTH from perifused equine anterior pituitary cells: 'permissive' roles for cortisol and CRH. Endocr Res 2000; 26: 445–63.
36 Grammatopoulos D, Thompson S, Hillhouse EW. The human myometrium expresses multiple isoforms of the corticotropin-releasing hormone receptor. J Clin Endocrinol Metab 1995; 80: 2388–93.
37 Grammatopoulos DK, Hillhouse EW. Role of corticotropin-releasing hormone in onset of labour. Lancet 1999; 354: 1546–9.
38 Nodwell A, Carmichael L, Fraser M, Challis J, Richardson B. Placental release of corticotrophin-releasing hormone across the umbilical circulation of the human newborn. Placenta 1999; 20: 197–202.
39 Asa SL, Kovacs K, Singer W. Human fetal adenohypophysis: morphologic and functional analysis in vitro. Neuroendocrinology 1991; 53: 562–72.
40 Smith R, Mesiano S, Chan EC, Brown S, Jaffe RB. Corticotropin-releasing hormone directly and preferentially stimulates dehydroepiandrosterone sulfate secretion by human fetal adrenal cortical cells. J Clin Endocrinol Metab 1998; 83: 2916–20.
41 Melamed M, Castaño E, Notides AC, Sasson S. Molecular and kinetic basis for the mixed agonist/antagonist activity of estriol. Mol Endocrinol 1997; 11: 1868–78.
42 Di WL, Lachelin GC, McGarrigle HH, Thomas NS, Becker DL. Oestriol and oestradiol increase cell to cell communication and connexin43 protein expression in human myometrium. Mol Hum Reprod 2001; 7: 671–9.
43 Challis JR, Lye SJ. Parturition. Oxf Rev Reprod Biol 1986; 8: 61–129.
44 Condon JC, Jeyasuria P, Faust JM, Wilson JW, Mendelson CR. A decline in the levels of progesterone receptor coactivators in the pregnant uterus at term may antagonize progesterone receptor function and contribute to the initiation of parturition. Proc Natl Acad Sci USA 2003; 100: 9518–23.
45 Sheehan PM, Rice GE, Moses EK, Brennecke SP. 5 Beta-dihydroprogesterone and steroid 5 beta-reductase decrease in association with human parturition at term. Mol Hum Reprod 2005; 11: 495–501.
46 Lindstrom TM, Bennett PR. The role of nuclear factor kappa B in human labour. Reproduction 2005; 130: 569–81.
47 Mesiano S, Chan EC, Fitter JT, Kwek K, Yeo G, Smith R. Progesterone withdrawal and estrogen activation in human parturition are coordinated by progesterone receptor A expression in the myometrium. J Clin Endocrinol Metab 2002; 87: 2924–30.

CHAPTER 9

Preventive Issues for All Gravidas

Priyadarshini Koduri
Division of Maternal-Fetal Medicine, and Department of Obstetrics and Gynecology, Thomas Jefferson University, Philadelphia, USA

Key points

- Primary preventive measures for preterm birth (PTB) remain poorly studied with few interventions shown to be effective.
- Risk factors for PTB, including medical conditions that may predispose a woman to PTB, should be identified at the first prenatal visit. Appropriate interventions should be applied depending on the risk factors identified.
- Avoiding extremes of age, aiming for at least a 6 month inter-pregnancy interval and insisting on responsible assisted reproductive technology (ART) can be helpful in preventing PTB.
- Women should be encouraged to maintain a healthy pre-pregnancy weight (>120 lb or a BMI > 19 kg/m^2).
- Encourage healthy balanced nutritional intake and avoidance of high protein diets.
- Daily folic acid supplementation for 1 year or longer prior to conception has been shown to reduce PTB risk.
- Bed rest is not recommended. In fact, women at low risk for PTB may safely engage in daily moderate exercise including light resistance training.
- Attempts should be made to modify the work environment avoiding prolonged standing >3 hours/day, long work hours >39 hours/week and shift work.
- All women should be encouraged to avoid smoking, illicit drug and alcohol use.
- Screen for domestic violence and offer appropriate resources and support.
- Screen for and treat sexually transmitted infections and asymptomatic bacteriuria.
- Women should be instructed to avoid douching.

Introduction

Prevention of spontaneous preterm birth (PTB) remains a challenge despite multiple interventions proposed and attempted. As described in Chapters 3 and 4, attempts at prediction have proven helpful, but prevention remains the ultimate goal. Many if not most women who deliver preterm have none of the **risk factors listed in Chapter 4**, and are **nulliparous**. Nonetheless, these risk factors **should be reviewed with every pregnant**

Table 9.1 Recommended primary prevention strategies to avoid preterm birth (PTB) in all gravidas. ART, assisted reproductive technologies. BMI, Body mass index.

Preconception
- Avoid extremes of age
- Aim for desirable inter-pregnancy interval (highest risk of PTB with interval <6 months)
- Avoid multiple gestations with an emphasis on responsible ART
- Folate supplementation
- Vaccinations (especially varicella, rubella, hepatitis B)
- Balanced diet
- Exercise
- Avoid <120 lb maternal weight or BMI < 19 kg/m^2
- Avoid illicit drug use and alcohol use
- Optimize any medical disease (e.g. diabetes)
- Stop or substitute any teratogenic medication with a safer alternative

Prenatal care
- Early ultrasound
- Screen for and treat asymptomatic bacteriuria
- Balanced diet
- Proper weight gain (at least 15 kg over 40 weeks for non-obese women)
- Avoid smoking, illicit drug use and alcohol
- Avoid prolonged standing >3 h/day
- Avoid long work hours >39 h/week
- Avoid shift work
- Avoid vaginal douching
- Screen for domestic violence and provide resources
- Screen and treat for sexually transmitted diseases (Chapter 15)
- Consider screening and treating women with prior PTB for BV (Chapter 14)

woman. **Primary prevention of both spontaneous and iatrogenic PTB encompasses interventions aimed at all pregnant women**, regardless of any identifiable risk factors, and has been shown to be **more efficacious** than secondary or tertiary prevention. A wide variety of interventions fall under primary prevention, keeping in mind that prevention of preeclampsia, intrauterine growth retardation (IUGR) and congenital anomalies also prevents PTB. This chapter will outline the evidence behind general preventative guidelines for all gravidas. Table 9.1 summarizes preventative guidelines applicable to all women while Table 9.2 summarizes guidelines for women with selected risk factors and Table 9.3 summarizes interventions that have not shown to be beneficial.

Preconception

Interventions to decrease PTB available for all women of reproductive age are described in **Table 9.1**. **Avoiding extremes of age, increasing**

Table 9.2 Recommended preconception interventions to decrease PTB in women with selected specific risk factors. PTB, preterm birth; *, especially iatrogenic PTB. LBW, low birth weight. IUGR, intrauterine growth restriction. NICU, neonatal intensive care unit. BMI, body mass index. NTD, neural tube defects. CD, Cesarean delivery. HTN, hypertension. VTE, venous thromboembolism. TSH, thyroid-stimulating hormone. FT4, free thyroxine. HIV, human immunodeficiency virus. RNA, ribonucleic acid.

Risk factor/population	Intervention	Prevention of
Smoking	Smoking cessation	PTB, LBW, etc. (Chapter 10)
Alcohol	Avoid all alcohol intake	PTB; congenital anomalies, mental retardation
Other drugs of abuse (cocaine, heroin, etc.)	Avoid all drugs of abuse	PTB, IUGR, neonatal withdrawal, etc. (effect depends on drug of abuse)
Diabetes	Hemoglobin A1C <7%; screening for asymptomatic bacteriuria	PTB*; congenital anomalies, length of NICU admission, perinatal mortality and long-term health consequences in infant; miscarriage; maternal hospitalizations, maternal renal disease
Obesity	Diet and exercise to achieve normal BMI; screening for diabetes	PTB*; infertility, fetal NTDs, PTB, CD, HTN-disorders, diabetes, VTE
Hypertension	Avoid angiotensin-converting enzyme inhibitors and angiotensin-receptor blockers. If long-standing HTN, assess for renal disease, ventricular hypertrophy, and retinopathy	PTB*; congenital anomalies, HTN complications, CD, IUGR, placental abruption, perinatal death.
Hypothyroidism	Thyroxine supplementation to maintain normal TSH (0.5–2.0 mcu/ml)	PTB*; infertility, maternal HTN, preeclampsia, abruption, anemia, PTB, LBW, fetal death, possibly neurological problems in infant
Hyperthyroidism	PTU (propylthiouracil) supplementation to maintain FT4 in high normal range, and TSH in low normal range	PTB*; spontaneous pregnancy loss, pre-eclampsia, fetal death, FGR, maternal congestive heart failure, and thyroid storm; neonatal Graves' disease
Asthma	Management following National Asthma Education and Prevention Program (NAEPP).	PTB*, LBW, preeclampsia, perinatal mortality
Systemic lupus erythematosus	≥6 months of quiescence on stable therapy	PTB*; HTN, preeclampsia, fetal death, IUGR, neonatal lupus
HIV	Initiate or modify antiviral agents with goals of: (1) HIV-1 RNA viral load level below the limit of detection of the assay (2) avoid teratogenic agents	PTB; perinatal HIV infection
Sexually-transmitted disease (e.g. Chlamydia)	Screen at risk populations	PTB; ectopic pregnancy (Chapter 15)
Social issues (e.g. abuse, etc.)	Counseling; referral to appropriate agency	PTB; physical and emotional trauma and their consequences

Table 9.3 Interventions currently *without* sufficient evidence to recommend them for prevention of preterm birth (PTB).

- Initiation of early prenatal care (<14 weeks gestation)
- Enhanced prenatal care (support)
- Bed rest (for either prophylaxis or therapy of PTB)
- Diet rich in omega 3 fatty acids
- High protein diet
- Vitamin supplementation other than folic acid
- Aspirin
- Organized social support to reduce stress
- Yoga or other forms of physical relaxation
- Treatment of periodontal disease
- Manual cervical exams
- Home uterine activity monitoring
- Screening for inherited or acquired thrombophilias
- Screening for cervico-vaginal group B streptococcus colonization

inter-pregnancy interval (highest risk of PTB with interval <6 months) **and avoiding multiple gestations with an emphasis on responsible ART** (confirming diagnosis of infertility, limiting number of embryos transferred and the use of multi-fetal reduction) are helpful in modifying risk [1–6]. **Preconception folate supplementation** (for 1 year or longer) is associated with a 70% decrease in risk of PTB between 20 and 28 weeks (OR 0.22, 95% confidence interval (CI) 0.08–0.61) and 50% decrease in PTB between 28 and 32 weeks (OR 0.45, 95% CI 0.24–0.83) [7]. Results from a double-blinded RCT **do not support inter-conception antibiotics** to prevent PTB in women with history of a prior PTB [8].

Early prenatal care

Early prenatal care is recommended for all gravidas, although there are no RCTs evaluating whether it is effective in preventing PTB. Retrospective data, however, suggests that in women living in the United States, early prenatal care is associated with fewer PTBs [9]. This relationship may not be causal but could be a marker for other risk factors for PTB. In a large RCT, enhanced prenatal care, characterized by more frequent visits, weekly pelvic exams starting after 20–24 weeks gestation and better patient education, did not result in lower PTB rates compared with standard prenatal care [10].

At an early visit, a comprehensive history should be obtained focusing on **identification of pre-existing medical conditions** which may place the woman at risk for PTB **(Table 9.2)**. Traditional **risk factors for PTB** listed in Chapter 4 should also be identified. While **many if not most women who experience spontaneous PTB have no identifiable risk factors, identifying any risk factors for which there is a known intervention is extremely important**. Several risk scoring systems have been described using the patient's history and other clinical findings to create an additive score in an attempt to predict PTB. The value of these systems, however, is uncertain because of their poor positive predictive value [11–15]. Moreover, several trials based on these scoring systems have demonstrated their inability to prevent PTB [16, 17].

An early ultrasound is typically performed as part of a woman's early prenatal care. It allows for accurate prediction of gestational age which is understandably key in management decisions and counseling regarding outcome should PTB become imminent later in the pregnancy. Early ultrasound also allows for identification of multiple gestations, fewer post-term inductions but no difference in the rate of low birth weight infant births (OR 0.96, 95% CI 0.82–1.12) [18].

Nutrition

All women should eat a well-balanced diet incorporating a variety of foods during pregnancy. **Low pre-pregnancy weight** (BMI < 19 kg/m^2 or body weight <120 lb) and **third-trimester rates of weight gain below the lower limit** of the Institute of Medicine recommended range (less than 0.38 kg/week with low BMI, less than 0.37 kg/week with normal BMI) are **associated with increased PTB** among all women (OR 2.46, 95% CI 1.53–3.92) [19, 20].

High protein diets or diets which involve balanced protein/energy supplementation do not have an effect on the length of gestation even in women who are nutritionally deprived, but **balanced supplementation** may be associated with improved fetal growth and a lower incidence of small for gestation age (SGA) births [21, 22]. The data on whether a diet rich in **omega-3-fatty acids** reduces the incidence of PTB is conflicting despite six trials, and until conclusive evidence is obtained such a diet cannot be recommended as a preventive measure [23–26].

Although daily prenatal vitamins are recommended for supplementation, they or any additional vitamin supplementation other than folate have not definitively been shown to improve PTB rates in all women. Of other vitamins/minerals/supplements studied in randomized trials,

magnesium was associated with prevention of PTB, but this result is based on poor quality trials [27]. **Zinc** supplementation is also associated in beneficial prevention of PTB in women of low income [28]. Supplementation with vitamin C has been associated with an increased risk of PTB [29].

In women at high risk for PTB, aspirin has shown promise. A meta-analysis investigating the effect and safety of acetylsalicylic acid in pregnancy demonstrated a small but significant effect on reducing the rates of PTB in high risk women (RR 0.92, 95% CI 0.86–0.98) which confirmed the results of Collaborative Low-Dose Aspirin Study in Pregnancy [30]. However, these results have not been replicated in women considered low risk for PTB.

Activity

Bed rest

There is **no evidence to suggest that bed rest prevents PTB** in singleton gestations even in women considered at high risk for PTB [31, 32]. Bed rest in pregnancy is associated with a 1–2% risk of thromboembolism in addition to lower patient morale, depression and physical deconditioning. Given these numerous adverse effects with no clear benefit, bed rest should not be recommended as a preventive measure.

Exercise

Mild to moderate exercise is recommended for all otherwise healthy gravidas. A RCT showed that previously sedentary healthy women with singleton gestations and an uncomplicated obstetrical history could safely engage in moderate supervised exercise programs involving toning and light resistance exercises during the last two trimesters of gestation without altering their risk of PTB [33]. Because there are no RCTs examining exercise in women at high risk for PTB, caution should be used in generalizing these findings to a high risk population.

Work environment

Prolonged standing >3 h/day, long work hours >39 h/week and shift work increase the risk of PTB (OR 1.16–1.29) [34]. These results are confirmed in a large case control study which also found that women who had low job satisfaction (OR 1.1–1.5) were at higher risk for PTB [35]. A case control study performed recently in the United States found that standing at least 30 hours per week and repeated lifting (up to 25 lb at least 13 times/week) were not associated with PTB [36]. This study also demonstrated a weak association between night shift work and PTB. No trials have been conducted assessing the efficacy of work place modifications on the rates of PTB. Regardless, it is still reasonable to consider the job description, weekly hours and the patient's ability to handle work-related stress or fatigue when making recommendations for adjustments in her work environment.

Sexual intercourse

Sexual intercourse is not considered a risk factor for PTB. Existing evidence does not suggest that sexual intercourse while pregnant, in women with singleton gestations, including those with a prior PTB < 32 weeks gestation, confers any additional risk of PTB [37–39].

Douching

There are no RCTs assessing the effect of douching on PTB. The existing evidence is inconclusive. In a prospective cohort study, douching in the 12 months prior to pregnancy, in the absence of bacterial vaginosis, was found to be **associated with an increased risk of PTB** (OR 1.29–3.75) [40]. Similarly, douching more than once per week was associated with an increased risk of PTB (OR 1.0–15.5) [41]. However, a cohort study of African-American women found that vaginal douching 6 months prior to pregnancy and <3 times per month was associated with a reduced risk of PTB (OR 0.42–0.95), while douching during pregnancy was associated with a trend towards increased PTB [42]. Until conclusive evidence is available, douching during pregnancy cannot be recommended as a preventive measure.

Lifestyle

Smoking cessation should be recommended for its general health benefits. Smoking cessation in pregnancy can prevent up to 15% of PTB, and as such is the single most successful intervention for preventing PTB. However, its effect on PTB is modest after adjustment for possible confounders such as abruption, placenta previa, premature rupture of membranes and intrauterine growth restriction [43]. Smoking, its relationship to PTB and intervention strategies in pregnancy will be extensively discussed in Chapter 10.

Heroin and amphetamines have also been linked to PTB while marijuana has not [44, 45]. Substances commonly used in pregnancy include cocaine, amphetamines, opioids, ethanol, marijuana and toluene-based solvents. Polysubstance abuse is common and is associated with a 25% risk of PTB. Cocaine is found in up to 60% of women in preterm labor who had a urine drug screen sent [46]. Limited data is available for the effects of ecstasy and LSD on pregnancy outcomes. Causation has been more difficult to prove given the numerous other risk factors for PTB women with drug addiction generally have. Although no RCTs have evaluated the effects of illicit drugs or alcohol on PTB, it is reasonable to counsel women against usage.

The association between low and moderate **alcohol consumption** and PTB is inconclusive. However, heavy drinking (>6.8 drinks/week or >68 g of alcohol/week) has recently been shown to be associated with an increased risk of PTB compared with those who abstained during pregnancy even if these women abstained before the second trimester (OR 1.73, 95% CI 1.01–3.14) [47].

Domestic violence has been associated with PTB in numerous studies, both prospective and retrospective, in addition to being associated with low birth weight and neonatal death [48–51]. No RCTs are available to evaluate the effect any intervention strategy may have. Nonetheless, women who experience intimate partner violence should be identified and **access to available interventions and social support** ensured.

Screening

Lower genital tract infections

Screening and treating sexually transmitted infections is recommended during pregnancy due to adverse maternal or neonatal sequelae which may follow untreated disease. These infections have been linked to PTB. However, there is limited level 1 evidence that treatment of these infections results in a reduced PTB rate [52]. Sexually transmitted infections are covered in detail in Chapter 15, while the relationship between bacterial vaginosis and PTB is discussed in Chapter 14. Antibiotic prophylaxis during pregnancy to unselected women is not associated with prevention of PTB [53].

Cervical screening

A program of **weekly digital cervical exams** in addition to patient education in women at high risk for PTB identified by an elevated Creasy score **has not been found to reduce the risk of PTB** [17, 54, 55] (see above under bedrest). Using transvaginal **cervical length** measurements to screen women at high risk for PTB will be reviewed in Chapter 12. Screening for cervico-vaginal group B streptococcus colonization before 30 weeks and treating with erythromycin is not associated with prevention of PTB [56].

Asymptomatic bacteriuria

Asymptomatic bacteriuria has been unequivocally linked to PTB. Screening with a urine culture during the first trimester and treatment of a culture with greater than 100 000 CFU/ml can **effectively reduce the incidence of PTB by 40%** in addition to reducing incidence of pyelonephritis [57]. Treatment with the narrowest spectrum sensitive antibiotic is recommended for 4–7 days although optimal length of treatment remains insufficiently studied [58]. Group B streptococcus bacteriuria should be treated regardless of colony counts for prevention of PTB [59].

Periodontal disease

Several studies have demonstrated an association between periodontal disease and PTB [60–62]. However, this association has been recently challenged by a recent prospective study [63]. In women with identified periodontal disease, progression of disease during pregnancy has not been shown to have an association with PTB [64] . Recent trials on intervention for periodontal disease have **not demonstrated a reduction in PTB** [65–67].

Home uterine activity monitoring (HUAM)

Self monitoring by teaching the patient to palpate and record her own contractions can be suggested, despite its subjectivity and poor sensitivity (89% of patients palpate less than 50% of their contractions) [68]. Randomized trials on HUAM devices employing outpatient tocography have suggested that compliance is poor and interpretation is subject to high inter-observer variability, thereby concluding that the method is **not clinically useful for predicting or preventing PTB** even when combined with a daily nursing contact [69–72].

Support and stress

Acute and chronic stress have been shown to be associated with PTB [73, 74]. Providing enhanced social support in the form of **emotional support and assistance**, while beneficial from a psychological standpoint, has **not been shown to reduce the incidence of PTB** [75]. Yoga, stress reduction and physical relaxation may result in a feeling of well being but similarly have not been proven to reduce rates of PTB [76].

Depression diagnosed either before or during the pregnancy, has been associated with PTB although risk factors for depression overlap with those for PTB. It is unclear whether professional intervention and medication alter birth outcome although they are recommended given maternal benefit.

Other risks

There are no RCTs to assess interventions for prevention of PTB in other at risk groups such as women with **multiple dilatations and evacuations, uterine anomalies, or cone biopsies** (Chapter 6). One recent approach is to follow these women with transvaginal ultrasound cervical length. No interventions have been shown to be beneficial in these women once the cervix shortens, so this approach deserves more research before widespread clinical use (Chapter 12). Other areas that deserve further study are screening for **inherited or acquired (antiphospholipid syndrome) thrombophilias**, which are associated with PTB, but for which there is no proven intervention aimed at preventing this outcome.

References

1 Nabukera SK, Wingate MS, Kirby RS, *et al.* Interpregnancy interval and subsequent perinatal outcomes among women delaying initiation of childbearing. J Obstet Gynaecol Res 2008; 34: 941–7.

2 Zhu BP, Rolfs RT, Nangle BE, *et al.* Effect of interval between pregnancies on perinatal outcomes. New Engl J Med 1999; 340: 589–94.

3 DeFranco EA, Stamilio DM, Boslaugh SE, *et al.* A short pregnancy interval is a risk factor for preterm birth and its recurrence. Am J Obstet Gynecol 2007; 197: 264. e1–6.

4 Khoshnood B, Lee KS, Wall S, Hsieh HL. Short interpregnancy intervals and the risk of adverse birth outcomes among five racial/ethnic groups in the United States. Am J Epidemiol 1998; 148: 798–805.

5 ACOG Practice Bulletin #56: Multiple Gestation: Complicated Twin, Triplet and High Order Multifetal Pregnancy. Obstet Gynecol 2004; 104: 869–83.

6 Kiely JL. What is the population based risk of preterm birth among twins and other multiples? Clin Obstet Gynecol 1998; 41: 3–11.

7 Bukowski R, Malone FD, Porter FT, *et al.* Preconceptional folate supplementation and the risk of spontaneous preterm birth: a cohort study. PLoS Med 2009;6: e1000061. doi: 10.1371/journal.pmed.100006.

8 Tita TN, Cliver SP, Geopfert AT, *et al.* Clinical trial of interconceptional antibiotics to prevent preterm birth: subgroup analyses and possible adverse anti-biotic-microbial interaction. Am J Obstet Gynecol 2007; 367.e1–6.

9 Vintzileos AM, Ananth CV, Smulian JC, *et al.* The impact of prenatal care in the United States on preterm births in the presence and absence of antenatal high risk conditions. Am J Obstet Gynecol 2002; 187: 1254–7.

10 Multicenter randomized controlled trial of a preterm birth prevention program. Collaborative Group on Preterm Birth Prevention. Am J Obstet Gynecol 1993; 169: 352–66.

11 Creasy RK, Gummer BA, Liggins GC. System for predicting spontaneous preterm birth. Obstet Gynecol 1980; 55: 692–5.

12 Nicholson W, Croughan-Minihane M, Posner S, *et al.* Preterm delivery in patients admitted with preterm labor: a prediction study. J Matern Fetal Med 2001; 10: 102–6.

13 Guinn DA, Wigton TR, Owen J, *et al.* Prediction of preterm birth in nulliparous patients. Am J Obstet Gynecol 1994; 171: 1111–5.
14 Mueller-Heubach E, Guzick DS. Evaluation of risk scoring in a preterm birth prevention study of indigent patients. Am J Obstet Gynecol 1989; 160: 829–35.
15 Honest H, Bachmann LM, Sundaram R, *et al.* The accuracy of risk scores in predicting preterm birth — a systematic review. J Obstet Gynaecol 2004; 24: 343–59.
16 Goldenberg RL, Davis RO, Cooper RL, *et al.* The Alabama preterm birth prevention project. Obstet Gynecol 1990; 75: 933–9.
17 Collaborative group on preterm birth prevention. Multicenter randomized controlled trial of a preterm birth prevention program. Am J Obstet Gynecol. 1993; 169: 352–66.
18 Neilson JP. Ultrasound for fetal assessment in early pregnancy. Cochrane Database Syst Rev 2000; (2): CD000182.
19 Schieve LA, Cogswell ME, Scanlon KS, *et al.* Pre-pregnancy body mass index and pregnancy weight gain: associations with preterm delivery. The NMIHS Collaborative Study Group. Obstet Gynecol 2000; 96: 194–200.
20 Hickey CA, Cliver SP, McNeal SF, *et al.* Prenatal weight gain patterns and spontaneous preterm birth among non-obese black and white women. Obstet Gynecol 1995; 85: 909–14.
21 Kramer MS, Kakuma R. Energy and protein intake in pregnancy. Cochrane Database Syst Rev 2007; 1.
22 Onwude JL, Lilford RJ, Hjartardottir H, *et al.* A randomized double blind placebo controlled trial of fish oil in high risk pregnancy. Br J Obstet Gynecol 1995; 102: 95.
23 Olsen SF, Secher NJ, Tabor A, *et al.* Randomized clinical trials of fish oil supplementation in high risk pregnancies. Fish Oil Trials in Pregnancy (FOTIP) Team. Br J Obstet Gynaecol 2000; 107: 382.
24 Olsen SF, Sorensen JD, Secher NJ, *et al.* Randomized controlled trial of effect of fish-oil supplementation on pregnancy duration. Lancet 1992; 339: 1003–7.
25 Smuts, CM. A randomized trial of docosahexaenoic acid supplementation during the third trimester of pregnancy. Obstet Gynecol 2003; 101: 469–79.
26 Makrides M, Duley L, Olsen SF. Marine oil, and other prostaglandin precursor, supplementation for pregnancy uncomplicated by pre-eclampsia or intra-uterine growth restriction. Cochrane Database Syst Rev 2006. Issue 3. Art. No.: CD003402. DOI: 10.1002/14651858. CD003402. Pub2.
27 Makrides M, Crowther CA. Magnesium supplementation in pregnancy. Cochrane Database Syst Rev 2001, Issue 4. Art. No.: CD000937. DOI: 10.1002/14651858. CD000937.
28 Mahomed K, Bhutta ZA, Middleton P. Zinc supplementation for improving pregnancy and infant outcome. Cochrane Database Syst Rev 2007, Issue 2. Art. No.: CD000230. DOI: 10.1002/14651858.CD000230.pub3.
29 Rumbold A, Crowther CA. Vitamin C supplementation in pregnancy. Cochrane Database Syst Rev 2005, Issue 1. Art. No.: CD004072. DOI: 10.1002/14651858. CD004072.pub2.
30 Krozer E, Costei AM, Boskovic R, *et al.* Effects of aspirin consumption during pregnancy on pregnancy outcomes: meta-analysis. Birth Defects Res (Part B) 2003; 68: 70–84.
31 Sosa C, Althabe F, Belizan J, *et al.* Bedrest in singleton pregnancies for preventing preterm birth. Cochrane Database Syst Rev 2004, Issue 1. Art. No. CD003581.
32 Hobel CJ, Ross MG, Bemis RL, *et al.* The West Los Angeles preterm birth prevention project. I. Program impact on high risk women. Am J Obstet Gynecol 1994; 170: 54–62.

33 Barakat R, Stirling JR, Lucia A. Does exercise training during pregnancy affect gestational age? A randomized controlled trial. Br J Sports Med 2008; 42; 674–87.
34 Mozurkevich EL, Luke B, Avni M, Wolf FM. Working conditions and adverse pregnancy outcome: a meta-analysis. Obstet Gynecol 2000; 95: 623–35.
35 Saurel-Cubizolles MJ, Zeitlin J, Lelong N, *et al.* Employment, working conditions and preterm birth: results from the Europop case-control survey. J Epidemio Community Health 2004;58: 395–401.
36 Pompeii LA, Savitz DA, Evenson KR, *et al.* Physical exertion at work and the risk of preterm delivery and small for gestational age birth. Am J Obstet Gynecol 2005; 106: 1279–88.
37 Yost NP, Owen J, Berghella V, *et al.* Effect of coitus on recurrent preterm birth. Obstet Gynecol 2006; 107: 793–7.
38 Berghella V, Klebanoff M, McPherson C, *et al.* Sexual intercourse association with asymptomatic bacterial vaginosis and Trichomas vaginalis treatment in relationship to preterm birth. Am J Obstet Gynecol 2002; 187: 1277–82.
39 Read JS, Klebanoff MA. Sexual intercourse during pregnancy and preterm delivery: effects of vaginal micro-organisms. The Vaginal Infections and Prematurity Study Group. Am J Obstet Gynecol 1993; 168: 514–9.
40 Thorp JM, Dole N, Herring AH, *et al.* Alteration in vaginal microflora, douching prior to pregnancy and preterm birth. Paediatr Perinat Epidemiol 2008; 22: 530–7.
41 Fiscella K, Franks P, Kendrick JS *et al.* Risk of preterm birth that is associated with vaginal douching. Am J Obstet Gynecol 2002; 186: 1345–50.
42 Misra DP, Trabert B. Vaginal douching and the risk of preterm birth among African American women. Am J Obstet Gynecol 2007; 196: 140.e1–8.
43 Kyrklund-Blomberg NB, Cnattinggius S. Preterm birth and maternal smoking: risks related to gestational age and onset of delivery. Am J Obstet Gynecol 1998; 179: 1051.
44 Ney JA, Dooley SL, Keith G, *et al.* The prevalence of substance abuse in patients with suspected preterm labor. Am J Obstet Gynecol 1990;162: 1562–5; discussion 1565–7.
45 Borges G, Lopez-Cervantes M, Medina-Mora ME, *et al.* Alcohol consumption, low birth weight and preterm delivery in the National Addiction Survey (Mexico). Int J Addict 1993; 28: 355–5.
46 Spence MR, Williams R, DiGregorio GJ, *et al.* The relationship between recent cocaine use and pregnancy outcome. Obstet Gynecol 1991; 78: 326–9.
47 O'Leary CM, Nassar N, Kurinczuk JJ, *et al.* The effect of maternal alcohol consumption on fetal growth and preterm birth. Br J Obstet Gynaecol 2009; 116: 390–400.
48 Lipsky S, Holt VL, Easterling TR, *et al.* Impact of police-reported intimate partner violence during pregnancy on birth outcomes. Obstet Gynecol 2003; 102: 557–64.
49 Rodrigues T, Rocha L, Barros H. Physical abuse during pregnancy and preterm delivery. Am J Obstet Gynecol 2008; 198: 171.e1–6.
50 Neggers Y, Goldenberg R, Cliver S, *et al.* Effects of domestic violence on preterm birth and low birth weight. Acta Obstet Gynecol Scand 2004; 83: 455–60.
51 Yost NP, Bloom SL, McIntire DD, *et al.* A prospective observational study of domestic violence during pregnancy. Obstet Gynecol 2005; 106: 61–5.
52 Goldenberg RL, Andrews WW, Yuan AC, *et al.* Sexually transmitted diseases and adverse outcomes of pregnancy. Clin Perinatol 1997; 24: 23–41.
53 Thinkhamrop J, Hofmeyr GJ, Adetoro O, Lumbiganon P. Prophylactic antibiotic administration in pregnancy to prevent infectious morbidity and mortality. Cochrane Database Syst Rev 2007, Issue 4. Art. No.: CD002250. DOI: 10.1002/14651858.CD002250.

54 Mueller-Heubach E, Reddick D, Barnett B, *et al.* Preterm birth prevention: evaluation of a prospective controlled trial. Am J Obstet Gynecol 1989; 160: 1172–8.
55 Main DM, Richardson DK, Hadley CB, *et al.* Controlled trial of a preterm labor detection program: efficacy and costs. Obstet Gynecol 1989; 74: 873–7.
56 Klebanoff MA, Regan JA, Rao AV, Nugent RP, Blackwelder WC, *et al.* Outcome of the vaginal infection and prematurity study: results of a clinical trial of erythromycin among pregnant women colonized with group B streptococcus. Am J Obstet Gynecol 1995; 172: 1540–5.
57 Smaill F. Antibiotics for asymptomatic bacteriuria in pregnancy. Cochrane Database Syst Rev 2001;(2): CD000490.
58 Villar J, Widmer M, Lydon-Rochelle M, Gulmezoglu AM, Roganti A. Duration of treatment for asymptomatic bacteriuria during pregnancy. Cochrane Library 2009, vol. 1.
59 Thompsen AC, Morup L, Hansen KB. Antibiotic elimination of group-B streptococci in urine in prevention of preterm labour. Lancet 1987; 591–3.
60 Xiong X, Buekens P, Vastardis S, *et al.* Periodontal disease and pregnancy outcomes: state of the science. Obstet Gynecol Surv 2007; 62: 605–15.
61 Jeffcoat MK, Geurs NC, Reddy MS, *et al.* Periodontal infection and preterm birth. J Am Dent Assoc 2001; 132: 875–88.
62 Offenbacher S, Katz V, Fertik G, *et al.* Periodontal disease as a possible risk factor for preterm low birth weight. J Periodontol 1996; 67: 1103–13.
63 Srinivas SK, Sammel MD, Stamilio DM, *et al.* Periodontal disease and adverse pregnancy outcome: is there an association? Am J Obstet Gynecol 2009; 200: 497.e1–497.e8.
64 Michalowicz BS, Hodges JS, Novak MJ, *et al.* Change in periodontitis during pregnancy and the risk of pre-term birth and low birthweight. J Clin Periodontol 2009; 36: 308–14.
65 Michalowicz BS, Hodges JS, Di Angelis AJ *et al.* Treatment of periodontal disease and the risk of PTB. N Engl J Med 2006; 355: 1885–94.
66 Offenbacher S, Beck J, Jared H *et al.* Maternal oral therapy to reduce obstetric risk (MOTOR): a report of a multi-centered periodontal therapy randomized-controlled trial on rate of preterm delivery. Am J Obstet Gynecol 2008: 199, Abstr 3. Page S2, DOI: 10.1016/j.ajog.2008.09.029.
67 Macones G, Jeffcoat M, Parry S *et al.* Screening and treating periodontal disease in pregnancy does not reduce the incidence of PTB: results from the PIPS study. Am J Obstet Gynecol 2008; 199, Abstr 5, Page S3, DOI: 10.1016/j.ajog.2008.09.031).
68 Newman RB, Gill PJ, Wittreich P, Katz M. Maternal perception of pre-labor uterine activity. Obstet Gynecol 1986; 68: 765–9.
69 Iams JD, Johnson FF, O'Shaughnessy RW.A prospective randomized trial of home uterine activity monitoring in pregnancies at risk for preterm labor. Part 2. Am J Obstet Gynecol 1988; 159: 595–603.
70 Colton T, Kayne HL, *et al.* A meta-analysis of home uterine activity monitoring. Am J Obstet Gynecol 1995; 173: 1499–505.
71 Grimes DA, Schulz KF. Randomized controlled trial of home uterine activity monitoring: a review and critique. Obstet Gynecol 1992; 79: 137–42.
72 Collaborative Home Uterine Activity Monitoring Group: A multicenter trial assessing a home uterine activity monitoring active versus sham device. Am J Obstet Gynecol 1995;173: 1120–7.
73 Dole N, Savitz DA, Hertz-Picciotto I, *et al.* Maternal stress and preterm birth. Am J Epidemiol 2003; 157: 14–24.

74 Rich-Edwards JW, Grizzard TA. Psychosocial stress and neuroendocrine mechanisms in preterm delivery. Am J Obstet Gynecol 2005; 192 (suppl): S30–35.
75 Hodnett Ed, Fredericks S. Support during pregnancy for women at increased risk of low birthweight babies. Cochrane Database Syst Rev, 2003; CD000198.
76 Hobel, CJ, Goldstein, A, Barrett, ES. Psychosocial stress and pregnancy outcome. Clin Obstet Gynecol 2008; 51: 333–9.

CHAPTER 10

Tobacco and Preterm Birth

Jeroen P. Vanderhoeven & Jorge E. Tolosa
Department of Obstetrics and Gynecology, Oregon Health and Sciences University, Oregon, USA

Key points

- Smoking is a modifiable risk factor associated with preterm birth (PTB), low birth weight and perinatal death.
- Smoking cessation in pregnancy reduces PTB, low birth weight, and perinatal death.
- Major compounds found in smoking tobacco affect placental pathophysiology.
- The use of a brief office-based intervention (the 5 A's) is an effective method to increase smoking cessation in pregnancy.
- Behavioral intervention is an effective method for increasing cessation rates.
- Smoking cessation in pregnancy can prevent up to 16% of PTB, and as such is the number one single, best evidence-based, successful intervention for the prevention of PTB.
- The use of nicotine replacement therapy or bupropion have yet to demonstrate sufficient safety and efficacy data to recommend routine use in pregnancy.
- The greatest risk of relapse is in the postpartum period. There is insufficient data to make recommendations for interventions.

Background

Tobacco use in pregnancy is one of the most important modifiable causes of preterm birth (PTB) and other complications in the United States [1]. Tobacco dependence is a chronic addictive condition that requires repeated intervention for cessation [2].

The predominant mode of consumption is via smoking cigarettes both worldwide and within the United States. There are a number of non-cigarette forms of tobacco consumption such as pipe smoking, chewed tobacco, and snuff. These, like cigarette users, have regional variations in terms of prevalence. Most studies typically define a light smoker as a cigarette smoker of fewer than 10 cigarettes per day and include infrequent smokers who may not smoke daily. In general, guidelines apply to all forms of tobacco consumption. Where research applies exclusively to cigarette smoking, the term *smoking* is used to replace the more general term *tobacco exposure*.

Epidemiology

Tobacco consumption among women is reported to vary between **9 and 22% worldwide** [3] and **18% in the United States** [4]. The prevalence of cigarette smoking is trending downwards in the United States. As of 2003, 10.2% of United States women reported smoking during pregnancy, a decrease from 11.2% reported in 2002 [5]. While smokeless tobacco use among women in the United States remains low (0.3%), there is a large range of regional differences with increased prevalence in rural communities (0.7%), the southern United States (0.7%), and is highest among Native Alaskan women (47–58%) [6, 7].

The highest prevalence among pregnant women who smoke occurs in those less than 18–19 years old (17.1%) and in those older than 40 (8.0%). American Indian women have the highest prevalence (18.1%), whereas Hispanic (2.7%) and Asian (2.2%) women have the lowest prevalence [5]. Women are more likely to smoke if they are of higher parity, have less than 12 years of education, a lower economic status, poor coping skills, or exposure to domestic violence [5, 8]. Among surveys including smokeless tobacco users, Native Alaskan women were noted to have high rates of use in pregnancy (16.9%) [7]. Worldwide, geographic areas with high prevalence of smokeless tobacco use included Lebanon (35.4%), Latvia (33.5%) and countries in the western Pacific such as the Northern Mariana Islands (38.3%) among women aged 13–15 [9]. One study of women from Mumbai, India reported a 17.1% tobacco use in pregnancy that was predominantly (99%) smokeless tobacco [10]. There is a paucity of epidemiologic data on smokeless tobacco users in pregnancy both worldwide and within the US.

Diagnosis and screening

Whereas the validity of self-reporting tobacco use is well described, research has indicated that this may not be generalizable to the pregnant population. There is **significant (14–23%) nondisclosure of self-reported smoking status during tobacco screening in pregnancy** [11]. In the research setting, biochemical markers have been used to validate smoking status. However, they are not part of screening owing to cost, time constraint, and unknown acceptability in the pregnant patient.

ASK about Tobacco use -- 1 minute

- Use a multi-choice questionnaire to elicit smoking status (Table 10.1)
- Document patient responses
    - o If the patient has stopped smoking before or after she found out she was pregnant (B or C)*, reinforce her decision to quit, congratulate her on success in quitting, and encourage her to remain smoke free throughout the pregnancy and postpartum
    - o If the patient is currently smoking (D or E)*, proceed to Advise, Assess, Assist, and Arrange

ADVISE current tobacco users to quit -- 1 minute

- Provide pregnancy specific educational materials
- Use a clear, strong, and personalized message specifically addressing the benefits of quitting on the woman, fetus, and newborn

ASSESS willingness to quit in the next 30 days -- 1 minute

- If the patient is willing to quit, continue to ASSIST
- If the patient is unwilling to quit, consider the 5 R's Framework (Figure 10.2)

ASSIST in quitting

- Set a quit date
- Enlist social supports in family and friends
- Anticipate the challenges of quitting
- Remove tobacco products from the home environment and create a smoke-free space
- Make recommendations for effective cessation

ARRANGE follow up appointment

- Ideally, soon after quit date
- Assess smoking status at subsequent prenatal visits
- Congratulate successes and provide encouragement

Figure 10.1 The 5A's brief counseling intervention for the patient willing to quit [2,12]. *, See Table 1. (Adapted with permission from BMJ Publishing Group Limited. Tobacco Control, Melvin CL, Dolan-Mullen P, Windsor RA, *et al.* Vol 9, pages 80–84, © 2000).

Successful interventions are dependent on effective screening and knowledge of the prevalence of exposure, among other factors. The **5 A's framework** (Figure 10.1) **is a useful screening tool** endorsed by the United States Department of Health and Human Services panel on treating tobacco use and dependence, the American College of Obstetricians and Gynecologists (ACOG), and the National Cancer Institute [1, 2, 8, 12]. A randomized trial demonstrated 40% improvement in biochemically validated disclosure rates by using a multiple choice questionnaire in comparison with oral or written 'yes or no' responses to the question 'Do you smoke' (Table 10.1) [11]. Even with improvements in screening, it is important to recognize that self-reporting remains an inadequate measure of tobacco use in pregnancy.

Pathophysiology

The major tobacco compounds causing harmful effects with smoking are **nicotine** and **carbon monoxide**. Other toxic compounds include

Table 10.1 Multiple choice questionnaire improves initial disclosure rates of smoking [11].

A	I have never smoked or I have smoked less than 100 cigarettes in my lifetime
B	I stopped smoking before I found out I was pregnant, and I am not smoking now
C	I stopped smoking after I found out I was pregnant, and I am not smoking now
D	I smoke some now, but I have cut down on the number of cigarettes I smoke since I found out I was pregnant
E	I smoke regularly now, about the same as before I found out I was pregnant

ammonia, polycyclic aromatic hydrocarbons, hydrogen cyanide, vinyl chloride, and nitrogen oxides.

Nicotine is classified as a Pregnancy Category D drug by the United States Food and Drug Administration (FDA). This is largely due to animal studies demonstrating toxicity to the developing central nervous system (CNS), a strong association with tobacco use and sudden infant death syndrome (SIDS), and concern for uteroplacental insufficiency caused by nicotine-mediated vasoconstriction. Pharmacologically, nicotine acts principally by binding to nicotinic cholinergic receptors mediating both psychoactive and vascular effects. Receptor activation triggers the release of a variety of neurotransmitters including dopamine, norepinephrine, epinephrine, acetylcholine, serotonin, γ-amniobutyric acid (GABA), glutamate, and endorphins. Nicotine is also a weak sympathomimetic drug. The cardiovascular effects of nicotine have demonstrated increases in heart rate, myocardial contractility, and transient increases in blood pressure. There is a flat dose response curve for these cardiovascular effects at the nicotine levels typically seen with tobacco consumption [13]. Cigarette smoking has been associated with an increase in platelet activation and coagulation abnormalities. Risk of thromboembolism in smokers is increased. Nicotine may increase plasminogen activator inhibitor-1, a major regulator of fibrinolysis, although the extent of nicotine activation in coagulation abnormalities is unresolved [14].

Nicotine crosses the placenta and can be detected in the fetal circulation at levels that exceed the maternal circulation by 15% and amniotic fluid levels are 88% higher than maternal plasma levels [15]. Nicotine has been postulated to cause uteroplacental insufficiency via vasoconstriction, produce neurotoxicity resulting in brain developmental delays, and inhibit the maturation of pulmonary cells.

Carbon monoxide (CO) also crosses the placenta and can be detected in the fetal circulation at levels exceeding those in the maternal circulation by 15% [15]. Exposure causes formation of carboxyhemoglobin (COHb) — a substance cleared slowly from the fetal circulation and which diminishes tissue oxygenation via competitive inhibition with oxyhemoglobin. The resulting left shift of the oxyhemoglobin dissociation curve causes decreased availability of oxygen to the fetus [15]. While this is a transient effect, there is a lag of up to seven hours before equilibration between fetal and maternal COHb levels occurs [13]. The long half life of CO and the lag between maternal–fetal equilibrium means that CO does not clear from the fetus during maternal sleep. Prolonged elevations in COHb stimulates erythrocyte production; this functional anemia is the etiology for elevated hematocrit in the newborn. The resulting increased blood viscosity is hypothesized to create suboptimal placental perfusion [13]. Carbon monoxide, through chronic cellular hypoxia, is a likely principal contributor to low birth weight among smokers [16].

Risks associated with smoking

Cigarette smoking has also been associated with increased risks during pregnancy including **intrauterine growth restriction, placenta previa, and abruptio placentae** in addition to other poor pregnancy outcomes such as **preterm premature rupture of membranes (PPROM), low birth weight, and perinatal mortality/SIDS** [1]. Smoking may result in damage to fetal genetic material which results in deletions and translocations at the chromosome 11q23 region [8, 17]. There are multiple proposed mechanisms for these outcomes perhaps reflecting the likelihood of a multifaceted pathway. Smoking is associated with impaired fetal oxygen delivery resulting in vasoconstriction and changes in intervillous blood flow that contribute to abnormal gas exchange within the placenta [18]. Cigarette smoking is also associated with precursors of PPROM such as lowered local immunity, decreased macrophage capability, and low ascorbic acid levels which may increase the possibility of inflammation and infection. Low maternal blood zinc and copper levels are noted in women with PPROM or PROM and are also associated with maternal smoking [13]. Nitric oxide, a potent myometrial relaxant, is reduced secondary to the effect of maternal smoking on nitric oxide synthetase activity [13].

Epidemiologic data suggests children born to women who smoked in pregnancy are at increased risk for developing **obesity and hypertension** [19], **asthma, otitis media, short stature, and hyperactivity** [8].

Smokeless tobacco has been associated with **low birth weight, PTB, preeclampsia, and perinatal mortality** [10, 20, 21]. However, there remains a paucity of data on the risks of smokeless tobacco use in pregnancy.

Primary prevention for the community

Community-based interventions such as **tobacco taxes, limiting access of tobacco products to minors, and prohibiting smoking in public spaces are important in promoting primary prevention attempts** [8].

Individual management

A higher proportion of women stop smoking in pregnancy than at any other time in their lives (43% of women) [5, 22]. **Pregnant women who smoke are identified at 81% of physician visits but fewer than 23% receive counseling** [2, 23]. **Up to 40% of women who quit in pregnancy achieve cessation prior to their first prenatal appointment**. Further, **another 20–30% of all smoking women will attempt to stop smoking in pregnancy** [8, 22]. This presents a unique opportunity to introduce interventions during the initiation of prenatal care as this may be the only time some women seek medical attention. Women are more likely to experience higher sustained levels of social and family support for quit attempts during pregnancy. **It is estimated that successful smoking cessation in pregnancy can prevent up to 16% of PTBs** [24].

Counseling

After screening for tobacco use with a multiple choice questionnaire (Table 10.1), current smokers should be assessed for desire to discontinue smoking. **Cessation attempts should be motivated by providing education of the risk of tobacco use on maternal and fetal health**. Former tobacco users should be congratulated and encouraged. Documentation of smoking status is recommended. **For women who are open to smoking cessation, the 5 A's and the 5 R's are recommended in clinical practice to help pregnant women quit smoking** [2]. Simple interventions such as the 5A's and 5R's increased long-term cessation rates (>5 months) in the general population from 5% to 15–20% [2]. 'The **5A's** for Patients Who Are Willing To Quit Smoking' is endorsed by the American College of Obstetricians and Gynecologists (ACOG) (**Figure 10.1**). Alternatively, for patients who are reluctant or unable to quit smoking during pregnancy may refer to 'The **5 R's** For Smokers Who Are Unwilling to Quit Smoking' [25] (**Figure 10.2**).

RELEVANCE
- Identify motivational factors
- Explore impact on her pregnancy, other children at home, health concerns and prior quitting experience

RISKS
- Stress the acute and long-term risks of smoking to the patient, her fetus, and her newborn

	Maternal risks	Fetal risks
Acute	• Shortness of breath • Asthma exacerbation • Harm to pregnancy (see text) • Future infertility	• Intrauterine growth restriction • Preterm birth • Placenta previa • Placental abruption • Premature rupture of membranes • Low birth weight • Perinatal mortality/SIDS
Long term	• Cardiovascular (CVA/MI) • Lung and other cancers • Pulmonary (COPD) • Osteoporosis • Long-term disability	• Pulmonary (asthma and increased respiratory tract infections) • Obesity • Otitis • Short stature • Hyperactivity

REWARDS
- Help the patient identify potential health, societal, and financial benefits to cessation
  - o Health (whiter teeth, improved feeling of well being, healthier baby)
  - o Financial (saving money)
  - o Moral and social (better role modeling for children)

ROADBLOCKS
- Identify barriers to quitting and note options that address these barriers
  - o Concern regarding withdrawal symptoms
  - o Fear of failure
  - o Lack of support
  - o Depression
  - o Being around other tobacco users

REPETITION
- Assess smoking status at every prenatal visit
- Tobacco users who have failed previous attempts should be reminded that most people make repeated quit attempts before they are successful

Figure 10.2 The 5R's brief counseling intervention for the patient unwilling to quit [2]. (Adapted with permission from Fiore MC, Jaén CR, Baker TB, *et al.* Treating Tobacco Use and Dependence: 2008 Update. Clinical Practice Guideline. Rockville, MD: US Department of Health and Human Services. Public Health Service. May 2008).

Studies of smoking cessation programs in pregnancy using randomized trials are based mostly on **oral and written advice at each prenatal visit regarding the risk of smoking for mother and baby, and a plan to quit**. These programs are associated with a 6% increase in smoking cessation, a substantial **16% decrease in PTB** and 19% **decrease in** low birth weight and **perinatal morbidity and mortality**. Support and reward techniques to help quit smoking are **one of the best** ***forms of evidence-based medicine***, based on a great number (>48) of good quality studies in >20 000 smoking pregnant women [22].

Smoking cessation programs are both clinically effective and cost-effective [2]. **All health care providers should strongly advise every patient who smokes to quit because evidence shows that physician advice to quit smoking increases abstinence rates.** A meta-analysis of seven studies evaluating the effectiveness of a brief intervention of physician advice (modal length of intervention of 3 minutes or less), increased abstinence rates from 7.9% to 10.2% (95% CI 8.5–12.0) in non-pregnant smokers [2]. A meta-analysis of eight studies comparing minimal intervention of less than 3 minutes of person-to-person psychosocial smoking cessation to 'usual care' interventions on pregnant smoking women noted that cessation rates increased from 7.6% to 13.3% (95% CI 9.0–19.4) [2]. **Advice should be clear, strong, and personalized** to the individual. An example might be, **'As your care provider, I need you to know that quitting smoking is the most important thing you can do to protect the health of your baby and your health'.** A 2005 Cochrane review evaluating whether more intensive counseling provided benefit found five trials which failed to demonstrate greater effect over brief counseling in the general population [26]. Until further evidence-based conclusions are available, **brief cognitive-behavioral interventions accompanied by pregnancy specific self-help materials are the most effective intervention** for pregnant smokers [2].

Preventive strategies for smoking cessation leading to reduction of PTB are summarized in Table 10.2.

Pharmacotherapy (Table 10.3)

Pharmaceutical cessation aids such as nicotine replacement therapy (NRT), varenicline, or bupropion SR have efficacy as first line agents in the general non-pregnant population. **The use of these medications is not yet routinely recommended in pregnancy**.

Nicotine replacement therapy (NRT)

NRT is available in **transdermal patch, nasal spray, chewing gum or lozenge**. There are known and theoretical risks to the developing fetus exposed to nicotine. In light of inconclusive data regarding the effectiveness of NRT in pregnancy, **NRT should be used with caution and women should be warned of uncertain side effects in pregnancy** [11].

Table 10.2 Actual management to prevent preterm birth with cessation interventions

Interventions at the individual level
- Screening questionnaire to help disclosure of smoking (Table 10.1)
- 5A's (Figure 10.1) for women willing to quit
- 5R's (Figure 10.2) for women unwilling to quit
- Written material
- Repeated counseling/monitoring each visit
- Document smoking status each visit
- Referral to smoking cessation professionals or quitline (1-800-QUIT-NOW)
- Congratulate successes, provide encouragement after failures
- Support and Reward programs

Community interventions
- Tobacco taxes
- Limiting access of tobacco products to minors
- Prohibiting smoking in public spaces

Table 10.3 Pharmacotherapy [2, 8, 25]

Agent	Effectiveness in non-pregnant adults	Safety in pregnancy	Effectiveness in pregnancy
Nicotine replacement therapy	**Proven**	Inadequate data	**Not proven**
Patch	**Proven**	Inadequate data	**Not proven**
Chewing gum	**Proven**	Inadequate data	**Not proven**
Inhaler	**Proven**	Inadequate data	No studies
Nasal spray	**Proven**	Inadequate data	No studies
Lozenges	Inadequate Data	Inadequate data	No studies
Bupropion SR	**Proven***	Inadequate data	No studies
Varenicline	**Proven***	No studies	No studies

* See text for details.

Four randomized controlled trials examining NRT in pregnancy have been published. Wisborg *et al.* randomized 250 >10 cigarettes per day smokers in the first trimester to 15 mg transdermal nicotine patches or placebo for 11 weeks. NRT was found to be no better than placebo at achieving cessation at the end of the intervention (OR 1.1; 95% CI 0.7–1.8). While no evidence of serious adverse effects of nicotine was noted, the birth weight adjusted for prematurity in the NRT group was on average 186 g greater than that of the placebo group [27]. Kapur *et al.* reported a smaller trial in which 30 women were randomized in the second trimester to 15 mg transdermal nicotine patches or placebo for 8 weeks followed by a taper; this trial also failed to reach statistically significant cessation rates [28]. Pollack *et al.* randomized 181 patients to cognitive behavioral therapy (CBT) with or without NRT in pregnant smokers. Women selected their NRT of choice upon entry. Combination NRT and CBT was associated with significantly higher quit rates. However, the Data Safety Monitoring Board (DSMB) halted the trial due to a significant higher incidence of adverse events (30% of the combination group compared with 17% of the CBT alone group). Notably, many of the adverse events were preterm labor in the combination group. Women randomized to the combination group were significantly more likely to have had prior PTB (32% vs 12%). The study concluded that the existing data could neither support nor oppose the safety of NRT in pregnancy [29]. Oncken *et al.* randomized 100 pregnant smokers prior to 24 weeks gestation to 2 mg nicotine gum and 94 to placebo [30]. Women were informed to take NRT or placebo for each cigarette smoked daily to a maximum of 20 pieces per day for 6 weeks followed by a taper. No significant difference was detected in cessation rates at 6 weeks of therapy or at 32–34 weeks gestation. However, birth weight significantly increased on average 337 g among NRT users compared with placebo. There were no significant differences in adverse events. These data suggest that the effectiveness of NRT in pregnancy is inconclusive.

A large prospective study using the Danish birth registry by Morales-Suarez-Varela *et al.* identified 250 former smokers exposed to NRT during the first trimester of pregnancy [31]. A slight increase in congenital malformation prevalence mostly limited to musculoskeletal defects was noted compared with mothers who smoked in the first trimester. Another study using the same Danish birth registry investigated the incidence of stillbirth among users of NRT and women who smoked in pregnancy [32]. Smoking in pregnancy increased the rate of stillbirth (HR 1.46, 95% CI 1.17–1.82) whereas NRT was not associated with increases in stillbirth in pregnancy [32]. The number of stillbirths in the NRT group was very small. Given the methodological limitations of these two studies, and the lack of adequately powered safety data, the safety of NRT in pregnancy also remains inconclusive.

The 2008 updated clinical practice guidelines from the United States Department of Health and Human Services cautions that 'concerns [of potential harms of tobacco as well as NRT] must be considered in the context of **inconclusive evidence that cessation medications boost abstinence rates in pregnant smokers'** [2].

Bupropion SR

Bupropion SR is an atypical antidepressant with both dopaminergic and noradrenergic central nervous system activity and has been approved by the FDA for use in smoking cessation. In the general population, an analysis of 24 studies comparing Bupropion with placebo demonstrated a near doubling in abstinence rates at 6 months post-quit (24.2% vs 13.8%) [2]. Bupropion is contraindicated in patients with known bulimia, anorexia nervosa, use of MAO inhibitor within the previous 14 days or a known or suspected history of seizure disorder [2]. The medication carries a **black box warning** due to association of antidepressant medications with suicidality in children, adolescents, and young adults under the age of 24. Bupropion is a FDA Category C medication in pregnancy.

Two prospective studies have evaluated the safety of this medication in pregnancy. Chun-Fai-Chan *et al.* evaluated 105 live births and noted no increase in rates of major malformations above baseline in women exposed to bupropion SR compared with women not exposed to this medication [33]. There was no difference in birth weight or neonatal death. Cole *et al.* compared data from the bupropion pregnancy registry and found no difference between pregnancies exposed in the first trimester compared with those exposed outside the first trimester or those exposed to another antidepressant in the prevalence of congenital malformation [34]. **No large trials have evaluated the effectiveness of bupropion SR in pregnancy for tobacco cessation**.

Varenicline

Varenicline remains an FDA Category C medication approved for smoking cessation in the general population. The drug blocks nicotine receptors resulting in reduction in nicotine cravings and withdrawal symptoms. Serious neuropsychiatric symptoms have been associated with varenicline including agitation, depression, and suicidality prompting the FDA to issue a public health advisory in 2008 precautioning the use of this medication in populations with a history of psychiatric illness [35]. **The safety and efficacy of varenicline in pregnancy has yet to be established** and therefore its use in pregnant and lactating women is not yet recommended for routine use in this population.

Postpartum prevention

Of the women who quit smoking during pregnancy, **50–90% will relapse within the first year after delivery** [22, 24]. Risk factors for relapse include **decreased sleep, concern about weight loss, and stresses of infant care**. Although there is insufficient evidence in recommending specific strategies to prevent relapse due to insufficient research, strategies for relapse prevention include ongoing counseling and support throughout the postpartum period using the 5A's framework [22].

References

1 American College of Obstetricians and Gynecologists. Smoking cessation during pregnancy. ACOG Committee Opinion No. 316. Washington (DC): ACOG; 2005.

2 Fiore MC, Jaén CR, Baker TB, *et al.* Treating Tobacco Use and Dependence: 2008 Update. Clinical Practice Guideline. Rockville, MD: US Department of Health and Human Services. Public Health Service. May 2008.

3 Mackay J, Eriksen M. The Tobacco Atlas. Geneva: World Health Organization; 2003.

4 Center for Disease Control. State-specific prevalence and trends in adult cigarette smoking — United States, 1998–2007. MMWR 2009; 58: 221–6.

5 Martin JA, Hamilton BE, Sutton PD, Ventura SJ, Manacker F, Munson ML. Births: Final Data for 2003. National Vital Statistics Reports; 54(2). Hyattsville, MD: National Center for Health Statistics; 2005. DHHS Publication (PHS) 2005–1120. http://www.cdc.gov/nchs/data/nvsr/nvsr54/nvsr54_02.pdf. Accessibility verified April 16, 2009.

6 Department of Health and Human Services. Women and Smoking: A Report of the Surgeon General. Rockville: US Department of Health and Human Services, Public Health Service, Office of the Surgeon General.

7 Kim SY, England L, Dietz PM, Morrow B, Perham-Hester KA. Prenatal cigarette smoking and smokeless tobacco use among Alaska native and white women in Alaska, 1996–2003. Matern Child Health J 2008; doi 10.1007/s10995-008-0402-9 (published 18 August 2008).

8 Crawford JT, Tolosa JE, Goldenberg RL. Smoking cessation in pregnancy: why, how, and what next ... Clin Obstet Gynecol 2008; 51: 419–35.

9 Warren CR, Jones NR, Peruga A, *et al.* Global youth tobacco surveillance, 2000–2007. MMWR 2008; 57(SS01): 1–21.

10 Gupta PC, Sreevidya S. Smokeless tobacco use, birth weight, and gestational age: population based, prospective cohort study of 1217 women in Mumbai, India. Br Med J 2004; 328: 1538.

11 Mullen PD, Carbonari JP, Tabak ER, Glenday MC. Improving disclosure of smoking by pregnant women. Am J Obstet Gynecol 1991; 165: 409–13.

12 Melvin CL, Dolan-Mullen P, Windsor RA, Whiteside HP Jr, Goldenberg RL. Recommended cessation counselling for pregnant women who smoke: a review of the evidence. Tob Control 2000; 9 Suppl 3: III80–4.

13 Dempsey DA, Benowitz NL. Risks and benefits of nicotine to aid smoking cessation in pregnancy. Drug Safety 2001; 24: 277–322.

14 Tapson VF. The role of smoking in coagulation and thromboembolism in chronic obstructive pulmonary disease. Proc Am Thorac Soc 2005; 2: 71–7.

15 Andres RL, Day MC. Perinatal complications associated with maternal tobacco use. Semin Neonatol 2000; 5: 231–41.

16 Carmines EL, Rajendran N. Evidence for carbon monoxide as a major factor contributing to the lower fetal weights in rats exposed to cigarette smoke. Toxicol Sci 2008; 102: 383–91.

17 de la Chica RA, Ribas I, Giraldo J, Egozcue J, Fuster C. Chromosomal instability in amniocytes from fetuses of mothers who smoke. JAMA 2005; 293: 1212.

18 Burton GJ, Palmer ME, Dalton KJ. Morphometric differences between the placental vasculature of non-smokers, smokers, and ex-smokers. Br J Obstet Gynaecol 1989; 96: 907.

19 Gao YJ, Holloway AC, Zeng ZH, *et al.* Prenatal exposure to nicotine causes postnatal obesity and altered perivascular adipose tissue function. Obes Res 2005; 13: 687–92.

20 England LJ, Levine RJ, Mills JL, Klebanoff MA, Yu KF, Cnattingius S. Adverse pregnancy outcomes in snuff users. Am J Obstet Gynecol 2003; 189: 939–43.
21 Gupta PC, Subramoney S. Smokeless tobacco use and risk of stillbirth: a cohort study in Mumbai, India. Epidemiology 2006; 17: 47–51.
22 Lumley J, Oliver SS, Chamberlain C, Oakley L. Interventions for promoting smoking cessation during pregnancy. Cochrane Database Syst Rev 2004.
23 Moran S, Thorndike AN, Armstrong K, Rigotti NA. Physicians' missed opportunities to address tobacco use during prenatal care. Nicotine Tob Res 2003; 5: 363–8.
24 Department of Health and Human Services. The Health Benefits of Smoking Cessation: US Department of Health and Human Services, Public Health Service, Centers for Disease Control, Center for Chronic Disease Prevention and Health Promotion, Office on Smoking and Health, 1990.
25 Fiore MC. The Tobacco Use and Dependence Clinical Practice Guideline Panel, Staff, and Consortium Representatives. Treating tobacco use and dependence: a US Public Health Service Report. JAMA 2000; 283: 3244–54.
26 Lancaster T, Stead AF. Individual behavioral counseling for smoking cessation. Cochrane Database Syst Rev, 2005.
27 Wisborg K, Henriksen TB, Jespersen LB, Secher NJ. Nicotine patches for pregnant smokers: a randomized controlled study. Obstet Gynecol 2000; 96: 967–71.
28 Kapur B, Hackman R, Selby P, Klein J, Koren G. Randomized, double-blind placebo-controlled trial of nicotine replacement therapy in pregnancy. Curr Ther Res 2001; 62: 274–8.
29 Pollack KI, Oncken CA, Lipkus IM, *et al.* Nicotine replacement and behavioral therapy for smoking cessation in pregnancy. Am J Prev Med 2007; 33: 297–305.
30 Oncken C, Dornelas E, Greene J *et al.* Nicotine gum for pregnant smokers: a randomized controlled trial. Obstet Gynecol 2008; 112: 859–67.
31 Morales-Suarez-Varela MM, Bille C, Christensen K, Olsen J. Smoking habits, nicotine use, and congenital malformations. Obstet Gynecol 2006; 107: 51–7.
32 Strandberg-Larsen K, Tinggaard M, Nybo Anderson AM, Olsen J, Grønbaek M. Use of nicotine replacement therapy during pregnancy and stillbirth: a cohort study. Br J Obstet Gynaecol 2008; 115: 1405–10.
33 Chun-Fai-Chan B, Koren G, Fayez I, *et al.* Pregnancy outcome of women exposed to buproprion during pregnancy: a prospective comparative study. Am J Obstet Gynecol 2005; 192: 932–6.
34 Cole JA, Modell JG, Haight BR, Cosmatos IS, Stoler JM, Walker AM. Bupropion in pregnancy and the prevalence of congenital malformations. Pharmacoepidemiol Drug Saf 2007; 16: 474–84.
35 Food and Drug Administration. Public health advisory: important information on Chantix (varenicline). http://www.fda.gov/cder/drug/advisory/varenicline.htm. Accessed April 16, 2009.

CHAPTER 11

Care for Women with Prior Preterm Birth

Jay D. Iams

Division of Maternal-Fetal Medicine, Department of Obstetrics and Gynecology, The Ohio State University Medical Center, Ohio, USA

Key points

- Obtain a thorough history and records for all prior pregnancies.
- Try to determine the pathways that led to the prior preterm birth (PTB), and to categorize it as *likely* or *unlikely* to recur.
- Estimate the woman's personal risk of another PTB.
- Identify and eliminate or minimize other risk factors (Chapters 4 and 9).
- Establish welcoming methods of communication between women with prior PTB and knowledgeable caregivers.
- Assess personal and family resources and barriers to receiving care.
- Apply evidence-based interventions aggressively for women whose likelihood of recurrent PTB is high:
  - Smoking cessation programs.
  - 17-α-hydroxy-progesterone caproate 250 mg IM weekly from 16 weeks until 36 weeks for women with prior spontaneous PTB at 20–36 6/7 weeks.
  - Cervical cerclage for women with short cervix (below 25 mm) or with visible membranes before 24 weeks and prior spontaneous PTB.
  - Screen for and treat bacteriuria >100 000 organisms/ml with appropriate antibiotics preconception, at the beginning of pregnancy, and later.
  - Corticosteroids (betamethasone 12 mg given IM and repeated in 24 hours) at 24–34 weeks should be considered for women with prior PTB who also manifest evidence of risk in the current pregnancy, e.g. spotting or bleeding, rapid cervical effacement to cervical length (CL) <15 mm, preterm labor (PTL), visible membranes. For women in whom PTB does not occur within 3 weeks, a single rescue course may be considered when PTB is deemed imminent.

Definition and description of a prior preterm birth

Components of a thorough history

The course, duration, and conclusion of all prior pregnancies should be reviewed with particular attention to the following (Chapter 4):

Preterm Birth. Edited by Vincenzo Berghella.

- A previous pregnancy ending between 16 and 36 6/7 weeks should be considered as a possible preterm birth (PTB), and the gestational age at the onset of symptoms and at delivery should be determined.
- Prior spontaneous abortions and elective terminations should be reviewed to determine the gestational age and methods of termination. Repeated elective terminations may increase the risk of early PTB [1–3].
- Pregnancies concluding between 16 and 20 weeks have traditionally been considered to be 'miscarriages' that have an etiology that differs from births after 20 weeks, but this is a custom not based in fact [4, 5]. Women whose prior pregnancy ended between 16 and 20 weeks have a risk of recurrent PTB that equals or exceeds that of women with prior PTB after 20 weeks [4], and should receive the same care.
- Preterm parturition is characterized by cervical ripening, decidual-membrane activation, and uterine contractions, any of which may predominate. The most common sequence is preterm cervical ripening followed by decidual-membrane activation and then contractions. This sequence is characterized by mild symptoms of pelvic pressure, premenstrual-like cramping and increased vaginal discharge, most often due to choriodecidual inflammation. This history is typically accompanied by preterm cervical effacement. The clinical presentation is usually advanced cervical effacement and dilation or ruptured membranes. Contractions are perceived as mild because the cervix is already effaced and slightly dilated. The risk of recurrent PTB for women who describe this scenario is high.
- When preterm parturition is initiated by membrane rupture or uterine contractions before cervical ripening has occurred, the cause, prognosis, and recurrence risk are variable. For example, when preterm ruptured membranes occurs after persistent spotting and/or an unexplained elevated maternal serum alpha-feto-protein, the etiology may be a blighted or vanishing twin, where the recurrence risk is likely to be low, or a uterine anomaly with abnormal placental implantation, where the recurrence risk will vary with the site of placental attachment.
- The circumstances of conception of a prior pregnancy ending in PTB are important. Assisted reproduction, including *in vitro* fertilization techniques and all levels of ovulation promotion (clomiphene) and stimulation (gonadotropins) is associated with a twofold increased risk of PTB [6, 7]. Super-ovulation followed by conception from fresh eggs in the same cycle has a greater risk of PTB than does use of frozen eggs [8].
- When the prior PTB was a twin pregnancy, the recurrence risk varies according to the gestational age of the twin birth [9]. The earlier the gestational age, the greater the risk of PTB in a subsequent singleton pregnancy, ranging from minimal increased risk for a twin birth after

34 weeks to as much as 40% when the prior twin birth occurred before 30 weeks.

- Although PTBs are commonly labeled as being *spontaneous* or *indicated*, these categories often overlap, can be difficult to distinguish, and may be misleading when caring for a subsequent pregnancy. Thus it is wise to review the records of any prior PTB, regardless of the clinical circumstances, when planning prenatal care. This is especially important for early PTBs between 16 and 26 weeks, where fetal anomalies, placental abnormalities, and spontaneous preterm parturition are easily confused.
- Pathology reports should be obtained and reviewed. Although the etiology of a prior PTB may not be evident, the exclusion of some conditions can be helpful, e.g. when cervical insufficiency is suggested by the absence of inflammation in the membranes.
- A history of treatment for CIN, especially cervical cone biopsy and LEEP (loop electrosurgical excision procedure), increases the risk of preterm delivery [10].

Recurrent vs non-recurrent PTB

Women with repeated PTBs are more likely to have a low pre-pregnancy weight (below 120 lb, with a body mass index less than 19.8 kg/m^2), and to be African-American than women with a single prior PTB [11–16]. Women with more than one PTB are also more likely to have a history of early PTB before 32 to 34 weeks and to demonstrate clinical and ultrasound evidence of short cervix (sonographic length <25 mm, and Bishop score >3), and a positive fFN at 22–24 weeks [17]. A study of CL and fibronectin in women with prior PTB found that rates of recurrent PTB varied substantially, from less than 10% in women with a CL > 35 mm and a negative fibronectin at 22–24 weeks, to more than 60% when the CL was <25 mm and the fibronectin test was positive at 22–24 weeks [18] (Chapter 12).

Estimation of individual risk of recurrent PTB

The risk of recurrent PTB is commonly reported to be increased by 1.5–2-fold to 4-fold or more, depending on the population (Figure 11.1). **The risk increases with the number of prior PTBs and as the gestational age of the PTB decreases**. Optimal clinical value can be derived by estimating an individual risk of recurrent PTB based on a combination of historical and current pregnancy risk factors, including maternal race/

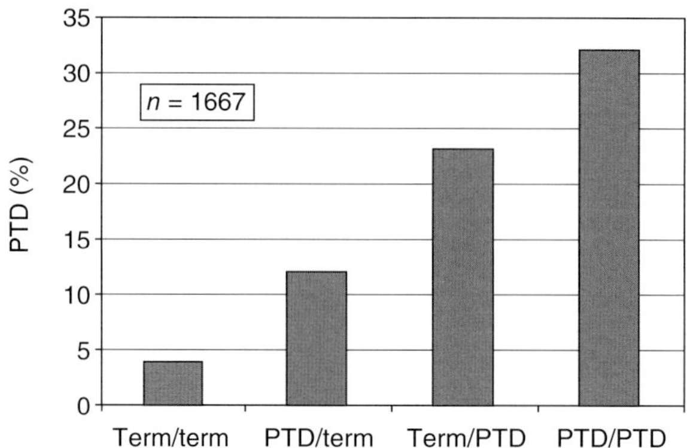

Figure 11.1 The risk of subsequent preterm birth is related to the outcome of the prior pregnancy, with the lowest risk occurring when a woman has had two prior preterm births and the highest risk when she has had two prior preterm births. PTD, preterm delivery. Data from Carr-Hill RA, Hall MH. The repetition of spontaneous preterm labour. Br J Obstet Gynaecol 1985; 92: 921–8 and Spong CY. Prediction and prevention of recurrent spontaneous preterm birth. Obstet Gynecol 2007; 110: 405–15.

ethnicity, the number, gestational age and sequence of prior births, and the results of tests such as fetal fibronectin (fFN) and digital or ultrasound assessment of the cervix.

Comparison of conservatively estimated personal recurrence risks for two hypothetical women, each with two prior PTBs, illustrates the utility of this approach:

- Patient A is a non-Hispanic white (NHW) woman whose first and second PTBs were at 34 weeks. Her baseline risk is ~11% (overall rate of PTB for NHW women), and increases by ~1.5 for each PTB: 11 × 1.5 = 17.25% × 1.5 = 26%.
- Patient B is a non-Hispanic black (NHB) woman with two prior PTBs at 28 and 26 weeks' gestation. Her baseline risk is 17% (the rate for NHB women in the United States), and increases by 1.5 fold because of the PTB, and then by another 1.5 fold because the birth was early, before 32 weeks. Her risk entering her second pregnancy was therefore ~35% (17 × 1.5 × 1.5). After a second PTB before 32 weeks, this same calculation yields a risk for her third pregnancy of more than 75 % (35 × 1.5 × 1.5 = 79%).

These relative risks are just estimates generated from published population risks, but they are consistent with observed rates reported in the literature [11, 14, 19–21]. More specific information has been reported from studies of various tests for PTB risk [18, 22–26], most usefully in the paper from Berghella *et al.* [24], as can be seen in Table 11.1. Antenatal care decisions,

Table 11.1 Predicted probability of preterm delivery before week 32, by cervical length (mm) and time of measurement (week of pregnancy), in women with singleton gestations and risk factors for preterm birth.

Cervical legnth (mm)	Week of pregnancy													
	15	16	17	18	19	20	21	22	23	24	25	26	27	28
0	76.3	73.7	70.9	67.9	64.7	61.4	58.0	54.5	51.0	47.5	44.0	40.5	37.2	33.9
5	67.9	64.8	61.5	58.1	54.6	51.1	47.6	44.0	40.6	37.2	34.0	30.9	28.0	25.2
10	58.1	54.7	51.2	47.6	44.1	40.7	37.3	34.1	31.0	28.0	25.3	22.7	20.3	18.1
15	47.7	44.2	40.7	37.4	34.1	31.0	28.1	25.3	22.7	20.4	18.2	16.2	14.3	12.7
20	37.4	34.2	31.1	28.1	25.4	22.8	20.4	18.2	16.2	14.4	12.7	11.2	9.9	8.7
25	28.2	25.4	22.8	20.4	18.2	16.2	14.4	12.7	11.3	9.9	8.7	7.7	6.7	5.9
30	20.5	18.3	16.3	14.4	12.8	11.3	9.9	8.7	7.7	6.7	5.9	5.2	4.5	3.9
35	14.5	12.8	11.3	10.0	8.8	7.7	6.8	5.9	5.2	4.5	4.0	3.5	3.0	2.6
40	10.0	8.8	7.7	6.8	5.9	5.2	4.5	4.0	3.5	3.0	2.6	2.3	2.0	1.7
45	6.8	5.9	5.2	4.5	3.9	3.4	3.0	2.6	2.3	2.0	1.7	1.5	1.3	1.1
50	4.6	4.0	3.5	3.0	2.6	2.3	2.0	1.7	1.5	1.3	1.2	1.0	0.9	0.8
55	3.0	2.7	2.3	2.0	1.8	1.5	1.3	1.2	1.0	0.9	0.8	0.7	0.6	0.5
60	2.0	1.8	1.5	1.3	1.2	1.0	0.9	0.8	0.7	0.6	0.5	0.4	0.4	0.3

e.g. the timing of administering antenatal steroids, might be influenced by the likelihood of PTB before 32 weeks shown in this table, and demonstrates the wide variation in the risk of recurrent PTB according to the length of the cervix at various points in pregnancy.

Interventions to reduce the risk of recurrent PTB

Numerous strategies and treatments have been proposed to reduce the risk of recurrent PTB, but few have been found effective when tested in clinical trials.

Interventions supported by firm evidence to support recommendations

Smoking Cessation Programs

Pregnant women are uniquely receptive to smoking cessation programs, especially when reinforced by physicians. A Cochrane Review concluded that smoking cessation programs in pregnancy reduce the rate of PTB (RR 0.84, 95% CI 0.72, 0.98) [27] (Chapter 10).

Screening and treatment for asymptomatic bacteriuria

Screening for asymptomatic bacteriuria reduces recurrent urinary tract infections and may also reduce the risk of recurrent PTB [28] (Chapter 9).

Prophylactic administration of progestational agents

There is now sufficient evidence from at least six trials to support the prophylactic use of progestational agents, particularly **17-alpha-hydroxy-progesterone caproate** (17P), 250 mg given intramuscularly, weekly between 16 and 36 weeks to women with **prior spontaneous PTB** between 20 and 36 6/7 weeks [21, 29, 30]. This therapy reduces the risk of recurrent PTB by approximately 35%. Treatment is especially effective for women with an early prior PTB [31]. 17P is ineffective in reducing the risk of PTB in women with twin or triplet pregnancies [32, 33]. This treatment appears to be safe for mothers and infants [29, 34]. Remaining unsettled questions surround the selection of the appropriate candidates for treatment, and the optimal pharmacological preparation. Common questions, with my answers based on non-level 1 evidence, are:

- Use in women with a twin pregnancy preceded by a spontaneous singleton PTB? *The indication is the obstetrical history, not the current multifetal pregnancy.*
- Use in women with a prior spontaneous PTB in a twin pregnancy? *The answer depends upon the gestational age of the prior twin pregnancy, and the circumstances leading to the PTB. Because a prior early (<30–32 weeks) PTB of twins confers an increased risk of singleton PTB in future pregnancies [9], a woman with a history of spontaneous PTB of twins before 30–32 weeks without complicating diagnoses such as hypertension or fetal growth restriction is a candidate for 17P at our center.*
- Use of oral progestational compounds? *No. There is only one randomized clinical trial [35] suggesting efficacy, so further studies are needed.*
- Use of vaginal progestational compounds? *No. Although some studies indicate a reduction in recurrent PTB in women treated with vaginal progestins [36, 37], there are other larger ones that do not [38]. Until more definitive evidence is available, we prefer injectable 17P because the many (at least six) trials confirm its efficacy [29, 30], the benefit was clear, and, because it was given as an injection, there is no question that the enrollees received the medication.*
- Use of 17P in women with suspected cervical insufficiency? *Yes. Because the clinical presentation of cervical insufficiency is indistinguishable from recurrent spontaneous PTB, we offer 17P prophylaxis to all women with prior early (16–20 weeks) spontaneous PT (Figure 11.2).*
- Use of 17P in women after arrested PTL? *No. There are no definitive studies to support this use.*

Cervical cerclage

Accumulated evidence from numerous studies that suggested a reduced risk of recurrent PTB for women with a **short cervix** in the current pregnancy treated with 'ultrasound-indicated' cerclage [39] has now been

Care algorithm for women with a history of birth at 16–34 weeks*

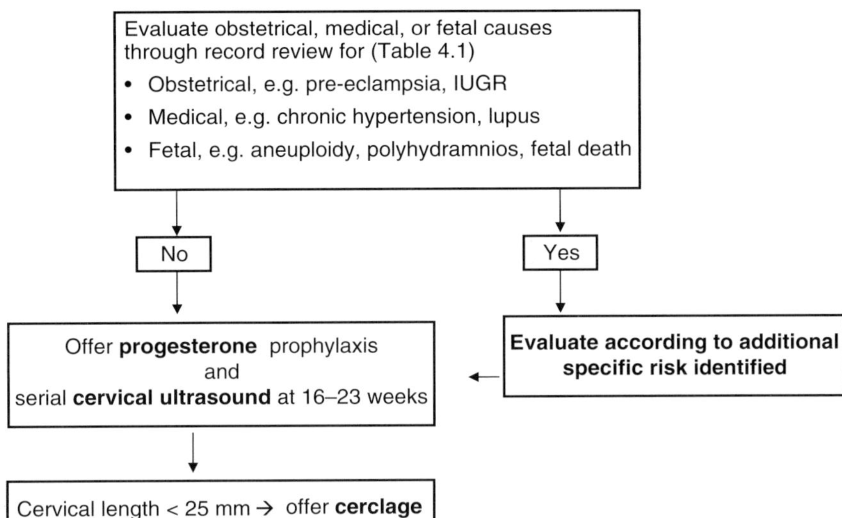

- All women receive nutritional and social work counseling at initial visit and as needed thereafter
- Smoking cessation education and program as needed
- All women receive nursing education and support at each visit, and invitation to call as needed between visits

Figure 11.2 Prematurity prevention program care algorithm. *See exceptions in Figure 11.3.

confirmed in a randomized clinical trial [40]. The rate of recurrent PTB before 35 weeks was significantly reduced in women with a prior PTB < 34 weeks and a CL less than 25 mm who were treated with a cervical cerclage (Chapter 12). Although the rate of recurrent PTB was not significantly reduced by cerclage among women with CL between 15 and 25 mm, their infants experienced significantly less morbidity in this study. As shown in the Care Algorithms (Figures 11.2 and 11.3), I recommend 17P prophylaxis to all with a history of apparent spontaneous PTB, and offer cerclage if the CL falls below 25 mm before 23 weeks gestation.

In women with ≥3 prior PTBs and/or second trimester losses (STLs), **history-indicated cerclage** at 12–14 weeks may decrease recurrent PTB, according to a subanalysis of a large trial [41]. It does not seem to be beneficial in women with less number or severity of prior PTBs or STLs [42, 43] Prior cerclage for indications other than the ones proven effective

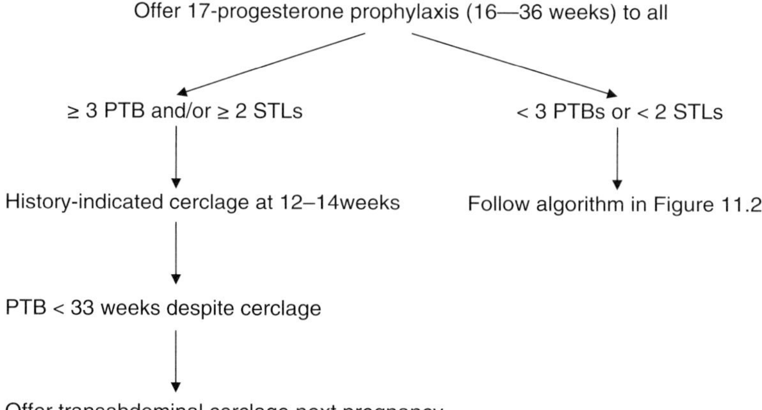

Figure 11.3 Clinical algorithm for care of asymptomatic women with multiple prior preterm birth (PTB) or second trimester losses (STLs).

by evidence-based medicine is not a reason for a history-indicated cerclage in subsequent pregnancies [44]. (Figure 11.3)

Transabdominal (TA) cerclage is a special kind of history-indicated cerclage, and has never been evaluated in a trial. A retrospective cohort study reported a lower incidence of recurrent PTB with TA cerclage at about 11–12 weeks in women with a prior transvaginal (TV) history-indicated cerclage who delivered <33 weeks anyway compared with placing another TV cerclage [45]. TA cerclage can now be safely performed laparoscopically, either before or during pregnancy at 11–12 weeks.

Therefore, **a woman with prior PTB(s) can be followed safely by TVU CL without placing in all of them a history-indicated cerclage** (Figures 11.2 and 11.3). This management is supported by at least four randomized trials, which show similar outcomes, including incidence of PTB, in women with prior PTBs who have a history-indicated cerclage compared with those followed by ultrasound and receiving the cerclage only in the minority (about 30–40%) of the cases, those in which the cervix shortens [46–49].

This approach of TVU CL screening is a 'first do no harm' approach, and not only improves outcomes, but decreases needless surgical intervention.

Antenatal administration of corticosteroids

This topic is considered in detail in Chapter 20. Evidence for improved outcomes for infants born preterm whose mothers received prenatal glucocorticoids is overwhelming. This treatment is included here because prenatal care for women with a prior PTB often includes a decision about whether and when antenatal corticosteroids (ANCS) should be administered. ANCS should be given when the clinical scenario suggests that PTB is imminent (within 7–14 days) before 34 weeks' gestation. Optimal protection against neonatal morbidity is achieved when ANCS treatment is given within 1–2 weeks of PTB, but prediction of imminent PTB has proved difficult [50]. I therefore give betamethasone or dexamethasone to women with a prior PTB as soon as there is current evidence of preterm parturition after 24 weeks, e.g. spotting or bleeding, cervical change demonstrated by digital or ultrasound examination, or a positive test for fFN. If delivery has not occurred within 3–4 weeks of this first course of ANCS, consider a second course if delivery appears to be imminent before 34 weeks' gestation [51].

Interventions suggested to reduce the risk of recurrent PTB for which evidence is absent, minimal, or mixed

- *Maternal activity restriction* is often recommended but there is insufficient evidence to support its use [52, 53]. It may cause harm by decreasing maternal muscle mass and increasing the risk of thromboembolism.
- *Maternal dietary fish consumption.* Omega-3 fatty acids (fish oil, Pikasol: 32% eicosapentaenoic acid (EPA), 23% docosahexaenoic acid (DHA), and 2 mg tocopherol/ml; four capsules/day: 1.3 g EPA and 0.9 g DHA, total 2.7 g/day; started ≥16 weeks — average 29–30 weeks) has been associated with prevention of PTB < 37 weeks by 46% and PTB < 34 weeks by 68% in women with a prior PTB < 37 weeks and a singleton gestation in one trial [54], but a recent much larger randomized trial in women with prior PTB who also received 17P found no added benefit from omega-3 fatty acid supplements [55].
- *Enhanced prenatal care and support,* in the form of provider-initiated care and nurse–family partnerships has been suggested to reduce the risk of PTB, but the evidence is inconsistent [56].
- *Weekly manual cervical exams* in addition to education for women at high-risk for PTB (≥10 on Creasy score) have not been associated with prevention of PTB [57–59].
- *Cerclage for dilated (> 1 cm) cervix* has been associated in a small randomized trial [60] and a larger observational study with a reduced risk of PTB [61] (Chapter 17).
- *Supplemental calcium* has not been studied in women with a prior PTB.
- *Energy and protein supplementation* may reduce the incidence of low birth weight but has no effect on PTB [62].
- *Antibiotic treatment* for women with a prior PTB and bacterial vaginosis has been suggested in secondary analyses to reduce the risk of recurrent PTB but evidence is inconsistent, and there are some trials in which an *increased risk* of PTB was reported (Chapter 14). Antibiotic treatment of women with a prior PTB and a positive fFN test [63] and

inter-conceptional antibiotics given to women with a prior PTB [64] were both associated with an increased rate of recurrent PTB. Other trials on women at high risk for PTB have shown that antibiotics are ineffective at reducing recurrent PTB [65–68].

Interventions that have been shown to be ineffective to reduce the risk of recurrent PTB

- *Nutritional supplements*. Randomized placebo-controlled trials of vitamins C and E [69, 70], have not found consistent reduction in PTB.
- *Early detection of PTL*. Some early trials suggested benefit but subsequent randomized trials of programs to detect PTL, including provider-initiated care, frequent nurse contact, and outpatient home uterine contraction monitoring (HUAM) did not reveal any reduction of recurrent PTB [71].
- *Contraction suppression* with various tocolytic drugs has been studied in women with prior PTB. This treatment reduces the frequency of contractions but has no effect on the rate of recurrent PTB or on neonatal outcomes [72–74].
- *Periodontal care for pregnant women* is apparently safe, but did not affect the rate of PTB in three recent randomized trials [75–77].

The context of prenatal care for women with a prior PTB

Women with a prior PTB may have lower rates of recurrent PTB when prenatal care includes specific attention to open communication between the patient and her caregivers. Lower rates of PTB have been reported in observational studies of provider-initiated contact [78], family nurse partnerships, and special programs for women with previous PTB [79]. Because the clinical presentation of preterm parturition is often more subtle than parturition at term, early signs and symptoms such as pelvic pressure and change in vaginal discharge may be easily dismissed unless patients and caregivers communicate easily.

The future of prenatal care for women with prior PTB

Current use of progestational agents and cerclage [80] is guided primarily by a clinical history of spontaneous PTB, or mid-pregnancy loss, and short cervix on ultrasound, respectively (Figures 11.2 and 11.3). Neither is fully effective in all women with these indications. As experience with progesterone supplementation grows, prophylaxis may be reserved for women with a prior PTB who also manifest another marker for PTB, such as a short cervix and/or a positive test for cervical inflammation, or who are found to have a genetic profile that suggests responsiveness to progesterone (Chapters 5, 6, 12, 13, 17, and 24).

References

1 Henriet L, Kaminski M. Impact of induced abortions on subsequent pregnancy outcome: the 1995 French national perinatal survey. Br J Obstet Gynaecol 2001; 108: 1036–42.
2 Ancel PY, Lelong N, Papiernik E, *et al.* for EUROPOP. History of induced abortion as a risk factor for PTB in European countries: results of the EUROPOP survey. Hum Reprod 2004; 19: 734–40.
3 Moreau C, Kaminski M, Ancel PY *et al.* for the EPIPAGE Group. Previous induced abortions and the risk of very preterm delivery: results of the EPIPAGE study. Br J Obstet Gynaecol 2005; 112: 430–7.
4 Edlow AG, Srinivas SK, Elovitz MA. Second trimester loss and subsequent pregnancy outcomes: what is the real risk? Am J Obstet Gynecol 2007; 197: 581.e1–e6.
5 Creinin M, Simhan HN. Can we communicate gravidity and parity better? Obstet Gynecol 2009; 113: 709–11.
6 Van Voorhis BJ. Outcomes from assisted reproductive technology. Obstet Gynecol 2006; 107: 183–200.
7 Reddy UM, Wapner RJ, Rebar RW, Tasca RJ. Infertility, assisted reproductive technology, and adverse pregnancy outcomes: executive summary of a National Institute of Child Health and Human Development workshop. Obstet Gynecol 2007; 109: 967–7.
8 Shih WG, Rushford DD, Bourne H, *et al.* Factors affecting low birthweight after assisted reproduction technology: difference between transfer of fresh and cryopreserved embryos suggests an adverse effect of oocyte collection. Human Reprod 2008; 23: 1644–53.
9 Menard MK, Newman RB, Keenan A, Ebeling M. Prognostic significance of prior preterm twin delivery on subsequent singleton pregnancy. Am J Obstet Gynecol 1996; 174: 1429–32.
10 Jakobsson M, Gissler M, Sainio S, *et al.* Preterm delivery after surgical treatment for cervical intraepithelial neoplasia. Obstet Gynecol 2007; 109: 309–13.
11 Adams MM, Elam-Evans LD, Wilson HG, *et al.* Rates of and factors associated with recurrence of preterm delivery. JAMA 2000; 283: 1591–6.
12 Esplin MS, O'Brien E, Fraser A, *et al.* Estimating recurrence risk of spontaneous preterm delivery. Obstet Gynecol 2008; 112: 516–23.
13 Kistka ZAF, Palomar L, Lee KA, Boslaugh SE, Wangler MF, Cole FS, *et al.* Racial disparity in the frequency of recurrence of PTB. Am J Obstet Gynecol 2007; 196: 131.e1–e6.
14 Mercer BM, Goldenberg RL, Moawad A, *et al.* The preterm prediction study: effect of gestational age and cause of PTB on subsequent pregnancy outcome. Am J Obstet Gynecol 1999; 181: 1216–21.

15 Mercer B, Milluzzi B, Collin M. Periviable birth at 20–26 weeks of gestation: proximate causes, previous obstetric history and recurrence risk. Am J Obstet Gynecol 2005; 193: 1175–80.

16 Mercer BM, Macpherson CA, Goldenberg RL, *et al.* Are women with recurrent spontaneous PTBs different from those without such history? Am J Obstet Gynecol 2006; 194: 1176–85.

17 Goldenberg RL, Iams JD, Mercer BM, *et al.* The preterm prediction study: the value of new vs standard risk factors in predicting early and all spontaneous PTBs. NICHD MFMU Network. Am J Public Health 1998; 88: 233–8.

18 Iams JD, Goldenberg RL, Mercer BM, *et al.* The preterm prediction study: recurrence risk of spontaneous PTB. Am J Obstet Gynecol 1998; 178: 1035–40.

19 Kaltreider DF, Kohl S. Epidemiology of preterm delivery. Clin Obstet Gynecol 1980; 23: 17–31.

20 Carr-Hill RA, Hall MH. The repetition of spontaneous preterm labour. Br J Obstet Gynaecol 1985; 92: 921–8.

21 Meis PJ, Klebanoff M, Thom E, *et al.* Prevention of recurrent preterm delivery by 17-alpha-hydroxyprogesterone caproate. N Eng J Med 2003; 348: 2379–85.

22 Kagan KO, To M, Tsoi E, Nicolaides KH. PTB: the value of sonographic measurement of CL. Br J Obstet Gynaecol 2006; 113 Suppl 3: 52–6. Review. Erratum in: Br J Obstet Gynaecol 2008; 115: 674–5.

23 Celik E, To M, Gajewska K, Smith GCS, Nicolaides KH. CL and obstetric history predict spontaneous PTB: development and validation of a model to provide individualized assessment. Ultrasound Obstet Gynecol 2008; 31: 549–54.

24 Berghella V, Roman A, Daskalakis C, *et al.* Gestational age at CL measurement and incidence of PTB. Obstet Gynecol 2007; 110: 311–7.

25 Durnwald CP, Walker H, Lundy JC, Iams JD. Rates of recurrent PTB by obstetrical history and CL. Am J Obstet Gynecol 2005;193:1170–4.

26 Crane JMG, Hutchens D. Use of transvaginal ultrasonography to predict PTB in women with a history of PTB. Ultrasound Obstet Gynecol 2008; 32: 640–5.

27 Lumley J, Oliver SS, Chamberlain C, Oakley L. Interventions for promoting smoking cessation during pregnancy. Cochrane Database Syst Rev 2004, Issue 4. Art. No.: CD001055. DOI: 10.1002/14651858.CD001055.pub2.

28 Smaill F. Antibiotics for asymptomatic bacteriuria in pregnancy. Cochrane Database Syst Rev 2001, Issue 2. Art. No.: CD000490. DOI: 10.1002/14651858.CD000490.

29 Meis PJ; Society for Maternal-Fetal Medicine. 17 hydroxyprogesterone for the prevention of preterm delivery. Obstet Gynecol 2005;105: 1128–35.

30 Dodd JM, Flenady V, Cincotta R, Crowther CA. Prenatal administration of progesterone for preventing PTB. Cochrane Database Syst Rev 2006, Issue 1. Art. No.: CD004947. DOI: 10.1002/14651858.CD004947.pub2.

31 Spong CY. Prediction and prevention of recurrent spontaneous PTB. Obstet Gynecol 2007; 110: 405–15.

32 Rouse DJ, Caritis SN, Peaceman AM, *et al.* A trial of 17 alpha-hydroxyprogesterone caproate to prevent prematurity in twins. N Engl J Med 2007; 357: 454–61.

33 Caritis SN, Rouse DJ, Peaceman AM, *et al.* Prevention of PTB in triplets using 17 alpha-hydroxyprogesterone caproate: a randomized controlled trial. Obstet Gynecol 2009; 113: 285–92.

34 Northen AT, Norman GS, Anderson K, *et al.* Follow-up of children exposed in utero to 17 alpha-hydroxyprogesterone caproate compared with placebo. Obstet Gynecol 2007; 110: 865–72.

35 Rai P, Rajaram S, Goel N, Gopalakrishnan RA, Agarwal R, Mehta S. Oral micronized progesterone for prevention of preterm birth. Internat J Gynecol Obstet 2009; 104: 40–3.

36 Fonseca EB, Bittar RE, Carvalho MH, Zugaib M. Prophylactic administration of progesterone by vaginal suppository to reduce the incidence of spontaneous PTB in women at increased risk: a randomized placebo-controlled double-blind study. Am J Obstet Gynecol 2003; 188: 419–24.
37 Fonseca EB, Celik E, Parra M, *et al.* Progesterone and the risk of PTB among women with a short cervix. N Engl J Med 2007; 357: 462–9.
38 O'Brien JM, Adair CD, Lewis DF, *et al.* Progesterone vaginal gel for the reduction of recurrent PTB: primary results from a randomized, double-blind, placebo-controlled trial. Ultrasound Obstet Gynecol 2007; 30: 687–96.
39 Berghella V, Odibo AO, To MS, Rust OA, Althuisius SM. Cerclage for short cervix on ultrasonography: meta-analysis of trials using individual patient-level data. Obstet Gynecol 2005; 106: 181–9.
40 Owen J, Hankins G, Iams JD, *et al.* Multicenter randomized trial of cerclage for PTB prevention in high-risk women with shortened mid-trimester cervical length. Am J Obstet Gynecol 2009; 201: 375. e1–8.
41 MCR/RCOG Working Party on Cervical Cerlage. Final report of the Medical Research Council/Royal College of Obstetricians and Gynaecologists multicentre randomized trial of cervical cerclage. Br J Obstet Gynaecol 1993; 100: 516–23.
42 Rush RW, Issacs S, McPherson K, Jones L, Chalmers I, Grant A. A randomized controlled trial of cervical cerclage in women at high risk of preterm delivery. Br J Obstet Gynaecol 1984; 91: 724–30.
43 Lazar P, Gueguen S, Dreyfus J, Renaud R, Pontonnier G, Papiernik E. Multicentre controlled trial of cervical cerclage in women at moderate risk of preterm delivey. Br J Obstet Gynaecol 1984; 91: 731–5.
44 Pelham J, Lewis D, Berghella V. Prior cerclage: to repeat or not to repeat? Am J Perinat 2008; 25: 417–20.
45 Davis G, Berghella V, Talucci M, Wapner RJ. Patients with a prior failed transvaginal cerclage: a comparison of obstetric outcomes with either transabdominal or transvaginal cerclage. Am J Obstet Gynecol 2000; 183: 836–9.
46 Althuisius SM, Dekker GA, van Geijn HP, Bekedam DJ, Hummel P. Cervical incompetence prevention randomized cerclage trial (CIPRACT): study design and preliminary results. Am J Obstet Gynecol 2000; 183: 823–9.
47 Beigi A, Zarrinkoub F. Elective versus ultrasound-indicated cervical cerclage in women at risk for cervical incompetence. Med J Islamic Rep Iran 2005; 19: 103–7.
48 Simcox R, Bennett F, Teoh G, Shennan AH. A randomized controlled trial of cervical scanning vs history to determine cerclage in high risk women (circle trial). J Obstet Gynecol 2007; 27 (suppl. 1): S18.
49 Kassanos D, Salamalekis E, Vitoratos N, Panayotopoulos N, Loghis C, Creatsas C. The value of transvaginal ultrasonography in diagnosis and management of cervical incompetence. Clin Exc Obstet Gynecol 2001; 28: 266–8.
50 Mercer B, Egerman R, Beazley D, *et al.* Antenatal corticosteroids in women at risk for PTB: a randomized trial. Am J Obstet Gynecol 2001; 184: S6.
51 Garite TJ, Kurtzman J, Maurel K, *et al.* Impact of a 'rescue course' of antenatal corticosteroids: a multicenter randomized placebo-controlled trial. Am J Obstet Gynecol 2009; 200: 248.e1–248.e9.
52 Sosa C, Althabe F, Belizán J, Bergel E. Bed rest in singleton pregnancies for preventing PTB. Cochrane Database Syst Rev 2004, Issue 1. Art. No.: CD003581. DOI: 10.1002/14651858.CD003581.pub2.
53 Hobel CJ, Ross MG, Bermis RL, Bragonier JR, Nessim S, Sandhu M, *et al.* The West Los Angeles preterm birth prevention project. I. Program impact on high-risk women. Am J Obstet Gynecol 1994; 170: 54–62.

54 Olsen SF, Secher NJ, Tabor A, Weber T, Walker JJ, Gluud C. Randomized clinical trials of fish oil supplementation in high risk pregnancies. Br J Obstet Gynaecol 2000; 107: 382–95.
55 Harper M, *et al.* for NICHD MFMU Network. Randomized controlled trial of omega-3 fatty acid supplementaiton for recurrent preterm birth prevention. Am J Obstet Gynecol 2008; 197: s2.
56 Hodnett ED, Fredericks S. Support during pregnancy for women at increased risk of low birthweight babies. Cochrane Database Syst Rev 2003, Issue 3. Art. No.: CD000198. DOI: 10.1002/14651858.CD000198.
57 Mueller-Heubach E, Riddick D, Barnett B, Bente R. Preterm birth prevention: evaluation of a prospective controlled trial. Am J Obstet Gynecol 1989; 160: 1172–8.
58 Main DM, Richardson DK, Hadley CB, Gabbe SG. Controlled trial of a preterm labor detection program: efficacy and costs. Obstet Gynecol 1989; 74: 873–7.
59 Collaborative group on preterm birth prevention. Multicenter randomized controlled trial of a preterm birth prevention program. Am J Obstet Gynecol 1993; 169: 352–66.
60 Althuisius SM, Dekker GA, Hummel P, van Geijn HP. Cervical incompetence prevention randomized cerclage trial: emergency cerclage with bed rest versus bed rest alone. Am J Obstet Gynecol 2003; 189: 907–10.
61 Pereira L, Cotter A, Gómez R, *et al.* Expectant management compared with physical examination-indicated cerclage (EM-PEC) in selected women with a dilated cervix at 14(0/7)-25(6/7) weeks: results from the EM-PEC international cohort study. Am J Obstet Gynecol 2007; 197: 483.e1–8.
62 Kramer MS, Kakuma R. Energy and protein intake in pregnancy. Cochrane Database Syst Rev 2003, Issue 4. Art. No.: CD000032. DOI: 10.1002/14651858.CD000032.
63 Shennan A, Crawshaw S, Briley A, *et al.* A randomised controlled trial of metronidazole for the prevention of PTB in women positive for cervicovaginal fFN: the PREMET Study. Br J Obstet Gynaecol 2006; 113: 65–74.
64 Andrews WW, Goldenberg RL, Hauth JC, Cliver SP, Copper R, Conner M. Interconceptional antibiotics to prevent spontaneous preterm birth: a randomized clinical trial. Am J Obstet Gynecol 2006; 194: 617–23.
65 Vermeulen GM, Bruinse HW. Prophylactic administration of clindamycin 2% vaginal cream to reduce the incidence of spontaneous preterm birth in women with an increased recurrence risk: a randomized placebo-controlled double-blind trial. Br J Obstet Gynaecol 1999; 106: 652–7.
66 Gighangi PB, Ndinya-Achola JO, Ombete J, Nagelkerke NJ, Temmerman M. Antimicrobial prophylaxis in pregnancy: a randomized, placebo-controlled trial with cefetamet-pivoxil in pregnant women with poor obstetrical history. Am J Obstet Gynecol 1997; 177: 680–4.
67 Hauth JC, Goldenberg RL, Andrews WW, DuBard MB, Copper RL. Reduced incidence of preterm delivery with metronidazole and erythromycin in women with bacterial vaginosis. N Engl J Med 1995; 333: 1732–6.
68 Thinkhamrop J, Hofmeyr GJ, Adetoro O, Lumbiganon P. Prophylactic antibiotic administration in pregnancy to prevent infectious morbidity and mortality. Cochrane Database Syst Rev 4, 2005.
69 Rumbold AR, Crowther CA, Haslam RR *et al.* Vitamins C and E and the risks of preeclampsia and perinatal complications. N Engl J Med 2006; 354: 1796–806.
70 Poston L, Briley AL, Seed PT, Kelly FJ, Shennan AH. Vitamins in Pre-eclampsia (VIP) Trial Consortium. Vitamin C and vitamin E in pregnant women at risk for pre-

eclampsia (VIP trial): randomised placebo-controlled trial. Lancet 2006; 367: 1145–54.

71 Dyson DC, Danbe KH, Bamber JA, *et al.* Monitoring women at risk for PTL. N Engl J Med 1998; 338: 15–19.

72 Dodd JM, Crowther CA, Dare MR, Middleton P. Oral betamimetics for maintenance therapy after threatened preterm labour. Cochrane Database Syst Rev 2006, Issue 1. Art. No.: CD003927. DOI: 10.1002/14651858.CD003927.pub2

73 Whitworth M, Quenby S. Prophylactic oral betamimetics for preventing preterm labour in singleton pregnancies. Cochrane Database Syst Rev 2008, Issue 1. Art. No.: CD006395. DOI: 10.1002/14651858.CD006395.pub2.

74 Gaunekar NN, Crowther CA. Maintenance therapy with calcium channel blockers for preventing PTB after threatened preterm labour. Cochrane Database Syst Rev 2004, Issue 3. Art. No.: CD004071. DOI: 10.1002/14651858.CD004071.pub2

75 Michalowicz BS, Hodges JS, Di Angelis AJ, *et al.* Treatment of periodontal disease and the risk of PTB. N Engl J Med 2006; 355: 1885–94.

76 Offenbacher S, Beck J, Jared H, *et al.* Maternal oral therapy to reduce obstetric risk (MOTOR): a report of a multi-centered periodontal therapy randomized-controlled trial on rate of preterm delivery. Am J Obstet Gynecol 2008: 199, Abstr 3. Page S2, DOI: 10.1016/j.ajog.2008.09.029.

77 Macones G, Jeffcoat M, Parry S, *et al.* Screening and treating periodontal disease in pregnancy does not reduce the incidence of PTB: results from the PIPS study. Am J Obstet Gynecol 2008;199, Abstr 5, Page S3, DOI: 10.1016/j.ajog.2008.09.031.

78 Moore ML, Meis PJ, Ernest JM, *et al.* A randomized trial of nurse intervention to reduce preterm and low birth weight births. Obstet Gynecol 1998; 91: 656–61.

79 Newman RB, Sullivan SA, Menard MK, *et al.* South Carolina Partners for PTB prevention: a regional perinatal initiative for the reduction of premature birth in a Medicaid population. Am J Obstet Gynecol 2008; 199: 393.e1–8.

80 Berghella V. Novel developments on CL screening and progesterone for preventing PTB. Br J Obstet Gynaecol 2009; 116: 182–7.

CHAPTER 12

Short Cervical Length

Timothy J. Rafael

Division of Maternal-Fetal Medicine and Department of Obstetrics and Gynecology, Thomas Jefferson University, Jefferson Medical College, Philadelphia, USA

Key points

- The parameter found in most populations to have the best predictive accuracy for preterm birth (PTB) < 35 weeks is a cervical length (CL) <25 mm by transvaginal ultrasound (TVU).
- The shorter the CL, and the earlier in gestational age it is detected, the higher the risk of PTB.
- Other factors that must be carefully considered when using CL for prediction and prevention of PTB are number of fetuses and other risk factors for PTB.
- In women with a prior PTB and CL of <15 mm between 14 and 24 weeks, the risk of PTB < 32 weeks is as high as 50%.
- Women with CL of >30 mm up to 24 weeks have only a 1% chance of delivering <26 weeks, and only a 9% risk of delivering before 35 weeks, regardless of previous history.
- In women with a normal CL (CL ≥ 25 mm), funneling does not seem to confer a clinically significant increased risk of PTB.
- In a low-risk singleton population (e.g. without a prior PTB), an ultrasound-indicated cerclage for a short CL found between 16–24 weeks has not been shown to be of significant benefit in prolonging gestation, or reducing rates of PTB < 35 weeks.
- In women with a previous spontaneous PTB at 16–34 weeks, performing an ultrasound-indicated cerclage for a CL < 25 mm found at 14–24 weeks is associated with a significant 29% decrease in PTB < 35 weeks.
- Therefore TVU CL screening is recommended in women with prior PTB, as it can also reassure the >60% of these pregnancies destined to have a normal (≥25 mm) CL and deliver at term without intervention.
- There appears to be no difference in outcomes when using a McDonald versus Shirodkar cerclage. McDonald is most commonly used given its ease of placement and removal compared with Shirodkar.
- As there is only one large randomized trial showing that micronized vaginal progesterone prevents PTB in women with short CL ≤ 15 mm, there are no current recommendations for its routine use in this population. This is an area of active investigation.

(Continued)

Preterm Birth. Edited by Vincenzo Berghella.

- Therefore currently there is insufficient evidence to recommend routine screening with TVU CL in low-risk singleton gestations or in multiple gestations (Chapter 16).
- Currently, routine repeated CL measurements following any cerclage are not recommended in that no intervention has been shown to affect outcome.
- There is insufficient evidence to routinely recommend the use of indomethacin, pessaries, and/or bed rest in women with short CL.
- Women with preterm labor at 23–34 weeks who are found to have a TVU CL ≥ 30 mm and negative fetal fibronectin (FFN) have less than a 1% chance of delivering within 1 week. Therefore no intervention should be used in this clinical setting, and reassurance provided (Chapter 18).
- In women with preterm labor, knowledge of CL and FFN is associated with a reduction in triage time (when compared with not having knowledge of results), as well as a reduction in the incidence of PTB (Chapter 18).

Introduction

Transvaginal ultrasound (TVU) examination of the cervix has emerged in the last 25 years as an **effective screening method for predicting those pregnancies which will spontaneously deliver preterm** (Table 12.1). Sensitivities and specificities of this test vary depending on the woman being studied [1], and interventions such as cerclage and progesterone differ in efficacy in different populations. Therefore, to be used effectively for prevention of preterm birth (PTB), the practitioner should know, through this chapter:

1. Proper techniques for performing cervical length (CL);
2. Stratification of risk for PTB based on CL, gestational age (GA) at screening, patient's previous history, number of fetuses, and other factors;
3. Interventions available to prolong gestation.

Table 12.1 Transvaginal ultrasound cervical length fulfills all criteria for an effective screening test.

- Screens for an important condition (preterm birth) (see Chapters 1–4)
- The technique is well-described (Table 12.2)
- It is safe and acceptable
- It recognizes early asymptomatic phase
- It is reliable (reproducible)
- It is valid (accurate in prediction)
- 'Early' treatment is effective at prevention of preterm birth

Table 12.2 Technique of transvaginal ultrasound for visualization of cervical length to aim at predicting and preventing preterm birth [1].

1	Has the patient emptied her bladder
2	Prepare a clean probe covered by a condom
3	Insert the probe (probe can be inserted by the patient for more comfort)
4	Place the probe in the anterior fornix of the vagina
5	Obtain a sagittal view of the cervix, with the long axis view of echogenic endocervical mucosa along the length of the canal (see Figures 12.1 and 12.2)
6	Withdraw the probe until the image is blurred and reapply just enough pressure to restore the image (to avoid excessive pressure on the cervix which can elongate it)
7	Enlarge the image so that the cervix occupies at least 2/3 of the image, and external and internal os are well seen
8	Measure the cervical length from the internal to the external os along the endocervical canal
9	Obtain at least three measurements, and record the shortest best measurement in millimeters over a period of at least three minutes, to allow time for development of a funnel
10	Apply transfundal pressure for 15 seconds, and record any changes in cervical length or funneling

Method

How

TVU examination of the cervix has emerged as the gold standard for evaluating CL. When it comes to predicting PTB, it has consistently demonstrated better diagnostic accuracy when compared with digital examination, regardless of patient population [2, 3]. It is also more reliable than transabdominal and translabial (transperineal) measurement [4]. Current recommendations for the performance of transvaginal ultrasound exam (TVU) of the cervix are described in Table 12.2 [1].

When

Most women destined to deliver preterm, especially if already at high risk for PTB by history, develop a CL < 25 mm at a mean gestational age of 19 weeks, usually between **16 and 24 weeks**, and not earlier [5]. Serial screening is more sensitive than a one-time measurement, but not currently cost-effective in most populations (Table 12.3) [6].

What

The parameter found in most populations to have the best predictive accuracy for PTB is a **CL < 25 mm**. The most common primary outcome studied is spontaneous PTB < 35 weeks. The shorter the CL, the higher is the risk of PTB (Figures 12.1–12.3). A normal CL is ≥25 mm, and usually

Table 12.3 Management suggestions for using cervical length (CL) for prediction and prevention of preterm birth (PTB) [6]. GA, gestational age. *Not recommended for clinical use yet. †If transvaginal ultrasound (TVU) CL is 25–29 mm, repeat in 1 week.

- Always use **TVU**
- Screen at **15–24 weeks** gestational age (the earlier the shorter CL, the higher the risk)
- Use shortest best **CL** in mm (normal is ≥25 mm)
- Be aware most and best data is for the outcome PTB < 35 weeks
- Frequency of TVU CL:
  - low-risk women: 1 at around 18–22 weeks*
  - high risk women (e.g. prior PTB): 2, at 14–18 and 18–22 weeks†
  - very high risk women (e.g. prior second trimester loss or very early spontaneous PTB): serial every 2 weeks from 14 to 24 weeks†
- Calculate individualized risk of PTB based on:
  - **CL** (the shorter, the higher the PTB risk)
  - **Gestational age** at measurements (Table 12.4) (the earlier the short CL is detected, the higher the PTB risk)
  - **Prior history**
  - **Singleton vs multiple** gestation (Table 12.5)

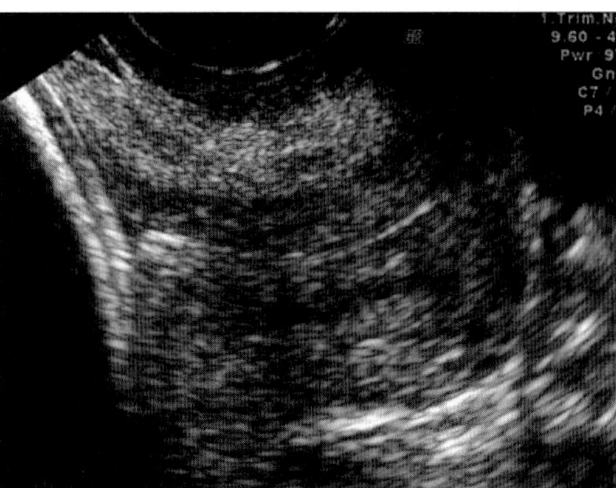

Figure 12.1 Transvaginal ultrasonography of closed normal cervix (cervical length >25 mm; exactly 34 mm).

<50 mm, before 30 weeks. After 30 weeks, physiologic shortening occurs even in women who deliver >37 weeks. CL before 14 weeks is usually normal, and not helpful clinically, except in rare women with large (or repeated) cone biopsies and recurrent second trimester losses [5]. For the purposes of simplicity, for the remainder of the chapter, CL will be assumed to mean 'functional cervical length', defined as the closed portion of the endocervical canal only [1].

In about 10% of low-risk and 25–33% of high-risk women, the internal os is open and **funneling** is present in the second trimester (Figures 12.2

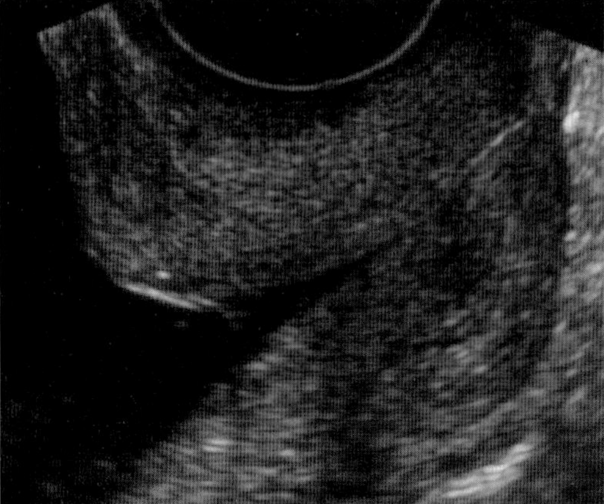

Figure 12.2 Transvaginal ultrasonography of a short cervix (cervical length 12 mm), with V-shaped funneling.

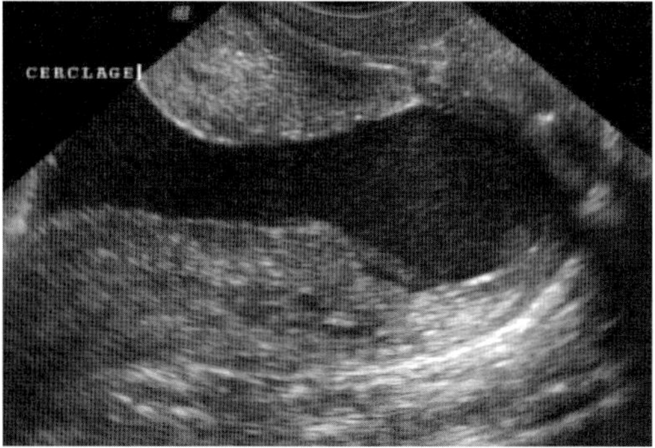

Figure 12.3 Transvaginal ultrasonography of a short cervix (cervical length 2 mm), with U-shaped funneling, despite cerclage.

and 12.3) [2, 7, 8]. In these cases, the funnel length (open portion of the cervix) and funnel width (internal os diameter) can be measured. The percent of funneling is defined as the funnel length divided by the total CL, where total CL is the funnel length and functional CL (Figure 12.4) [8]. If it is present, the shape of the funnel can be documented (although it can be a subjective finding), going from a normal T shape, to Y, then V, and finally a U shape (in progressing order of severity) [9]. Of note, in women with a normal CL, funneling does not seem to confer an increased risk of PTB [10]. Findings related to funneling in the presence of short CL vary, with some finding that women with funneling have an increase risk of PTB and worse outcomes compared with those with short CL alone [10, 11], while others, including a more recent study, found that funneling in

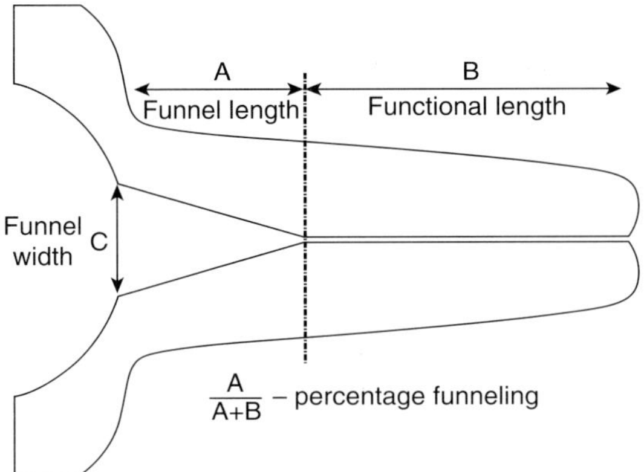

Figure 12.4 Measurements of the cervix with funneling [10].

the presence of a short functional CL does not add appreciably to the risk of early gestational age at delivery [12, 13]. Overall, the functional CL is the preferred method to assess risk for PTB, keeping in mind that if funneling is present, the cervix is almost always short.

Several other parameters could be measured, such as endocervical canal dilatation, anterior and posterior cervical width, cervical position (horizontal versus vertical), lower uterine segment thickness, cervical angle, visibility of chorion at internal os, cervical index (funnel length +1/functional length) and vascularity. As they add little to prediction by CL alone, we do not recommend them for clinical use. Sludge, or debris (see Figure 6.1) has been shown to be predictive of PTB, but it is unclear if the presence of sludge improves the predictive accuracy already provided by CL [14]. Three-dimensional ultrasonography is also currently more a research tool than a clinical one for TVU CL [15].

PTB prediction by CL in clinical care

Accurate prediction of PTB allows the best management. Prediction of PTB using TVU CL must also account for many other factors that influence PTB (Table 12.3) [6]. Other factors that must be carefully considered when using CL for prediction of PTB are: gestational age at measurement, population studied (obstetrical-gynecological risk factors for PTB, number of fetuses, e.g. singleton vs multiple — see also Chapter 6), FFN, contractions, and infection.

Gestational age

The earlier the short CL is detected, the higher is the risk of PTB, so a CL of 20 mm first detected at 16 weeks has a much higher incidence

Table 12.4 Predicted probability of preterm delivery before week 35, by cervical length (mm) and time of measurement (week of pregnancy) in women with risk factors for PTB. Adapted from Berghella *et al.* [20].

	Week of pregnancy													
Cervical length (mm)	15	16	17	18	19	20	21	22	23	24	25	26	27	28
0	69.8	68.7	67.5	66.3	65.2	64.0	62.7	61.5	60.2	59.0	57.7	56.4	55.1	53.8
5	62.5	61.3	60.0	58.7	57.5	56.2	54.9	53.6	52.2	50.9	49.6	48.3	47.0	45.7
10	54.6	53.3	52.0	50.7	49.4	48.1	46.7	45.4	44.1	42.8	41.6	40.3	39.0	37.8
15	46.5	45.2	43.9	42.6	41.3	40.1	38.8	37.6	36.3	35.1	33.9	32.8	31.6	30.5
20	38.6	37.3	36.1	34.9	33.7	32.5	31.4	30.3	29.2	28.1	27.0	26.0	25.0	24.0
25	31.2	30.1	29.0	27.9	26.9	25.8	24.8	23.9	22.9	22.0	21.1	20.3	19.4	18.6
30	24.7	23.7	22.8	21.8	21.0	20.1	19.3	18.5	17.7	16.9	16.2	15.5	14.8	14.2
35	19.1	18.3	17.5	16.8	16.1	15.4	14.7	14.1	13.4	12.8	12.2	11.7	11.2	10.6
40	14.6	13.9	13.3	12.7	12.1	11.6	11.1	10.6	10.1	9.6	9.2	8.7	8.3	7.9
45	11.0	10.5	10.0	9.6	9.1	8.7	8.3	7.9	7.5	7.2	6.8	6.5	6.2	5.9
50	8.2	7.8	7.4	7.1	6.7	6.4	6.1	5.8	5.5	5.2	5.0	4.7	4.5	4.3
55	6.0	5.7	5.5	5.2	4.9	4.7	4.5	4.3	4.0	3.8	3.7	3.5	3.3	3.1

of PTB than the same short CL of 20 mm detected at 20 weeks (but normal at 16 weeks) (Table 12.4) [10]. Screening for PTB by TVU CL is not very effective when done before 14 weeks, as even women at highest risk for PTB usually maintain a closed and long (>25 mm) cervix on TVU [5]. This is because the endocervical canal is continuous with the lower uterine segment, which gets falsely measured as CL.

Population (Table 12.5)

Asymptomatic singleton gestations: low risk

A woman at lowest risk of PTB should have none of the risks listed in Table 4.1. In a low risk population, at least with no prior PTB, CL is a normally distributed variable, with mean CL being 34.0 and 32.6 mm for nulliparous women at 24 and 28 weeks, respectively. After 30 weeks, a progressive physiologic shortening of CL is noticed in most women destined to deliver at term. For multiparous women, CL means are approximately 36.1 and 34.5 mm at 24 and 28 weeks, respectively. The 10th percentile at 24 weeks for both low-risk populations has been noted to be 25 mm. While the differences between nulliparous and multiparous women regarding CL has been noted to be statistically significant, these differences have not been of clinical importance [16,17]. Unfortunately, for this low risk population, because the incidence of PTB is low, the sensitivities and positive predictive values are low (37.3% and 17.8% at 24 weeks, respectively, and 49.4% and 11.3% at 28 weeks, respectively) [16].

Table 12.5 Prediction of preterm birth by CL based on obstetric-gynecologic risk factors.

Singleton gestations	*n*	PTB (%)*	Primary outcome (GA in weeks)	GA (weeks)	CL	Sens	Spec	PPV	NPV	RR
Low risk Iams [16]	2915	4.3	<35	22–25	<25	47	84	35	90	3.4
Prior preterm birth Owen [7]	183	26	<35	16–24	<25	69	80	55	88	4.5
Prior LEEP Berghella [22]	55	6	<35	16–24	<25	67	87	22	98	10.2
Prior cold knife cone Berghellla [22]	45	22	<35	16–24	<25	60	69	35	86	2.5
Prior multiple D&Es Visintine [23]	131	30	<35	14–24	<25	53	75	48	78	2.2
Uterine anomalies Airoldi [21]	64	11	<35	14–23$^{6/7}$	<25	71	91	50	95	13.5
Twin Goldenberg [25]	147	32	<35	22–24	<25	30	88	54	74	3.2
Triplet Guzman [61]	47	34	<32	15–20	<25	25	100	100	72	N/A

*as it relates to primary outcome.

In fact, the overwhelming majority of low risk women found to have a cervical length less than 25 mm at 24 weeks of gestation actually deliver after 35 weeks.

Prior PTB

In this high risk population CL is quite predictive of PTB. In a well-designed prospective blinded observational study, it was found that not only is a CL < 25 mm predictive of PTB when found between 16 and 18 6/7 weeks' gestation (Relative Risk 3.3, Positive Predictive Value 75%), but also by continuing measurements up to a gestational age of 23 6/7 weeks, the sensitivity for detecting PTB < 35 weeks' gestation could be increased to as high as 70% [7]. In women with extremely shortened CL of <15 mm found between 14 and 24 weeks gestation, the risk of PTB < 32 weeks is 50% [18]. Providing reassurance to an anxiety-filled population, a CL of >30 at 24 weeks is associated with only a 1% chance of delivering <26 weeks, and only a 9% risk of delivering before 35 weeks [19]. A useful

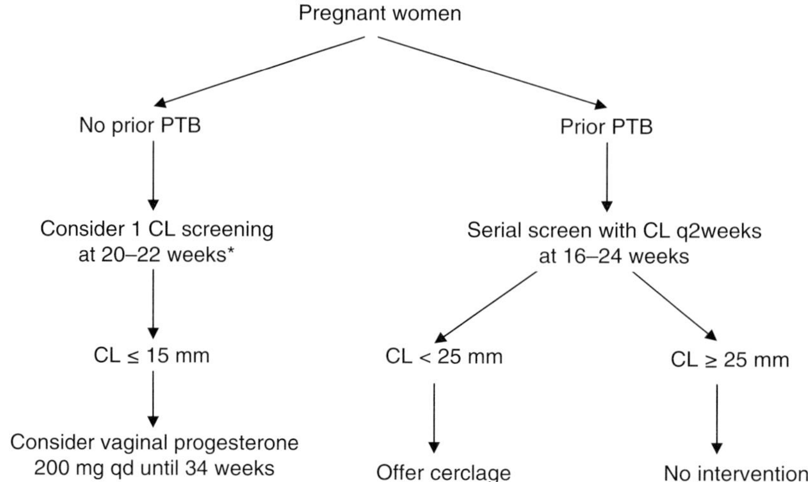

Figure 12.5 Clinical algorithm for screening with transvaginal ultrasound cervical length (CL) in women without symptoms of preterm labor. PTB, preterm birth. Qd, once every day. *Not yet confirmed by multiple trials.

tool for quantifying percentage risk of PTB < 35 weeks in this population is summarized in Table 12.4 [20], and a proposed algorithm for screening is summarized in Figure 12.5.

Uterine anomalies, prior cervical surgery, multiple dilation and curettages

In women with known uterine anomalies (bicornuate uterus, septate uterus, uterine didelphys, unicornuate uterus), a CL < 25 mm (measured up until 23 6/7 weeks' gestation) carries a 13-fold risk of PTB < 35 weeks compared with those not having short CL. Among those groups, women with a unicornuate uterus have been shown to have the highest rate of cervical shortening and PTB [21]. Short CL has also been shown to be predictive of PTB < 35 weeks in both women who have had a prior cone biopsy [22], as well as those with more than one dilation and curettage [23].

Multiple gestations

Although twin pregnancies currently represent only 2% of live births, they represent a substantial portion of PTB (Chapter 16). Only 1.6% of singletons deliver before 32 weeks as compared with 11.9% of twins [24]. While the mechanism underlying the premature onset of labor in multiple gestations may differ from that in singleton gestations (e.g. uterine stretch), CL also plays a role in PTB in this population. Several studies have looked at CL in twin gestations, with a preterm prediction study finding that a CL ≤ 25 mm at 24 weeks is the best of all the predictors of PTB evaluated, including fetal fibronectin (FFN) and bacterial vaginosis. At 24 weeks, a CL ≤ 25 mm gave a rate of PTB < 35 weeks of approximately 50% [25]. Again, for reassurance purposes, a CL >35 mm is associated with a very low risk (4%) of PTB [26]. Additional studies have also shown that the prediction of spontaneous PTB by CL is not significantly improved by certain other maternal characteristics (e.g. ethnic origin, BMI, age) [27]. While the median CL in twin gestations is similar to that in singleton pregnancies, not only do twin gestations have a higher proportion of CL < 25 mm at 24 weeks' gestation (12.9% in twins compared with 8–10% in singletons) [28], but also twin gestations have been shown to have a progressively much shorter cervix starting after 20 weeks' gestation [29]. The sensitivity for PTB when performed before 24 weeks is low, only 25–30% in twins and triplets (Table 12.5), making early interventions such as cerclage unlikely to be effective. It is possible that screening up to 28 weeks and use of interventions safe at that gestational age such as progesterone or anti-inflammatory agents may prove cost-effective in the future. Currently, the lack of effective interventions to prolong gestation precludes a recommendation of CL screening in twin gestations.

Women with cerclage

Evaluation of CL pre- and post-cerclage placement has shown that not only does CL increase post-cerclage, but also the increase in CL is associated with a higher rate of term delivery [30,31]. Currently, routine repeated CL measurements following an ultrasound-indicated or physical exam-indicated cerclage are not recommended in that no intervention has been studied to affect outcome. In women who have had a history-indicated cerclage, with subsequent CL shortening <25 mm, placing a reinforcement cerclage has been associated with worse prognosis and should not be done [32].

Preterm labor

An episode of preterm labor (PTL) increases a woman's risk of having a PTB, although the majority go on to deliver at term [33]. As will be reviewed in more details in Chapter 18, TVU CL is very useful in the management of PTL and intact membranes (see Figure 18.1).

FFN

Having both tests (CL and FFN) positive does increase the risk of PTB over having just one positive test, as described in Chapter 13.

Uterine contractions

Women with a short CL often have asymptomatic contractions [34]. The presence of contractions predictably increases the risk of PTB [35].

Infections

As seen in Chapter 6, a short CL is associated with a higher risk of intra-amniotic infection; the shorter the CL, the higher the incidence of infection. The incidence is 1–2% in singleton gestations with a poor obstetrical history and a TVU CL < 25 mm in the second trimester [11], so there is usually no need to do an amniocentesis before placing an ultrasound-indicated cerclage. The presence of bacterial vaginosis further increases the risk of PTB in women with a short CL. There are no studies on any association between other infections that contribute to PTB (e.g. Chlamydia, gonorrhea, etc.) and TVU CL.

Interventions for short CL

With the advent of TVU CL, the obstetrician was given a mighty tool in being able to predict those at high and low-risk for sustaining a spontaneous PTB (Tables 12.4 and 12.5) [20]. Unfortunately, without the benefit of a proven intervention, many obstetricians are left with the question, 'Well, what do I do now with the results that I have?' Here are the most up to date level 1 recommendations when faced with a mid-trimester short CL < 25 mm. A summary of evidence for screening with TVU CL for prevention of PTB is given in Table 12.6.

Cerclage

Low risk singleton population

An ultrasound-indicated cerclage for a short CL found between 16 and 24 weeks has not been shown in randomized trials to be of benefit in reducing rates of PTB < 35 weeks [36–38]. This leads to the **recommendation of not routinely screening this population for short CL**. Nonetheless, a meta-analysis showed that there is a trend for a 24% reduction in PTB from 33% to 26% in women with a CL < 25 mm, singleton gestations and no prior PTB, cone biopsy, Mullerian anomaly or multiple D&Es [37]. Further studies are needed.

Previous PTB singleton population

In a meta-analysis of four randomized trials with 208 such women, cerclage for CL < 25 mm found up until 24 weeks was associated with a 39% decrease in PTB < 35 weeks [37]. A recent multi-centered randomized NICHD-sponsored trial with 301 women with prior PTB and 16–22 6/7 week CL < 25 mm also found a 23% decrease in PTB < 35 weeks [39]. Together, these five trials on 509 similar women (**prior PTB and second trimester CL < 25 mm**) report a significant **decrease of 29% in PTB < 35**

Table 12.6 Summary of evidence for screening with transvaginal ultrasound (TVU) cervical length (CL) for prevention of preterm birth (PTB). *See also text. RCT, randomized controlled trial. LEEP, loop electrosurgical excision procedure. D&E, dilatation and evacuation. PTL, preterm labor. PPROM, preterm premature rupture of membranes.

Population	Prediction of PTB	Evidence for prevention	Future research
Singletons			
Low-risk	Yes	Yes (but limited: one RCT with **vaginal progesterone** if **CL ≤ 15 mm** at 22–24 weeks [50])	Other RCTs testing interventions such as cerclage, progesterone, etc.
Prior PTB	Yes	Yes (**cerclage** if **CL < 25 mm** at 16–23 weeks)	Other RCTs testing interventions (and combinations) such as cerclage, progesterone, etc.
Cervical surgery (e.g. cone biopsy, LEEP, etc)	Yes	No	RCTs testing interventions
Uterine anomalies	Yes	No	RCTs testing interventions
Multiple D&Es	Yes	No	RCTs testing interventions
Multiple gestations			
Twins	Yes	No (Chapter 16)	RCTs testing interventions
Triplets	Yes	No	RCTs testing interventions
PTL	Yes	Yes (Chapter 20)	RCTs testing interventions
PPROM	Yes	No (Chapter 21)	RCTs testing interventions

weeks, from 41% in the no cerclage to 29% in the cerclage group. Previable (<24 weeks) and perinatal mortality are also significantly decreased [39].

In women with a prior history-indicated cerclage (Chapter 11), placing a **reinforcing cerclage** in those with short CL has been associated with a **worse prognosis** [32]. Placing the 'ultrasound-indicated' cerclage **as high as possible**, at least 2 cm from the external os, has been associated with greater reduction of PTB compared with placing the cerclage in the lower third of the cervix [40]. Regarding which **type** of cerclage to use, secondary analysis from published randomized controlled trials has revealed no difference in outcomes when using a McDonald versus Shirodkar cerclage [41]. We use mersilene tape as **suture**, but no prospective study has compared different sutures for cerclage. In this population it appears **reasonable to follow with serial CL measurements (at 1–2 week intervals) up until 24 weeks**, offering ultrasound-indicated cerclage for CL < 25 mm up until that gestational age (Figure 12.5). This management prevents unnecessary history-indicated cerclages (Chapter 11), and has decreased the overall incidence of cerclage at our institution from about 3% (1998–2003) to about 0.5–1% (2006–08). This evidence confirms what McDonald [42] and Shirodkar [43] had postulated, i.e. that **cerclage is indicated for women with *both* a prior preterm birth *and* a cervix that is shortening and/or dilating in the second trimester**.

Other high-risk singletons

While we have discussed the increased risk of PTB in women such as those with prior cone biopsy, uterine anomalies, prior multiple dilation and curettages (Chapter 6), as of yet there is insufficient evidence to recommend placement of any kind of cerclage in this population [37]. Randomized trials targeting these high-risk populations, especially once they develop a short CL, are needed.

Multiple gestations

Cerclage for CL < 25 mm has been associated with a 215% increase in PTB compared with no cerclage in a population of 49 twin pregnancies reported in a meta-analysis of trials [37]. Therefore cerclage should be placed in multiple gestations only under research trials, and **not in clinical care**.

Other notes on cerclage

For a full description of the technique and other aspects of cerclage, please refer to other literature [44,45]. We prefer McDonald cerclage, as it is as efficacious as Shirodkar [41], and easier to place and remove. Suture type has not been studied extensively, but we do place a Mersilene tape 5 mm as high as safely possible on the cervix. There is limited information on using indomethacin [46], which, if used, should be given for ≤48 hours peri-cerclage. No information is present in the literature regarding the additional use of antibiotics, which we do not use as many other studies on antibiotics have not shown prevention of PTB in women with intact membranes.

The benefits of TVU CL screening are also that women with prior multiple PTBs or second trimester losses who would previously be offered a history-indicated cerclage at 12–14 weeks can now safely be followed by ultrasound [46–49]. In fact, about 60% of these women maintain a

CL ≥ 25 weeks until past 24 weeks, have a low risk of PTB, and can forgo all interventions (Chapter 11).

Progesterone

Two randomized trials have been published so far on the efficacy of progesterone supplementation in women with short CL. In a randomized, double-blind, placebo-controlled trial, the use of daily 200 mg of micronized vaginal progesterone until 34 weeks in the small percentage (1.6%) of mostly low-risk women identified to have a short CL ≤ 15 mm at 22–24 weeks was found to be associated with a 44% reduction in the rates of PTB < 34 weeks. Of note, women with a previous PTB comprised only 12% and 18.4% of the progesterone and placebo groups, respectively. A small number of twin gestations with a short CL were also included in the study, and a non-significant reduction in PTB < 34 weeks was noted in this population [50].

In a secondary analysis from another randomized, double-blind, placebo-controlled trial, daily doses of 90 mg of vaginal progesterone gel showed a trend toward reduction of PTB < 32 weeks, as well as improvement in neonatal outcome in 46 women with a short CL < 28 mm [51].

As the evidence that vaginal progesterone prevents PTB in women with short CL ≤ 15 mm is only from one large trial, there are no current recommendations for its use. At least four other on-going placebo-controlled trials are evaluating the effect of progesterone supplementation in the general population screened and identified to have a short CL (NICHD; Columbia Labs; Netherlands; Fetal Medicine Foundation). It is currently unknown if combined interventions for short CL, such as both cerclage and progesterone, are more efficacious than just one such intervention.

Indomethacin

As it has been shown that women with short CL also have painless uterine contractions [34], the rationale for using a tocolytic agent to affect outcome is apparent. Indomethacin in women with short CL was associated with prevention of PTB < 24 weeks and PPROM, but not PTB < 35 weeks [52]. However, in women with an ultrasound-indicated cerclage, administration of indomethacin around the time of cerclage placement has not been associated with a decrease in spontaneous PTB < 35 weeks [53]. As none of these data comes from randomized trials, further research should be of level 1 quality.

Antibiotics

As mentioned in Chapter 6, a short CL has been associated with infection. It seems reasonable to assume that antibiotics could be efficacious when used in this population. Unfortunately, just as antibiotics failed to prevent

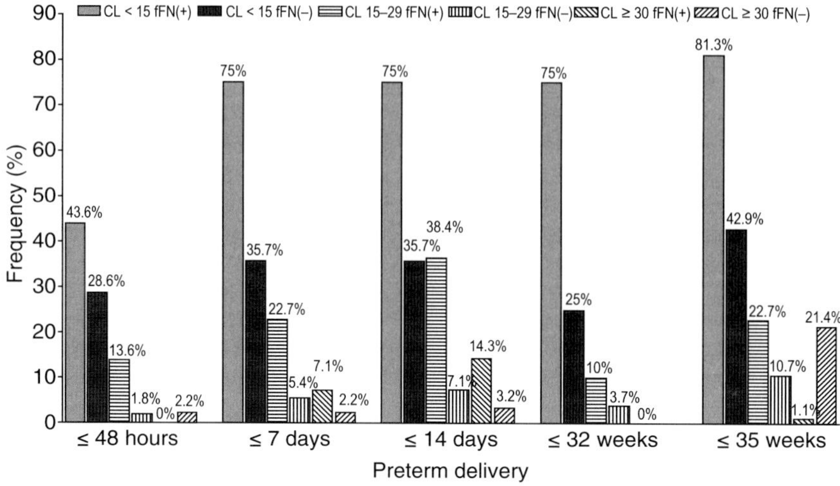

Figure 12.6 Frequency of spontaneous preterm birth in women with preterm labour according to cervical length (CL) results (categorized as <15 mm, 15–29 mm, and ≥30 mm) and vaginal fetal fibronectin (fFN) determination [58].

PTB in other at risk populations with intact membranes, the only data (non-randomized) so far failed to demonstrate prevention of PTB in women with a short CL < 25 mm [54].

Pessary

Although a few studies have demonstrated the possible benefit of pessary placement in women with short CL [55,56], there have been no randomized controlled studies evaluating pessary versus no pessary. Two are currently on-going. As of yet, it is not currently recommended for use in this population [57].

Bed rest

There are no randomized controlled trials comparing bed rest versus routine activity in women with short CL. A well-designed prospective trial evaluating this is needed before specific recommendations for bed rest can be made.

Preterm labor and short CL

TVU measurement of CL is very useful in the management of PTL with intact membranes (Chapter 18). Despite symptomatic women with PTL being at high risk for PTB, many of them are destined to deliver at term (>70%) [33].

In fact, **women with PTL who are found to have a TVU CL ≥ 30 mm and negative fetal fibronectin have less than a 1% chance of delivering within 1 week** [33]. A useful graph describing percentage risk for PTB for women with a diagnosis of PTL, incorporating both CL and FFN, is depicted in Figure 12.6 [58]. Ideally, one would like to triage and/or treat women with suspected PTL in an efficient, yet thorough and complete manner.

Interestingly, **a clinician's knowledge of both CL and FFN has been shown to reduce the length of evaluation time in this very population, as well as incidences of PTB**, when compared with clinicians blinded to these results [59]. A suggested algorithm for the use of TVU CL and FFN in women with preterm labor symptoms is shown in **Figure 18.1** [59].

In one small randomized controlled trial, women with singleton gestations and PTL treated with 17P had less significant shortening of the cervix at days 7 and 21 compared with women who did not receive progesterone, and subsequently had a reduction in their rates of PTB (prior to 37 weeks) as high as 85% [60]. To date, however, progesterone in any form is not recommended for use in women with PTL.

References

1 Berghella V, Bega G, Tolosa J, Berghella M. Ultrasound assessment of the cervix. Clin Obstet Gynecol 2003; 46: 947–62.

2 Berghella V, Tolosa JE, Kuhlman K, Weiner S, Bolognese RJ, Wapner RJ. Cervical ultrasonography compared to manual examination as a predictor of preterm delivery. Am J Obstet Gynecol 1997; 177: 723–30.

3 Matijevic R, Grgic O, Vasilj O. Is sonographic assessment of cervical length better than digital examination in screening for preterm delivery in a low-risk population? Acta Obstet Gynecol 2006; 85: 1342–7.

4 Owen J, Neely C, Northen A. Transperineal versus endovaginal ultrasonographic examination of the cervix in the midtrimester: a blinded comparison. Am J Obstet Gynecol 1999; 181: 780–3.

5 Berghella V, Talucci M, Desai A. Does transvaginal sonographic measurement of cervical length before 14 weeks predict preterm delivery in high-risk pregnancies? Ultrasound Obstet Gynecol 2003; 21: 140–4.

6 Mella MT, Berghella V. Prediction of preterm birth: cervical sonography. Sem Perinatol 2009; 33: 317–24.

7 Owen J, Yost N, Berghella V, *et al.* Mid-trimester endovaginal sonography in women at high risk for spontaneous preterm birth. JAMA 2001; 286: 1340–8.

8 Berghella V, Kuhlman K, Weiner S, *et al.* Cervical funneling: sonographic criteria predictive of preterm delivery. Ultrasound Obstet Gynecol 1997; 10: 161–6.

9 Zilianti M, Azuaga A, Calderon F, *et al.* Transperineal sonography in second trimester to term pregnancy and early labor. J Ultrasound Med 1991; 10: 481–5.

10 Berghella V, Roman A. Does funneling increase the incidence of preterm birth in women with normal cervical length? Am J Obstet Gynecol 2005; 193: s147.

11 Rust OA, *et al.* Does the presence of a funnel increase the risk of adverse perinatal outcome in a patient with a short cervix? Am J Obstet Gynecol 2005; 192: 1060–6.

12 Berghella V, Owen J, MacPherson C, *et al.* Natural history of cervical funneling in women at high risk for spontaneous preterm birth. Obstet Gynecol 2007; 109: 863–9.

13 To MS, Skentou A, Liao W, Cacho A, Nicolaides KH. Cervical length and funneling at 23 weeks of gestation in the prediction of spontaneous early preterm delivery. Ultrasound Obstet Gynecol 2001; 18: 200–3.

14 Kusanovic JP, Espinoza J, Romero R, *et al.* Clinical significance of the presence of amniotic fluid 'sludge' in asymptomatic patients at high risk for spontaneous preterm delivery. Ultrasound Obstet Gynecol 2007; 30: 706–14.

15 Berghella V, Bega G. Ultrasound evaluation of the cervix. In: Callen PW (ed), *Ultrasonography in Obstetrics and Gynecology*, 5th Edn. Philadelphia, PA: Saunders Elsevier, 2008: 698–720.

16 Iams JD, Goldenberg RL, Meis PJ, *et al.* The length of the cervix and the risk of spontaneous premature delivery. National Institute of Child Health and Human Development Maternal Fetal Medicine Unit Network. N Engl J Med 1996; 334: 567–72.

17 Iams JD, Johnson FF, Sonek J, Sachs L, Gebauer C, Samuels P. Cervical competence as a continuum: a study of ultrasonographic cervical length and obstetric performance. Am J Obstet Gynecol 1995; 172: 1097–103.

18 Hassan SS, Romero R, Berry SM, *et al.* Patients with an ultrasonographic cervical length </=15 mm have nearly a 50% risk of early spontaneous preterm delivery. Am J Obstet Gynecol 2000; 182: 1458–67.

19 Owen J, Yost N, Berghella V, *et al.* Can shortened midtrimester cervical length predict very early spontaneous preterm birth? Am J Obstet Gynecol 2004; 191: 298–303.

20 Berghella V, Roman A, Daskalakis C, Ness A, Baxter JK. Gestational age at cervical length measurement and incidence of preterm birth. Obstet Gynecol 2007; 110: 311–17.

21 Airoldi J, Berghella V. Transvaginal ultrasound of the cervix to predict preterm birth in women with uterine anomalies. Obstet Gynecol 2005; 106: 553–6.

22 Berghella V, Pereira L, Gariepy A, *et al.* Prior cone biopsy: prediction of preterm birth by cervical ultrasound. Am J Obstet Gynecol 2004; 191: 1393–7.

23 Visintine J, Berghella V, Henning, D, Baxter J. Cervical length for prediction of preterm birth in women with multiple prior induced abortions. Ultrasound Obstet Gynecol 2008; 31: 198–200.

24 Martin JA, Hamilton BE, Sutton PD, *et al.* Births: final data for 2004. National vital statistics reports. Vol. 55. No. 1. Hyattsville, MD: National Center for Health Statistics, 2006.

25 Goldenberg RL, Iams J, Miodovnik M, *et al.* The preterm prediction study: risk factors in twin gestation. Am J Obstet Gynecol 1996; 175: 1047–53.

26 Yang JH, Kuhlman K, Daly S, Berghella V. Prediction of preterm birth by second trimester cervical sonography in twin pregnancies. Ultrasound Obstet Gynecol 2000; 15: 288–91.

27 To MS, Fonseca EB, Molina FS, *et al.* Maternal characteristics and cervical length in the prediction of spontaneous early preterm delivery in twins. Am J Obstet Gynecol 2006; 194: 1360–5.

28 Skentou C, Souka A, To MS, Nicolaides KH. Prediction of preterm delivery in twins by cervical assessment at 23 weeks. Ultrasound Obstet Gynecol 2001; 17: 7–10.

29 Kushnir O, Izquierdo LA, Smith JF, *et al.* Transvaginal sonographic measurement of cervical length: evaluation of twin pregnancies. J Rep Med 1995; 40: 380–2.
30 Guzman ER, Houlihan C, Vintzileos A, *et al.* The significance of transvaginal ultrasonographic evaluation of the cervix in women treated with emergency cerclage. Am J Obstet Gynecol 1996; 175: 471–6.
31 Althuisius SM, Dekkar GA, van Geijn HP, *et al.* The effect of therapeutic McDonald cerclage on cervical length as assessed by transvaginal ultrasonography. Am J Obstet Gynecol 1999; 180: 366–9.
32 Baxter J, Airoldi J, Berghella V. Short cervical length after history indicated cerclage: is a reinforcing cerclage beneficial? Am J Obstet Gynecol 2005; 193: 1204–7.
33 Berghella V, Ness A, Bega G, Berghella M. Cervical sonography in women with symptoms of preterm labor. Obstet Gynecol Clin North Am 2005; 32: 383–96.
34 Lewis D, Pelham J, Sawhney H, *et al.* Uterine contractions in asymptomatic pregnant women with a short cervix on ultrasound. J Mat Fetal Neonatal Med 2005; 18: 325–8.
35 Berghella V, Iams JD, Newman RB, *et al.* Frequency of uterine contractions in asymptomatic pregnant women with or without a short cervix on transvaginal ultrasound. Am J Obstet Gynecol 2004; 191: 1253–6.
36 To MS, Alfirevic Z, Heath VCF, *et al.* Cervical cerclage for prevention of preterm delivery in women with short cervix: randomized controlled trial. Lancet 2004; 363: 1849–53.
37 Berghella V, Odibo AO, To MS, *et al.* Cerclage for short cervix on ultrasound: meta-analysis of trials using individual patient-level data. Obstet Gynecol 2005; 106: 181–9.
38 Rust OA, Atlas R, Reed J, Van Gaalen J, Balducci J. Revisiting the short cervix detected by transvaginal ultrasound in the second trimester: why cerclage therapy may not help. Am J Obstet Gynecol 2001; 185: 1098–105.
39 Owen J, Vaginal Ultrasound Trial Consortium. Multicenter randomized trial of cerclage for preterm birth prevention in high-risk women with shortened mid-trimester cervical length. Am J Obstet Gynecol 2008; 199: S3.
40 Scheib S, Visintine JF, Miroshnichenko G, Harvey C, Rychlak K, Berghella V. Is cerclage height associated with the incidence of preterm birth in women with an ultrasound-indicated cerclage? Am J Obstet Gynecol 2009; 200: e12–5.
41 Odibo AO, Berghella V, To MS, Rust OA, Althuisius SM, Nicolaides KH. Shirodkar versus McDonald cerclage for the prevention of preterm birth in women with short cervical length. Am J Perinatol 2007; 24: 55–60.
42 McDonald IA. Suture of the cervix for inevitable miscarriage. J Obstet Gynaecol Br Emp 1957; 64: 346–50.
43 Shirodkar VN. A new method of operative treatment for habitual abortion in the second trimester of pregnancy. Antiseptic 1955; 52: 299–303.
44 Berghella V, Baxter J, Berghella M. Cervical insufficiency. In: Apuzzio JJ, Vintzileos AM, Iffy L, *Operative Obstetrics,* 3rd Edn. New York, NY: Taylor & Francis, 2006: 157–72.
45 Berghella V, Seibel-Seamon J. Contemporary use of cervical cerclage. Clin Obstet Gynecol 2007; 2: 468–77.
46 Althuisius SM, Dekker GA, van Geijn HP, *et al.* Cervical Incompetence Prevention Randomized Cerclage Trial (CIPRACT): study design and preliminary results. Am J Obstet Gynecol 2000; 183: 823–9.
47 Kassanos D, Salamalekis E, Vitoratos N, *et al.* The value of transvaginal ultrasonography in diagnosis and management of cervical incompetence. Clin Exp Obstet Gynecol 2001; 28: 266–8.

48 Beigi A, Zarrinkoub F. Elective versus ultrasound-indicated cervical cerclage in women at risk for cervical incompetence. Med J Islamic Rep Iran 2005: 19: 103–17.

49 Simcox R, Bennett F, Teoh TG, Shennan AH. A randomized controlled trial of cervical scanning vs history to determine cerclage in high risk women (circle trial). J Obstet Gynaecol 2007; 27; Supplement 1, S18–S19.

50 Fonseca E, Celik E, Parra M, Singh M, Nicolaides KH. Progesterone and the risk of preterm birth among women with a short cervix. N Eng J Med 2007; 357: 462–9.

51 DeFranco EA, O'Brien JM, Adair CD, *et al.* Vaginal progesterone is associated with a decrease in risk for early preterm birth and improved neonatal outcome in women with a short cervix: a secondary analysis from a randomized, double-blind, placebo-controlled trial. Ultrasound Obstet Gynecol 2007; 30: 697–705.

52 Berghella V, Rust OA, Althuisius SM. Short cervix on ultrasound: does indomethacin prevent preterm birth? Am J Obstet Gynecol 2006; 195: 809–13.

53 Visintine J, Airoldi J, Berghella V. Indomethacin administration at the time of ultrasound-indicated cerclage: is there an association with a reduction in spontaneous preterm birth? Am J Obstet Gynecol 2008; 198: 643.e1–e3.

54 Berghella V, Rust O, Althuisius S, To M. Short cervix on ultrasound: do antibiotics prevent preterm birth? Am J Obstet Gynecol 2005; 193: S48.

55 Acharya G, Eschler B, Grønberg M, *et al.* Noninvasive cerclage for the management of cervical incompetence: a prospective study. Arch Gynecol Obstet 2006; 273: 283–7.

56 Arabin B, Halbesma J, *et al.* Is treatment with vaginal pessaries an option in patients with a sonographically detected short cervix? J Perinat Med 2003; 31: 122–33.

57 Dharan VB, Ludmir J. Alternative treatment for a short cervix: the cervical pessary. Sem Perinatol 2009: 33: 338–42.

58 Gomez R, Romero R, Medina L, *et al.* Cervicovaginal fibronectin improves the prediction of preterm delivery based on sonographic cervical length in patients with preterm uterine contractions and intact membranes. Am J Obstet Gynecol 2005; 192: 350–9.

59 Ness A, Visintine J, Ricci E, Berghella V. Does knowledge of cervical length and fetal fibronectin affect management of women with threatened preterm labor? A randomized trial. Am J Obstet Gynecol 2007; 197: 426.e1–7.

60 Facchinetti F, Paganelli S, Comitini G, Dante G, Volpe, A. Cervical length changes during preterm cervical ripening: effects of 17-α-hydroxyprogesterone caproate. Am J Obstet Gynecol 2007; 196; 453.e1–4.

61 Guzman ER, Walters C, O'Reilly-Green C, *et al.* Use of cervical ultrasonography in prediction of spontaneous preterm birth in triplet gestations. Am J Obstet Gynecol 2000; 183: 1108–13.

CHAPTER 13
Fetal Fibronectin

Maria Bisulli
Department of Obstetrics and Gynecology, St. Orsola Malpighi Hospital, Universita of Bologna, Bologna, Italy

Key points

- Fetal fibronectin (FFN) is one of the screening tests currently available which is most predictive of preterm birth (PTB).
- The most accurate prediction is achieved when FFN results are combined with transvaginal ultrasound (TVU) cervical length (CL).
- Until there is a treatment with clear benefit, there is not enough evidence for screening with FFN any *asymptomatic* woman, including low- or high-risk singletons, or multiple gestations.
- In *symptomatic* women with threatened preterm labor (PTL), the negative predictive value (NPV) approaches 100%, allowing no treatment in women with a negative FFN study. Instead, the PPV for delivering within 7 days is very low (<20%), making this test of limited value to decide which symptomatic woman with positive FFN to treat with steroids for fetal maturity, tocolysis, and admission.
- FFN, in combination with TVU CL, may decrease PTB in symptomatic women with PTL (Chapter 18).

Description of fetal fibronectin

Fetal fibronectin (FFN) is a viscous **glycoprotein** that is secreted by fetal membranes and helps attach the chorion to the uterine decidua, and it is concentrated in this area (Figure 13.1). It acts as a 'glue' between the pregnancy and the uterus. In normal conditions it is detectable in cervico-vaginal secretions up to 20–22 weeks (probably because of the absence of a complete fusion between fetal membranes and the decidua), and after 37 weeks (because the process of labor is starting) (Figure 13.2). Even at the early gestational ages (GA), it can be used for prediction of PTB by quantitative analysis. FFN is present at only very low levels between 22 and 35 weeks (<50 ng/ml). Its presence in the cervico-vaginal secretions during this interval is associated with PTB.

Preterm Birth. Edited by Vincenzo Berghella.

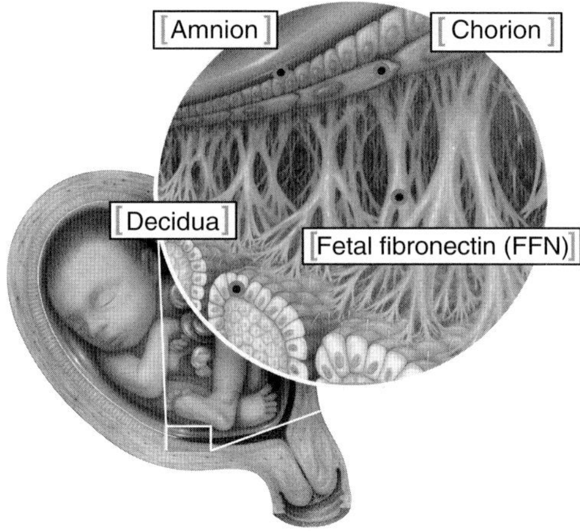

Figure 13.1 Location of fetal fibronectin concentration in normal pregnant women.

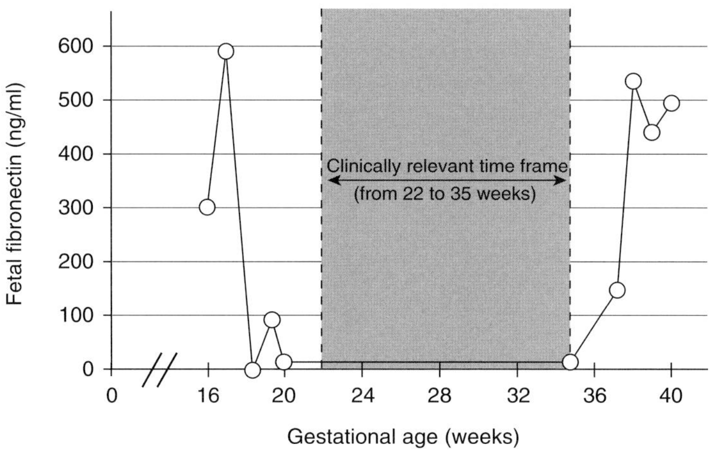

Figure 13.2 Presence of fetal fibronectin in cervico-vaginal fluid at each gestational age.

Historic notes

Lockwood in 1991 was the first to report the association between positive FFN and PTB [1]. His hypothesis was that the presence of FFN in vaginal secretions may reflect the separation of the chorion from the decidual layer of the uterus, with the release of intact or degraded chorionic components of the extracellular matrix into the cervical and vaginal secretions.

Chorio-decidual inflammation and infection appear to be the major causes of this disruption and of the subsequent presence of FFN in cervico-vaginal secretion [1]. In 1995 the Food and Drug Administration (FDA) approved the FFN ELISA test for assessing PTB risk in symptomatic women between 24 and 35 weeks. Now FFN is considered one of the best predictor of spontaneous PTB (SPTB) in all populations studied so far, including low and high-risk singletons, multiple gestations, asymptomatic and symptomatic women [2, 3].

Technical aspects

Method of collection

The current recommended (by the manufacturer and the FDA) collection method for cervico-vaginal FFN involves direct visualization and sampling with a sterile **swab**, completely submerged for 10 seconds in the posterior fornix using a vaginal **speculum**. There is a 95% agreement between this standard collection technique and 'blind' methods in which a speculum is not used [4, 5]. An assay for detecting the presence of vaginal FFN is now commercially available and the results can be **ready within 1 hour** from testing. Samples are defined as **positive if the fibronectin concentration is ≥ 50 ng/ml between 22 and 34 6/7 weeks** [6].

False positives

The test can be affected (false positive result) by:

- gel (e.g. for vaginal ultrasound probe);
- sexual intercourse (sperm contains an epitope similar to FFN that may cross react);
- previous digital cervical examination [7];
- blood presence in the sample;
- amniotic fluid.

For the first three above, the issue must occur within 24 hours before sampling to affect results. Candidates for testing should meet the following criteria: intact fetal membranes, cervical dilatation less than 3 cm, and gestational age between 22 and 34 weeks. Therefore, **in women in whom both FFN and transvaginal ultrasound (TVU) cervical length (CL) screening is being obtained, FFN must be done first**.

Frequency of screening

After a positive result the FFN test does not usually need to be repeated, because the risk of PTB stays elevated anyway even in asymptomatic women [8].

Prediction of PTB

In clinical practice the FFN assay has been used as a screening test to identify women who would eventually deliver preterm in both low and high risk populations (Tables 13.1 and 13.2) [9–14]. Clinical use should be discussed separately for two different populations: asymptomatic women, and women with symptoms of PTB such as preterm labour (PTL). This is because the FFN test has very different characteristics in these populations.

Table 13.1 Delivery before 35 weeks in *asymptomatic* women if positive fetal fibronectin. GA, gestational age. PTB, preterm birth. PPV, positive predictive value. NPN, negative predictive value. NA, not available. *Outcome: delivery at <34 weeks.

		GA at testing (weeks)	Incidence of PTB (%) (<35 weeks)	Sensitivity (%)	Specificity (%)	PPV (%)	NPV (%)
Singleton	*Low risk*						
	Iams [9] (*n* = 2107)	22–24	3.04	23.4	97.0	19.7	98.0
	Goldenberg [10] (*n* = 10,456)	8–22	NA	30.4	90.5	14.7	NA
	High risk						
	Morrison [11] (*n* = 85)	26–28	16.5	48	89	43	89
	Kurzman [12] (*n* = 563)*	24	6.7*	15.7	96.7	32.0	92.0
Twins							
	Goldenberg [13] (*n* = 147)	24	32.0	6.7	96.0	42.8	68.6

Table 13.2 Delivery within 7 days in *symptomatic* women with 725 singleton pregnancies if positive fetal fibronectin [14]. GA, gestational age. PTB, preterm birth. PPV, positive predictive value. NPN, negative predictive value.

	GA at testing	Incidence of PTB < 7 days (%)	Sensitivity (%)	Specificity (%)	PPV (%)	NPV (%)
Delivery within 7 days	24+0/ 34+6	2.9	90.5	83	13.4	99.7
Delivery within 14 days	24+0/ 34+6	3.9	88.5	99.2	16.2	99.5

Asymptomatic

One of the largest studies on the use of FFN in asymptomatic pregnant women was the NICHD (National Institute of Child Health and Human Development) Preterm Prediction Study performed from 1992 to 1994 [15]. Almost 3000 asymptomatic women were enrolled. This study showed that the best predictor for spontaneous PTB (at <32 weeks) was a positive FFN (adjusted RR 14.1; 95% CI 9.3–21.4), the second was a short CL (<25 mm) (adjusted RR 7.7; 95% CI 4.5–13.4), and the third was a prior spontaneous PTB (adjusted RR 7.1; 95% CI 3.8–13.2). A positive FFN test and TVU CL < 25 mm increased the risk of PTB at less than 32 weeks of gestation 35.3-fold for nulliparas, compared with nulliparas with a normal CL and negative FFN.

Predictive accuracy for SPTB < 35 weeks in asymptomatic patients from some of the largest and best performed (e.g. blind) studies are reported in Table 13.1 [9–13]. These studies establish these main conclusions:

- The highest prediction is achieved in high-risk pregnant women.
- A most accurate prediction of PTB is achieved in asymptomatic women with the combination of FFN and CL (Table 13.3) [9, 16].
- The positive predictive value (PPV), which is of most use clinically, is generally very low if the a priori risk of PTB is < 10%.
- The well-publicized high NPV is usually 90% or more, but this is the same or worse than the a priori NPV in populations with PTB risk < 10%.
- The best study in twins [13] reports a very low sensitivity, i.e. most twin gestations which deliver preterm do not have a prior positive FFN. A most accurate prediction of PTB is achieved in asymptomatic women with the combination of FFN and CL (Table 13.3) [9, 16]. In the largest study of asymptomatic twin pregnancies, the best predictive factor at 24 weeks was a CL < 25 mm, while at 28 weeks FFN was the only statistically significant predictor of SPTB at <32 weeks [13].

Unfortunately, until there is a treatment with clear benefit, **there is not enough evidence for screening with FFN any asymptomatic women**, either low- or high-risk singletons, or multiple gestations.

Symptomatic PTL

The main challenge for the physician who has to take care of a woman with symptoms of PTB, is to figure out her real risk of actually delivering preterm. In fact, 90% of women with threatened PTL will not deliver within 7 days, and up to 75% will deliver at term [17]. Therefore, in this population the NPV for delivery within 7 days is already 90% without doing any costly tests of prediction. By increasing this NPV, the FFN test could avoid useless treatment and anxiety for the woman with symptoms of PTL but destined to deliver at term, as well as for her physician.

Table 13.3 Prediction of preterm birth before 35 weeks of gestation of a positive fetal fibronectin test and cervical length ≤25 mm in asymptomatic and symptomatic women. GA, gestational age. PTB, preterm birth. PPV, positive predictive value. NPV, negative predictive value.

	GA at testing		Sensitivity (%)	Specificity (%)	PPV (%)	NPV (%)
Asymptomatic		Incidence of PTB < 35 weeks (%)				
Iams [9] (*n* = 2107)	22–24	3.04	15.6	99.5	50.0	94.4
Symptomatic		Delivery within 48 hours (%)				
Gomez [16] (*n* = 215)	22–35	7.9	41.2	95.4	43.7	95.0
		Delivery within 7 days (%)				
Gomez [16] (*n* = 215)		13.0	42.8	97.9	75.0	91.9

Leitich *et al.* in their systematic review of 40 prospective studies illustrates that FFN is an effective short term marker to predict PTB, especially in women with PTB, with sensitivity of 54% (95% CI 43–65) and specificity of 85% (95% CI 81–89) [2, 18]. Another systematic review of Honest *et al.* emphasizes that the test is most accurate in predicting SPTB within 7–10 days among women with threatened PTL before advanced cervical dilatation, with median likelihood ratios of 5.42 (95% CI 4.36–6.74) for a positive result, and 0.25 (95% CI 0.20–0.31) for a negative result [19].

Sensitivity, specificity, negative and positive predictive values for SPTB within 7 days in symptomatic women in the largest blind study are reported in Table 13.2. As can be seen, the NPV approaches 100%, allowing no treatment in women with symptoms of PTL who have a negative FFN study. Instead, the PPV for delivering within 7 days is very low (<20%), making this test of limited value to decide which symptomatic woman with positive FFN to treat with steroids for fetal maturity, tocolysis and admission [14].

The ability of FFN in predicting SPTB improves if this test is associated with TVU CL (Table 13.3). Many centers now use a combination of these two tests. A prospective cohort study performed by Gomez *et al.* showed that the combined use of sonographic CL and vaginal FFN test improves the prediction of SPTB more than that provided by each test alone [16]. This effect was observed with CL < 30 mm; in fact **in women with a CL ≥ 30 mm the risk of PTB within 1 week is**

about < 2%, and FFN is probably not beneficial. Symptomatic women with CL < 25 mm and positive FFN have a 75% (12/16) chance of being delivered within 7 days (Table 13.3) [16]. Hinkz proposed a two-step testing in which first FFN and then a TVU CL were performed. A FFN test was sent only in women with a CL between 21 and 30 mm. The overall sensitivity, specificity, positive and NPVs were of 86, 90, 63 and 97% for delivery within 28 days [20].

Limited information is available in symptomatic twin pregnancies, where FFN has been reported to have a positive and negative predictive value of 54% and 93.7% respectively [21].

Prevention of PTB

Asymptomatic women

FFN has not been shown to reduce PTB when screening occurs in asymptomatic women. While predictive of PTB to some extent (Table 13.1), there are no large randomized trials in asymptomatic women to demonstrate that knowledge of FFN results affects the incidence of PTB [22]. More research is needed in this area (Table 13.4). We would speculate that interventions should be tried first in asymptomatic women with risk factors for PTB, as the predictive accuracy of FFN is best in this population. Other research areas include the use of more aggressive steroid for fetal maturity therapy in asymptomatic women with positive FFN, a practice that has not yet been proven effective by trials. Cost-effectiveness

Table 13.4 When might fetal fibronectin testing be helpful to you? Evidence for effectiveness of fetal fibronectin testing in prevention of preterm birth. *When performed in conjunction with TVU CL. PTB, preterm birth. RCT, randomized controlled trials. PTL, preterm labor.

Population	Prediction of PTB	Possible benefit in prevention of PTB shown by limited *prospective* data	Prevention of PTB proven by *level I data in multiple RCTs*
Asymptomatic			
Singleton			
Low-risk	Yes	No	No
Prior PTB	Yes	No	No
Cerclage in place	Yes	No	No
Multiple	Yes	No	No
Symptomatic (PTL)			
Singleton	Yes	Yes*	No
Multiple	Yes	No	No

studies should be performed, as each test is billed at around $200 in the US, and limited data is available regarding cost–benefit [23–25].

Antibiotics have been the only interventions studied so far for prevention of PTB in asymptomatic pregnant women with positive FFN. Some authors hypothesize that since FFN presence in cervical vaginal secretion can be associated with infection, antibiotic therapy could be beneficial in prevention of SPTB in women with a positive FFN test. Two randomized trials have shown that the use of **metronidazole does not decrease the risk of SPTB**, and does not improve neonatal outcomes in asymptomatic low risk women with a positive FFN test [26], and it is likely to increase PTB in high risk women with a positive FFN test [27].

Moreover **bacterial vaginosis** (BV) is present in up to 15–42% of pregnant women, and is associated with as much as a fourfold increase in SPTB and preterm premature rupture of membranes [28]. The coexistence of BV and positive FFN may represent a subpopulation of women who have two markers of infection and those have a better chance to benefit from antibiotic treatment. A study on 215 women with positive FFN and BV treated with metronidazole or placebo, shows that patients in which the BV was resolved had a lower rate of SPTB at < 34 weeks. The authors speculate that this is not due to the therapy but to spontaneous BV resolution [29]. A small subanalysis of another trial showed a non-significant reduction in PTB in women with positive FFN and BV treated with metronidazole compared with placebo [30]. Currently, there is no mandate to screen or treat women with asymptomatic BV or positive FFN for purpose of decreasing PTB.

In asymptomatic women between 18 and 24 weeks with a short CL (<25 mm), FFN has been assessed to identify women more likely to benefit from ultrasound-indicated **cerclage**. A recent non-randomized study doesn't support this hypothesis and demonstrated no difference in the incidence of PTB < 35 weeks [31].

Symptomatic women

As shown above, the best feature of FFN is its NPV, which was found to be up to 99.5% even in symptomatic women [32]. Thus a negative test can be clinically useful to avoid unnecessary potentially harmful and expensive interventions like corticosteroid administration, tocolysis, admission to the hospital and sometimes transfer to a level III hospital with a maternal fetal medicine unit and intensive care nursery. Corticosteroids for fetal maturity have most beneficial effects if administered at least 48 hours before but within 7 days of delivery [33].

In a systematic review, Honest *et al.* reported that if steroids were to be used for all symptomatic women without FFN testing, then we would need to treat 109 women to prevent one case of respiratory distress syndrome. If we treated only those women with a positive FFN test result we would need to treat 17, a number considerably lower than that without testing [19]. Moreover, although tocolysis therapy may prolong pregnancy for 48–72 hours, it is not without potential for serious side effects for mother and baby [34]. In one cost analysis, the use of FFN reduced PTL admission, length to stay and prescription of tocolysis, without any impact on neonatal outcome. The overall cost of managing women with threatened PTB was reduced by 50% [35]. In a prospective study, the use of FFN test was associated with a 90% reduction in maternal transfer to a MFM unit and with a reduction of all the costs [23].

Does knowledge of the FFN result affect the incidence of PTB in symptomatic women? There are five randomized control trials on this topic, enrolling 235 women assigned to knowledge, and 249 to no knowledge of FFN [36–40]. They have been analyzed in a recent Cochrane review [22]. This meta-analysis shows that knowledge of FFN results in the management of women with symptoms of PTL is associated with a lower incidence of PTB < 37 weeks (Table 13.4). Only one study [36] proposed a **protocol** of management, based mostly on TVU CL but also FFN, that could be replicated (**see Figure 18.1**).

Unfortunately it is still **unclear which interventions are more beneficial when FFN (and/or TVU CL) results are known**. For example, in symptomatic women with a short CL and/or a positive FFN result, there are no studies to assess the efficacy for prevention of SPTB of common traditional interventions such as tocolysis, hospitalization, etc.

One trial randomized women with PTL and positive FFN as well as women with PPROM to either glyceryl nitrate (GTN) or beta-mimetic (salbutamol or ritodrine) tocolysis [41]. Beta-mimetic tocolysis was found to be more efficacious than GTN tocolysis. This was not a placebo-controlled study, and therefore does not answer the question on effectiveness of tocolysis in general in women with PTL screened with FFN.

One randomized multicenter study on activity restriction in women treated for PTL and testing **negative for FFN** has shown that there was no difference in incidence of PTB before 37 weeks between the group of bed rest except bathroom and shower privileges, compared with controls who resumed normal activities, including home and work responsibilities [42]. In this study they did not consider TVU CL as a predictive factor.

In a sample of both asymptomatic and symptomatic women at 23–31 weeks, the incidences of intra-amniotic infection and inflammation if FFN was positive were 1.8% and 5.3%, respectively [43]. It is **important to consider intra-amniotic infection especially in women symptomatic for PTL with positive FFN**.

Suggested management algorithm

Figure 18.1 shows our proposed algorithm for use of FFN in women with PTL [36]. Women with threatened PTL are those who present with these symptoms: > 6 contraction/hour, cramping, pressure, cervical vaginal dilatation less then 3 cm with intact membrane, between 24 and 34 weeks. A careful history, physical examination, FFN sampling (first!) and (then) TVU CL should be obtained.

(1) If CL is >30 mm, the woman can be reassured that the delivery is not imminent and she can be managed expectantly as an outpatient.

(2) If CL is 20–30 mm, the FFN results can be used to further triage these patients. Women with this CL but with a negative FFN result can also usually be managed expectantly and do not require hospitalization. If the FFN is positive, they should be treated as women with a CL < 20 mm.

(3) If CL is <20 mm, or 20–30 mm with positive FFN, these women warrant close observation and consideration for additional intervention. The decision for corticosteroid administration, transfer to a tertiary care center (depending on gestation age), and tocolytic therapy in these women should be made on an individual basis, but is generally recommended.

References

1 Lockwood CJ, Senyei AE, Dische MR, *et al.* Fetal fibronectin in cervical and vaginal secretions as a predictor of preterm delivery. N Engl J Med 1991; 5; 325: 669–74.

2 Leitich H, Egarter C, Kaider A, *et al.* Cervico-vaginal fetal fibronectin as a marker for preterm delivery: a meta-analysis. Am J Obstet Gynecol 1999; 180: 1169–76.

3 Goldenberg RL, Iams JD, Miodovnik M, *et al.* The preterm prediction study: risk factors in twin gestations. National Institute of Child Health and Human Development Maternal-Fetal Medicine Units Network. Am J Obstet Gynecol 1996; 175: 1047–53.

4 Stafford IP, Garite TJ, Dildy GA, *et al.* A comparison of speculum and non speculum collection of cervicovaginal specimens for fetal fibronectin testing. Am J Obstet Gynecol 2008; 199: e1–e4.

5 Roman AS, Koklanaris N, Paidas MJ, *et al.* 'Blind' vaginal fetal fibronectin as a predictor of spontaneous preterm delivery. Obstet Gynecol 2005; 105: 285–9.

6 Lu GC, Goldenberg RL, Cliver SP, *et al.* Vaginal fetal fibronectin levels and spontaneous preterm birth in symptomatic women. Obstet Gynecol 2001; 97: 225–8.

7 McKenna DS, Chung K, Iams JD. Effect of digital cervical examination on the expression of fetal fibronectin. J Reprod Med 1999; 44: 796–800.

8 Goldenberg RL, Mercer BM, Iams JD, *et al.* The preterm prediction study: patterns of cervicovaginal fetal fibronectin as predictors of spontaneous preterm delivery. Am J Obstet Gynecol 1997; 177: 8–12.

9 Iams JD, Goldenberg RL, Mercer BM, *et al.* The preterm prediction study: can low-risk women destined for spontaneous preterm birth be identified? Am J Obstet Gynecol 2001; 184: 652–5.

10 Goldenberg RL, Klebanoff M, Carey JC, *et al.* Vaginal fetal fibronectin measurements from 8 to 22 weeks' gestation and subsequent spontaneous preterm birth. Am J Obstet Gynecol 2000; 183: 469–75.
11 Morrison JC, Allbert JR, McLaughlin BN. Oncofetal fibronectin in patients with false labor as a predictor of preterm delivery. Am J Obstet Gynecol 1993; 168: 538–42.
12 Kurtzman J, Chandiramani M, Briley A, *et al.* A quantitative fetal fibronectin screening in asymptomatic high-risk patients and the spectrum of risk for recurrent preterm delivery. Am J Obstet Gynecol 2009; 200: 263.e1–6.
13 Goldenberg RL, Iams JD, Miodovnik M, *et al.* The preterm prediction study: risk factors in twin gestations. National Institute of Child Health and Human Development Maternal-Fetal Medicine Units Network. Am J Obstet Gynecol 1996; 175: 1047–53.
14 Peaceman A, Andrews W, Thorp J, *et al.* Fetal fibronectin as a predictor of preterm birth in patients with symptoms: a multicenter trial. Am J Obstet Gynecol 1997; 177: 13–18.
15 Goldenberg RL, Mercer BM, Meis PJ, *et al.* NICHD Maternal Fetal Medicine Units Network. The preterm prediction study: fetal fibronectin testing and spontaneous preterm birth. Obstet Gynecol 1996; 87: 643–8.
16 Gomez R, Romero R, Medina L, *et al.* Cervicovaginal fibronectin improves the prediction of preterm delivery based on sonographic cervical length in patients with preterm uterine contractions and intact membranes. Am J Obstet Gynecol 2005; 192: 350–9. Erratum in: Am J Obstet Gynecol 2005; 193: 308–9.
17 Guinn DA, Goepfert AR, Owen J, *et al.* Management options in women with preterm uterine contractions: a randomized trial. Am J Obstet Gynecol 1997; 177: 814–8.
18 Leitich H, Kaider A. Fetal fibronectin: how useful is it in the prediction of preterm birth? Br J Obstet Gynaecol 2003; 110 (Suppl. 20): 66–70.
19 Honest H, Bachmann LM, Gupta JK, *et al.* Accuracy of cervicovaginal fetal fibronectin test: predicting risk of spontaneous preterm birth. Systematic review. BMJ 2002; 325: 301.
20 Hincz P, Wilczynski J, Kozarzewski M, *et al.* Two-step test: the combined use of fetal fibronectin and sonographic examination of the uterine cervix for prediction of preterm delivery in symptomatic patients. Acta Obstet Gynecol Scand 2002; 81: 58–63.
21 Terrone DA, Rinehart BK, Kraeden U, *et al.* Fetal fibronectin in symptomatic twin gestations. Prim Care Update Ob Gyns 1998; 5: 179.
22 Berghella V, Hayes E, Visintine J, *et al.* Fetal fibronectin testing for reducing the risk of preterm birth. Cochrane Database System Rev 2008; 4: CD006843.
23 Giles W, Bisits A, Knox M, *et al.* The effect of fetal fibronectin testing on admissions to a tertiary maternal-fetal medicine unit and cost savings. Am J Obstet Gynecol 2000; 182: 439–42.
24 Joffe GM, Jacques D, Bemis-Heys R, Burton R, Skram B, Shelburne P. Impact of the fetal fibronectin assay on admissions for preterm labor. Am J Obstet Gynecol 1999;180: 581–6.
25 Swamy GK, Simhan HN, Gammill HS, *et al.* Clinical utility of fetal fibronectin for predicting preterm birth. J Reprod Med 2005; 50: 851–6.
26 Andrews WW, Sibai BM, Thom EA, *et al.* National Institute of Child Health & Human Development Maternal-Fetal Medicine Units Network. Randomized clinical trial of metronidazole plus erythromycin to prevent spontaneous preterm delivery in fetal fibronectin-positive women. Obstet Gynecol 2003; 101: 847–55.
27 Shennan A, Crawshaw S, Briley A, *et al.* A randomised controlled trial of metronidazole for the prevention of preterm birth in women positive for cervicovaginal fetal fibronectin: the PREMET Study. Br J Obstet Gynaecol 2006; 113: 65–74.

28 Leitich H, Bodner-Adler B, Brunbauer M, *et al.* Bacterial vaginosis as a risk factor for preterm delivery: a meta-analysis. Am J Obstet Gynecol 2003; 189: 139–47.
29 Hendler I, Andrews WW, Carey CJ, *et al.* The relationship between resolution of asymptomatic bacterial vaginosis and spontaneous preterm birth in fetal fibronectin-positive women. Am J Obstet Gynecol 2007; 197: 488.e1–5.
30 Goldenberg RL, Klebanoff M, Carey C, *et al.* Metronidazole treatment of women with a positive fetal fibronectin result. Am J Obstet Gynecol 2001; 185: 485–6.
31 Keeler SM, Roman AS, Coletta JM, *et al.* Fetal fibronectin testing in patients with shortcervix in the midtrimester: can it identify optimal candidates for ultrasound-indicated cerclage? Am J Obstet Gynecol 2009; 200: 158.e1–6.
32 Iams JD, Casal D, McGregor JA, *et al.* Fetal fibronectin improves the accuracy of diagnosis of preterm labor. Am J Obstet Gynecol 1995; 173: 141–5.
33 Guinn DA, Atkinson MW, Sullivan L, *et al.* Single vs weekly courses of antenatal corticosteroids for women at risk of preterm delivery: a randomized controlled trial. JAMA 2001; 286: 1581–7.
34 Kiefer DG, Vintzileos AM. The utility of fetal fibronectin in the prediction and prevention of spontaneous preterm birth. Rev Obstet Gynecol 2008; 1: 106–12.
35 Joffe GM, Jacques D, Bemis-Heys R, *et al.* Impact of the fetal fibronectin assay on admissions for preterm labor. Am J Obstet Gynecol 1999; 180: 581–6.
36 Ness A, Visintine J, Ricci E, *et al.* Does knowledge of cervical length and fetal fibronectin affect management of women with threatened preterm labor? A randomized trial. Am J Obstet Gynecol 2007; 197: 426.e1–7.
37 Lowe MP, Zimmerman B, Hansen W. Prospective randomized controlled trial of fetal fibronectin on preterm labor management in a tertiary care center. Am J Obstet Gynecol 2004; 190: 358–62.
38 Grobman WA, Welshman EE, Calhoun EA. Does fetal fibronectin use in the diagnosis of preterm labor affect physician behavior and health care costs? A randomized trial. Am J Obstet Gynecol 2004; 191: 235–40.
39 Nguyen TCQ, Toy EC, Baker B. The cost-effectiveness of fetal ?bronectin testing in suspected preterm labor: a randomized trial. Obstet Gynecol 2002; 99(4 Suppl): 97S.
40 Plaut MM, Smith W, Kennedy K. Fetal ?bronectin: the impact of a rapid test on the treatment of women with preterm labor symptoms. Am J Obstet Gynecol 2003; 188: 1588–95.
41 Bisits A, Madsen G, Knox M, *et al.* The Randomized Nitric Oxide Tocolysis Trial (RNOTT) for the treatment of preterm labor. Am J Obstet Gynecol 2004; 191: 683–90.
42 Elliott JP, Miller HS, Coleman S, *et al.* A randomized multicenter study to determine the efficacy of activity restriction for preterm labor management in patients testing negative for fetal fibronectin. J Perinatol 2005; 25: 626–30.
43 Yoon BH, Romero R, Moon JB, *et al.* The frequency and clinical significance of intra-amniotic inflammation in patients with a positive cervical fetal fibronectin. Am J Obstet Gynecol 2001; 185: 1137–42.

CHAPTER 14
Bacterial Vaginosis

Nancy W. Hendrix
Department of Obstetrics and Gyneology, Thomas Jefferson University, Philadelphia, USA

Key points
- Screening and treating for bacterial vaginosis (BV) for prevention of preterm birth (PTB) is not beneficial in the general population.
- In women with a prior PTB, data is conflicting as to the efficacy of screening and treating for BV to prevent PTB, with most meta-analyses not showing significant prevention of PTB.

Introduction

Bacterial vaginosis (BV) is regarded as the most common cause of vaginal discharge in reproductive-aged women. In the United States, the estimated prevalence of BV is 29% among women aged 14–49 [1]. The prevalence of BV in the United Kingdom, France and Sweden is 23–27% [2–7], which correlates with the world-wide prevalence range of 11–48% [8].

Microbiology

Although BV is considered the most common vaginal infection of sexually active women, it is **not actually an infection, hence the term vaginosis**. BV is a condition defined by a **change in the microbial ecosystem of the vagina [9]**, resulting from an **increase in facultative and anaerobic bacteria with a concomitant decrease in *Lactobacillus* species** which are a normal part of the vaginal microflora. The amplified numbers of multiple microorganisms include the following major constituents: *Gardnerella vaginalis*, *Mobiluncus* species, *Mycoplasma hominis*, *Peptostreptococcus*, *Prevotella* species (formerly *Bacteroides*), and *Ureaplasma urealyticum* [10]. The origin of the imbalance in vaginal flora is poorly understood.

As *Lactobacillus* organisms decrease, vaginal pH increases and overgrowth of anaerobes occurs. These anaerobes break down vaginal

Table 14.1 Risk factors for bacterial vaginosis.

Douching
Genetic factors
African-American and African-Caribbean race
Multiple/new sexual partners
Smoking

peptides into amines which are malodorous and cause vaginal discharge by transudation and epithelial cell exfoliation.

Risk factors

Various risk factors for BV include **new or multiple sexual partners, cigarette smoking, douching, and genetic/racial factors** [11–13] (Table 14.1). **African-American** women in the United States and **Afro-Caribbean** women in Great Britain are three times more likely to have BV than white women and this difference may explain 50% of the PTBs in their infants [14].

It is not clear whether BV is sexually transmitted since BV can occur in women who have never been sexually active [15]. A high prevalence of BV has been noted in lesbians [16]. This may support the hypothesis of sexual transmission, but it has also been postulated that one type of sexual activity, such as oral–genital sex, may be a more important factor than coitus.

Studies among nonpregnant women demonstrate that **BV resolves spontaneously among two-thirds or more of patients within a 3–6 month period** [10–17]. Unfortunately, BV **also regularly recurs over time regardless of initial successful treatment** [6]. Some predictors of recurrence include absence of *Lactobacillus* species and persistence of at least one abnormal BV-associated microbiologic or vaginal fluid biochemical factor [6, 18].

Diagnosis

Clinical diagnosis requires that at least **three of four Amsel criteria be met** [9] (Table 14.2). The presence of **clue cells** has been found to be the single most reliable predictor of BV [19]. Clue cells are vaginal epithelial cells covered with coccobacilli and polymorphonuclear cells and should comprise at least 20% of the epithelial cells of the discharge with saline solution on a microscope slide. **For research purposes, BV is defined**

Table 14.2 Amsel clinical criteria for diagnosing bacterial vaginosis[9].

Adherent, thin, homogeneous discharge
Vaginal pH > 4.5
Positive amine test
>20% clue cells on wet mount

by the Nugent criteria in which **Gram-stain**ed smears are scored based on the number of lactobacilli, which tend to be low, and the presence of organisms resembling *Mobiluncus* and *Bacteroides*, which tend to be high [20]. A score of 7–10 (usually ≥ 7) is used to diagnose BV and this finding has been associated with a 1.5 to 3-fold increase in PTB [21, 22].

It is important to note that **half or more of women with BV are asymptomatic** [23]. Those women who do have symptoms usually complain of a malodorous vaginal discharge that is more noticeable after intercourse.

Laboratory tests

The pap smear should not be used as an indicator for infection due to its low sensitivity [24]. A vaginal culture is typically not employed because no single microorganism is specific for BV. *Gardnerella vaginalis* is virtually always present in symptomatic infection but it is also present in half or more of asymptomatic women and is not considered diagnostic. DNA probes, such as Affirm TM VP III, are available but expensive and also specific for *Gardnerella vaginalis* only [25].

When compared with the Amsel criteria of BV diagnosis, a Gram stain of the discharge has been found to be highly sensitive (97%) and specific (79%) [19, 26]. This method (Gram stain) is considered the gold standard in laboratory testing but is primarily utilized in research due to the need for an experienced technician and/or microbiologist. Diagnostic kits which detect an elevated pH and trimethylamine or prolineaminopeptidase, such as FemExam, QuickVue Advance, and Pip Activity TestCard, are rapid, inexpensive, and commercially available tests that may aid those clinicians without access to a microscope [27, 28].

Obstetric complications

Numerous studies, of which only a few are cited here, have associated BV with obstetrical complications. These morbidities include spontaneous abortion, PTB, preterm labor (PTL), preterm premature rupture of membranes (PPROM), amniotic fluid infection, and postpartum endometritis [29–31]. **The diagnosis of BV is associated with a 6–49% chance of having a PTB, depending on PTB prevalence, other risk factors for PTB, and presence or absence of symptoms of PTL.**

Screening

Despite the correlation between BV and obstetric morbidities, **screening for BV during pregnancy is controversial**. Two meta-analyses have evaluated the effectiveness of antibiotics for BV in the *general obstetric population* and found no significant reduction in PTB or PPROM [32, 33]. Based upon this data, **screening and treating all pregnant women with asymptomatic BV to prevent PTB is not recommended**.

Several randomized trials and meta-analyses have been performed in women with *prior preterm birth.* The Cochrane meta-analysis (15 randomized controlled trials [RCT]; $n = 5888$), which is the largest and most recent, found that detection and treatment of asymptomatic BV appeared to reduce the presence of BV, PPROM and low birthweight, but not PTB (17–22% decrease, but not statistically significant) [32]. There was suggestion that screening and treating before 20 weeks is most effective, including in prevention of PTB, but this was driven by small studies, with the largest RCT still showing no benefit [34]. The United States Preventive Services Task Force (USPSTF) also performed a meta-analysis of women with a prior PTB and asymptomatic BV but results could not be pooled due to heterogeneity. The USPSTF found that three of four RCTs reduced PTB [35]. A Canadian meta-analysis in 2005 (14 trials on BV; 5500 women randomized) also concluded **against any significant benefit of screening and treating women with prior PTB for BV** [36].

Treatment

In non-pregnant women, BV should be treated to relieve symptomatic infection and reduce the risk of infectious morbidity after surgical procedures [37, 38]. Treatment of BV has also been shown to reduce the transmission of other sexually transmitted diseases [39–41] so that some experts recommend treating all nonpregnant women diagnosed with BV. Treatment of the sexual partner is not performed since no benefit has been

Table 14.3 Recommended medications for treatment of bacterial vaginosis in the obstetric patient[46].

Metronidazole 500 mg po BID × 7 d
Metronidazole 250 mg po TID × 7 d
Clindamycin 300 mg po BID × 7 d

demonstrated [42]. Follow up visits are unnecessary if symptoms resolve. However, as stated previously, recurrence is not uncommon.

In pregnant women, the indications for treatment are not as clear cut. **The sole accepted indication for treatment of BV in pregnancy is a symptomatic infection**. However, treatment of an asymptomatic infection in pregnancy is controversial, despite the association between BV and obstetric morbidities mentioned previously.

Effective treatments for BV consist of metronidazole, clindamycin or tinidazole. It should be noted that the optimal regimen is not known. All of these alternatives have been proven to be equally efficacious with high cure rates of ≥ 80% [43–45]. **Metronidazole and clindamycin are both pregnancy category B and the only two included in recommended treatment regimens** by the Centers for Disease Control and Prevention (CDC) in the United States [46]. It is **unclear which one is most effective, if at all, at prevention of PTB**. Tinidazole, a second generation nitroimidazole, is a pregnancy category C and not recommended at this time (Table 14.3).

Some physicians avoid prescribing metronidazole in the first trimester because of the potential for teratogenicity by crossing the placenta. However, no relationship was demonstrated between metronidazole use in the first trimester and increased teratogenic risk by two meta-analyses [47, 48].

It should also be mentioned that even though topical therapy has proven as effective as oral therapy in eradicating BV in gynecologic patients, **only oral antibiotic regimens have been found to reduce PTB**. Several trials of topical clindamycin did not reduce PTB even though it was found to adequately treat BV [49–51]. Because of an increase in neonatal adverse events such as low birth weight and neonatal infections in these trials when clindamycin cream was given between 16 and 32 weeks, the CDC recommends intravaginal use only during the first half of pregnancy [46].

Even with all of the information regarding treatment in pregnancy, the optimal antibiotic, time of therapy and duration of use have not been identified. **Earlier diagnosis and treatment appear to be more effective compared with late second trimester treatment when attempting to prevent PTB** [31, 52]. For this reason, **the CDC recommends screening (if conducted in women with prior PTB) be**

Table 14.4 Recommendations of selected organizations regarding screening and treating bacterial vaginosis during pregnancy. ACOG, American College of Obstetricians and Gynecologists. CDC, Centers for Disease Control and Prevention. RANZCOG, Royal Australian and New Zealand College of Obstetricians and Gynaecologists. RCOG, Royal College of Obstetricians and Gynaecologists. SOGC, Society of Obstetricians and Gynaecologists of Canada. USPSTF, United States Preventive Services Task Force.

General obstetric population (at low risk for preterm birth)
ACOG: Not beneficial (Level B) [53]
CDC: Unclear [46]
Cochrane Review: Not beneficial [32]
RANZCOG: No published guidelines
RCOG: Conflicting results (Grade C) [54]
SOGC: No routine screening or treatment (Level I-B) [55]
USPSTF: Not beneficial [35]
Women with prior preterm birth
ACOG: Insufficient data to support use (Level A) [53]
CDC: Consider evaluation and treatment [46]
Cochrane Review: Not beneficial [32]
RANZCOG: No published guidelines
RCOG: Treatment may reduce the risk of preterm birth (Grade C) [54]
SOGC: May benefit from routine screening and treatment (Level I-B) [55]
USPSTF: Insufficient evidence [35]

performed during the first prenatal visit [46]. Recommendations of selected organizations regarding screening and treating BV during pregnancy are shown in Table 14.4 [53–55].

Women with PTL

The presence of asymptomatic BV in women with symptoms of PTL between 24 and 34 weeks is associated with an increased risk of PTB compared with similar women without BV [56]. There are no trials to assess efficacy of screening and treating for BV in women with PTL for preventing PTB. Therefore this intervention cannot at present be recommended.

The future

Many other vaginal biomarkers have been identified that might better identify which woman with BV might be most at risk for PTB, and/or benefit from therapy. These include various cytokines (IL-1beta, IL-8, etc), sialidase, prolidase, neutrophil levels, etc. [57]. Further research on these co-markers, co-infections, host-immune response and gene-environment interactions [58] should shed more light on this controversial condition.

References

1 Allsworth JE, Peipert JF. Prevalence of bacterial vaginosis: 2001–2004 National Health and Nutrition Examination Survey Data. Obstet Gynecol 2007; 109: 114–20.
2 Lefevre JC, Averous S, Bauriaud R, Blanc C, Bertrand MA, Lareng MB. Lower genital tract infections in women: comparison of clinical and epidemiologic findings with microbiology. Sex Transm Dis 1988; 15: 110–3.
3 Hay PE, Taylor-Robinson D, Lamont RF. Diagnosis of bacterial vaginosis in a gynaecology clinic. Br J Obstet Gynaecol 1992; 99: 63–6.
4 Riordan T, Macaulay ME, James JM, *et al.* A prospective study of genital infections in a family planning clinic. 1. Microbiological findings and their association with vaginal symptoms. Epidemiol Infect 1990; 104: 47–53.
5 Larsson P-G, Platz-Christensen JJ. Enumeration of clue cells in rehydrated air-dried vaginal wet smears for the diagnosis of bacterial vaginosis. Obstet Gynecol 1990; 76: 727–30.
6 Cook RL, Redondo-Lopez V, Schmitt C, Meriwether C, Sobel JD. Clinical, microbiological and biochemical factors in recurrent bacterial vaginosis. J Clin Microbiol 1992; 30: 870–7.
7 Bump RC, Zuspan FP, Buesching WJ, Ayers LW, Stephens TJ. The prevalence, six month persistence and predictive values of laboratory indicators of bacterial vaginosis (nonspecific vaginitis) in asymptomatic women. Am J Obstet Gynecol 1984; 150: 917–24.
8 Tolosa JE, Chaitnongwongwatthana S, Daly S, *et al.* The International Infections in Pregnancy study: variations in the prevalence of bacterial vaginosis and distribution of morphotypes in vaginal smears among pregnant women. Am J Obstet Gynecol 2006; 195: 1198–204.
9 Amsel R, Totten PA, Speigel CA, Chen KCS, Eschenbach DA, Holmes KK. Nonspecific vaginitis: diagnostic criteria and microbial and epidemiologic associations. Am J Med 1983; 74: 14–22.
10 Hill GB. The microbiology of bacterial vaginosis. Am J Obstet Gynecol 1993; 169: 450–4.
11 Fethers KA, Fairley CK, Hocking JS, Gurrin LC, Bradshaw CS. Sexual risk factors and bacterial vaginosis: a systematic review and meta-analysis. Clin Infect Dis 2008; 47: 1426–35.
12 Ryckman KK, Simhan HN, Krohn MA, Williams SM. Predicting risk of bacterial vaginosis: the role of race, smoking and corticotropin-releasing hormone-related genes. Mol Hum Reprod. 2009; 15: 131–7.
13 Ness RB, Hillier SL, Richter HE, *et al.* Douching in relation to bacterial vaginosis, lactobacilli, and facultative bacteria in the vagina. Obstet Gynecol 2002; 100: 765–72.
14 Goldenberg RL, Klebanoff MA, Nugent R, *et al.* Bacterial colonization of the vagina during pregnancy in four ethnic groups. Am J Obstet Gynecol 1996; 175: 1317–24.

15 Yen S, Schafer MA, Moncada J, Campbell CJ, Flinn SD, Boyer CB. Bacterial vaginosis in sexually experienced and non-sexually experienced young women entering the military. Obstet Gynecol 2003; 102: 927–33.

16 Evans AL, Scally AJ, Wellard SJ, Wilson JD. Prevalence of bacterial vaginosis in lesbians and heterosexual women in a community setting. Sex Transm Infect 2007; 83: 470–5.

17 Bump RC, Buesching WJ. Bacterial vaginosis in virginal and sexually active adolescent females: evidence against exclusive sexual transmission. Am J Obstet Gynecol 1988; 158: 935–9.

18 Eschenbach DA, Davick PR, Williams BL, *et al.* Prevalence of hydrogen peroxide-producing *Lactobacillus* species in normal women and women with bacterial vaginosis. J Clin Microbiol 1989; 27: 251–6.

19 Eschenbach DA, Hillier S, Critchlow C, Stevens C, DeRouen T, Holmes KK. Diagnosis and clinical manifestations of bacterial vaginosis. Am J Obstet Gynecol 1988; 158: 819–28.

20 Nugent RP, Krohn MA, Hillier SL. Reliability of diagnosing bacterial vaginosis is improved by a standardized method of gram stain interpretation. J Clin Microbiol 1991; 29: 297–30.

21 Meis PJ, Goldenberg RL, Mercer B, *et al.* The preterm prediction study: significance of vaginal infections. Am J Obstet Gynecol 1995; 173: 123–5.

22 Hillier SL, Nugent RP, Eschenbach DA, *et al.* for the Vaginal Infections and Prematurity Study Group. Association between bacterial vaginosis and preterm delivery of a low-birthweight infant. N Eng J Med 1995; 333: 1737–42.

23 Klebanoff MA, Schwebke JR, Zhang J, Nansel TR, Yu KF, Andrews WW. Vulvovaginal symptoms in women with bacterial vaginosis. Obstet Gynecol 2004; 104: 267–72.

24 Lowe NK, Neal JL, Ryan-Wenger NA. Accuracy of the clinical diagnosis of vaginitis compared with a DNA probe Laboratory Standard. Obstet Gynecol 2009; 113: 89–95.

25 Greene JF, Kuehl TJ, Allen SR. The papanicolaou smear: inadequate screening test for bacterial vaginosis during pregnancy. Am J Obstet Gynecol 2000; 82: 1048–9.

26 Nugent RP, Rohn MA, Hillier SL. Reliability of diagnosing bacterial vaginosis is improved by a standardized method of gram stain interpretation. J Clin Microbiol 1991; 29: 297–301.

27 West B, Morison L, Schim van der Loeff M, *et al.* Evaluation of a new rapid diagnostic kit (FemExam) for bacterial vaginosis in patients with vaginal discharge syndrome in the Gambia. Sex Transm Dis 2003; 30: 483–9.

28 Gutman RE, Peipert JF, Weitzen S, Blume J. Evaluation of clinical methods for diagnosing bacterial vaginosis. Obstet Gynecol 2005; 105: 551–6.

29 Gravett MG, Nelson JP, DeRouen T, Critchlow C, Eschenbach DA, Holmes KK. Independent associations of bacterial vaginosis and *Chlamydia trachomatis* infection with adverse pregnancy outcome. JAMA 1986; 256: 1899–903.

30 Meis PG. Goldenberg RL, Mercer B, *et al.* The preterm prediction study: significance of vaginal infections. National Institute of Child Health and Human Development Maternal-Fetal Medicine Units Network. Am J Obstet Gynecol 1995; 173: 1231–5.

31 Leitich H, Bodner-Adler B, Brunbauer M, Kaider A, Egarter C, Husslein P. Bacterial vaginosis as a risk factor for preterm delivery: a meta-analysis. Am J Obstet Gynecol 2003; 189: 139–47.

32 McDonald HM, Brocklehurst P, Gordon A. Antibiotics for treating bacterial vaginosis in pregnancy. Cochrane Database Syst Rev 2009; 1: CD000262.

33 Nygren P, Fu R, Freeman M, Bougatsos C, Klebanoff M, Guise JM. US Preventive Services Task Force. Evidence on the benefits and harms of screening and treating

pregnant women who are asymptomatic for bacterial vaginosis: an update review for the US Preventive Services Task Force. Ann Intern Med 2008; 148: 220–33.

34 Carey JC, Klebanoff MA, Hauth JC, *et al.* Metronidazole to prevent preterm delivery in pregnant women with asymptomatic bacterial vaginosis. N Eng J Med 2000; 342: 534–40.

35 US Preventive Services Task Force. Screening for bacterial vaginosis in pregnancy to prevent preterm delivery: US Preventive Services Task Force recommendation statement. Ann Intern Med 2008; 148: 214–9.

36 Okun N, Gronau KA, Hannah ME. Antibiotics for bacterial vaginosis or trichomonas vaginalis in pregnancy: a systematic review. Obstet Gynecol 2005; 105: 857–68.

37 Miller L, Thomas K, Hughes JP, Holmes KK, Stout S, Eschenbach DA. Randomised treatment trial of bacterial vaginosis to prevent post-abortion complication. Br J Obstet Gynaecol 2004; 111: 982–8.

38 Larsson PG, Carlsson B. Does pre-and post-operative metronidazole treatment lower vaginal cuff infection rate after abdominal hysterectomy among women with bacterial vaginosis? Infect Dis Obstet Gynecol 2002; 10: 133–40.

39 Myer L, Denny L, Telerant R, Souza M, Wright TC, Kuhn L. Bacterial vaginosis and susceptibility to HIV infection in South African women: a nested case-control study. J Infect Dis 2005; 192: 1372–80.

40 Cherpes TL Meyn LA, Krohn MA, Lurie JG, Hillier SL. Association between acquisition of herpes simplex virus type 2 in women and bacterial vaginosis. Clin Infect Dis 2003; 37: 319–25.

41 Wiesenfeld HC, Hillier SL, Krohn MA, Landers DV, Sweet RL. Bacterial vaginosis is a strong predictor of Neisseria gonorrhoeae and Chlamydia trachomatis infection. Clin Infect Dis 2003; 36: 663–8.

42 Potter J. Should sexual partners of women with bacterial vaginosis receive treatment? Br J Gen Pract 1999; 49: 913–8.

43 Hanson JM, McGregor JA, Hillier SL, *et al.* Metronidazole for bacterial vaginosis: a comparison of vaginal versus oral therapy. J Reprod Med 2000; 45: 889–96.

44 Ferris DG, Litaker MS, Woodward L, Mathis D, Hendrich J. Treatment of bacterial vaginosis: a comparison of oral metronidazole, metronidazole vaginal gel, and clindamycin vaginal cream. J Fam Pract 1995; 41: 443–9.

45 Livengood CH, Ferris DG, Wiesenfeld HC, *et al.* Effectiveness of two tinidazole regimens in treatment of bacterial vaginosis: a randomized controlled trial. Obstet Gynecol 2007; 110: 302–9.

46 Sexually Transmitted Diseases Treatment Guidelines, 2006. MMWR Recomm Rep 2006; 55: 1–95. http: //www.cdc.gov/mmwr/

47 Burtin P, Taddio A, Ariburnu O, Einarson TR, Koren G. Safety of metronidazole in pregnancy: a meta-analysis. Am J Obstet Gynecol 1995; 172: 525–9.

48 Caro-Patón T, Carvajal A, Martin de Diego I, Martin-Arias LH, Alvarez Requejo A, Rodríguez Pinilla E. Is metronidazole teratogenic? A meta-analysis. Br J Clin Pharmacol 1997; 44: 179–82.

49 McGregor, JA, French JI, Jones W, *et al.* Bacterial vaginosis is associated with prematurity and vaginal fluid sialidase: results of a controlled trial of topical clindamycin cream. Am J Obstet Gynecol 1994; 170: 1048–60.

50 Joesoef MR, Hillier SL, Wiknjosastro G, *et al.* Intravaginal clindamycin treatment for bacterial vaginosis: effects on preterm delivery and low birth weight. Am J Obstet Gynecol 1995; 173: 1527–31.

51 Vermeulen GM, Bruinse HW. Prophylactic administration of clindamycin 2% vaginal cream to reduce the incidence of spontaneous preterm birth in women with an

increased recurrence risk: a randomized placebo-controlled double-blind trial. Br J Obstet Gynaecol 1999; 106: 652–7.

52 Ugwumadu A, Manyonda I, Reid F, Hay P. Effect of early oral clindamycin on late miscarriage and preterm delivery in asymptomatic women with abnormal vaginal flora and bacterial vaginosis: a randomized controlled trial. Lancet 2003; 361: 983–8.

53 American College of Obstetricians and Gynecologists. Assessment of risk factors for preterm birth. ACOG Practice Bulletin No. 31. Obstet Gynecol 2001; 98: 709–16.

54 Royal College of Obstetricians and Gynaecologists. Infection and pregnancy-study group statement. Consensus statement 2001. http: //www.rcog.org.uk/womens-health/clinical-guidance

55 Yudin MH, Money DM. Infectious Diseases Committee. Screening and management of bacterial vaginosis in pregnancy. J Obstet Gynecol Can 2008; 30: 702–8.

56 Goffinet F, Maillard F, Mihoubi N, *et al.* Bacterial vaginosis: prevalence and predictive value for premature delivery and neonatal infection in women with preterm labour and intact membranes. Eur J Obstet Gynecol Reprod Biol 2003; 108: 146–51.

57 Cauci S, Culhane JF. Modulation of vaginal immune response among pregnant women with bacterial vaginosis by *Trichomonas vaginalis, Chlamydia trachomatis, Neisseria gonorrhea,* and yeast. Am J Obstet Gynecol 2007; 196: 133.e1–133.e7.

58 Macones GA, Parry S, Elkousy M, Clothier B, Ural SH, Strauss JF. A polymorphism in the promoter region of TNF and bacterial vaginosis: preliminary evidence of gene-environment interaction in the etiology of spontaneous preterm birth. Am J Obstet Gynecol 2004; 190: 1504–8.

CHAPTER 15
Sexually Transmitted Infections

Neil S. Seligman
Division of Maternal-Fetal Medicine, Department of Obstetrics and Gynecology, Thomas Jefferson University, Philadelphia, USA

Key points

- Chorioamniotic infection, resulting in cytokine and prostaglandin production, causes 25–40% of all preterm births (PTBs).
- Several common sexually transmitted infections (STIs) are associated with an increased risk of PTB: syphilis; genital herpes (primary); gonorrhea; Chlamydia (IgM+); Trichomonas; HIV.
- All pregnant women should be screened for syphilis, Chlamydia, and HIV at the first prenatal visit. Women with risk factors should also be screened for hepatitis C and gonorrhea.
- Pregnancy does not alter the presentation of STIs.
- Standard antibiotic regimens are effective in treating sexually transmitted infections during pregnancy (Table 15.2).
- Consistent condom use can significantly lower the incidence and transmission of STIs.
- In women who would have been treated for cervical intraepithelial neoplasia grade 2 or 3, it is estimated that vaccination with the quadrivalent vaccine (Guardisil®) could reduce PTB by 60%.

Introduction

Infection is an important cause of preterm birth (PTB) [1, 2] (Chapter 7). **Chorioamniotic infection is associated with 25–40% of cases of PTB [1, 3]. Possible mechanisms for the link between bacterial infection and PTB include: (1) infection of maternal (decidua) or fetal (placenta, membranes, and amniotic fluid) tissues resulting in production of cytokines and prostaglandins directly by bacterial phospholiase A or indirectly as a result of bacterial endotoxin; (2) production of matrix degrading enzymes [1, 4, 5]; (3) antibiotic treatment causing bacterial cell lysis. The mechanism linking viral infection and PTB is unclear.** Bacterial and viral pathogens include several common sexually transmitted infections (STIs). In the

Preterm Birth. Edited by Vincenzo Berghella. © 2010 Blackwell Publishing

Infection	First antenatal care visit		Rescreen third trimester	Screening and diagnostic tests
	All women	High risk women		
Syphilis	ACOG, CDC[a]	NA	ACOG,CDC[a,b,c]	RPR, VDRL[d]
Genital herpes	No	No	No	Culture, PCR, HSV1/2 IgG
Gonorrhea	No	ACOG, CDC[e,f]	No	Culture, NAAT[e]
Chlamydia	CDC	ACOG[b,f]	CDC[b,f]	Culture, NAAT[e]
Trichomonas	No	No	No	Microscopy, culture
Hepatitis C	No	ACOG, CDC[g]	No	HCV IgG
HIV	CDC, ACOG[h]	NA	CDC[b]	ELISA

Table 15.1 Screening and diagnosis of common sexually transmitted infections in asymptomatic women. ACOG, American College of Obstetricians and Gynecologists. CDC, Centers for Disease Control and Prevention. NA, not applicable. a, laws vary by state. b, women living in high prevalence area. c, multiple sexual partners, unprotected sex, presence of other sexually transmitted infections (STI), African-American race, incarceration. d, serologic non-treponemal tests are not useful for diagnosing primary syphilis. e, NAAT, nucleic acid amplification tests. f, age <25 years old, prior STI, multiple sexual partners, having a partner with a past history of any STI, sex work, drug use, and inconsistent condom use. g, history of injection drug use, blood transfusion, or organ transplant. h, annual screening regardless of pregnancy for: injection drug user, partner uses injection drugs or is HIV+, exchanges sex for drugs or money, STI since last test, multiple sexual partners.

United States, 19 million individuals, mostly of reproductive age, contract a STI each year [6]. This chapter reviews the evidence for the association between STIs and PTB along with evidence for screening and treatment in pregnancy. **The American College of Obstetricians and Gynecologists (ACOG) and the Center for Disease Control and Prevention (CDC) provide evidence-based recommendations, which are summarized in Tables 15.1 and 15.2**. Electronic resources are listed in Table 15.3. These concepts can be used also for preconception counseling and preventive strategies. Consistent condom use can significantly lower the incidence and transmission of STIs.

Syphilis

Syphilis is caused by infection with the Gram negative spirochete *Treponema pallidum*. The primary stage is characterized by a painless indurated ulcer. Maternal syphilis is an important cause of prematurity. Worldwide, active syphilis affects nearly 1 million pregnancies and adverse pregnancy outcomes may occur in up to 80% of cases [7]. **Annually syphilis**

Table 15.2 Treatment of sexually transmitted infections in pregnancy. CSR, Cochrane Systematic Review[9] (efficacy of the treatment during pregnancy is supported by a Cochrane Systematic Review).

Infection	First line treatment	Alternative treatment	Additional considerations	CSR
Syphilis		None	Penicillin allergy Jarisch-Herxheimer reaction	✓[12]
• Primary, secondary, early latent	Benzathine penicillin G 2.4 million units IM in a single dose			
• Late latent and latent unknown duration	Benzathine penicillin G 2.4 million units IM × 3 doses at 1 week intervals (7.2 million units total)			
Granuloma inguinale	Azythromycin 1 g orally weekly for 3 weeks or until all lesions healed	Erythromycin base 500 mg orally four times a day for 21 days or until all lesions healed		
Lymphogranuloma venereum	Erythromycin base 500 mg orally four times a day for 21 days	None		
Chancroid	Azythromycin 1 g orally single dose	Ceftriaxone 250 mg IM single dose		
Genital herpes				
• First episode	Acyclovir 400 mg orally 3 times a day for 7–10 days/200 mg orally 5 times a day for 7–10days	Valacyclovir 1 g orally twice a day for 7–10 days		
• Chronic suppression	Acyclovir 400 mg orally twice a day	Valacyclovir 500 mg orally twice a day/1 g orally once a day		
• Episodic therapy for recurrence	Acyclovir 400 mg orally three times a day for 5 days/800 mg twice a day for 5 days/800 mg three times a day for 2 days	Valacyclovir 500 mg orally twice a day for 3 days/1 g orally once a day for 5 days		
Gonorrhea	Ceftriaxone 125 mg IM single dose (99.1% efficacy)[27]	Cefixime 400 mg orally single dose (97.4% efficacy)[27] or Spectimomycin 2 g IM single dose (98.2% efficacy)[27]	Antibiotic resistance Test of cure 4–6 weeks following treatment Treat for co-infection with Chlamydia	✓[49]
Chlamydia	Azythromycin 1 g orally single dose	Erythromycin base 500 mg orally four times a day for 7 days	Test of cure 4–6 weeks following treatment	✓[50]
Pelvic inflammatory disease	Clindamycin 900 mg IV every 8 hours PLUS Gentamycin 2 mg/kg IV loading dose then 1.5 mg/kg every 8 hours maintenance dose	None	Switch to enteral treatment after clinical improvement	
Trichomonas	Metronidazole 2 g orally single dose	Metronidazole 500 mg orally twice a day for 5–7 days	Treatment may increase the rate of preterm birth	✓[36]

Table 15.3 Key electronic resources.

- HIV Guidelines: http://www.aidsinfo.nih.gov/Guidelines/
- Sexually Transmitted Infection Treatment Guidelines: http://www.cdc.gov/std/treatment/default.htm
- Syphillis Elimination Effort: http://www.cdc.gov/stopsyphilis/
- Gonorrhea Antibiotic Resistance: http://www.cdc.gov/std/Gonorrhea/arg/default.htm
- Sexually Transmitted Infection Statistics: http://www.cdc.gov/std/stats/default.htm

infection is responsible for approximately 270,000 premature or low-birthweight neonates worldwide [8]. The relative risk of PTB is approximately 2.0 [1, 9] and is related to titer, i.e. new infection (380 previously unscreened women in Tanzania: titer ≥ 1 : 8 = 20% PTB [72.7% of which were ≥1 : 32] vs titer < 1 : 8 = 0% PTB; vs seronegative = 3% PTB) [10].

Screening

In the United States, the rate of primary and secondary syphilis in women has increased each year from 2004 to 2007, and the rate of congenital syphilis also increased in 2006 and 2007 [7]. Universal screening of pregnant women for syphilis is cost-effective even in countries with a low incidence of syphilis [11]. Screening is recommended for all pregnant women at the first antenatal care visit (Table 15.1). Women who are at high risk of infection should be rescreened in the third trimester. Laws regarding antenatal syphilis screening vary from state to state. Rescreening all high-risk women in the third trimester is mandated in only a few states.

Diagnosis

Non-treponemal tests (Venereal Disease Research Laboratory [VDRL] or rapid plasma reagin [RPR]) are used for screening but are not useful for primary syphilis (Table 15.1). Non-treponemal tests have a high false-positive rate. **A positive result from a screening test should be confirmed with a treponemal test such as the FTA-ABS** (fluorescent-treponemal antibody absorption test). Interpretation of a low non-treponemal titer (<1 : 8) can be difficult (does not differentiate between prior, recent, or treated infections), and should be coordinated with the local department of health.

Treatment

Benzathine penicillin G is the treatment for active syphilis during pregnancy, but the optimal treatment regimen is uncertain [12].

A single dose of benzathine penicillin G 2.4 million units was 98% effective in preventing congenital syphilis [13] in a study which included women that may not have been recently infected (persistent low titer). The same treatment was not effective in preventing PTB or congenital syphilis compared with no treatment in a study excluding women with a persistently low titer. However, the addition of a second dose one week later was associated with a favorable neonatal outcome [14]. Currently recommended regimens are based on stage of infection (Table 15.2). Women who are allergic to penicillin should be desensitized. Non-reassuring fetal testing and/or PTB can result from treatment during the second trimester if the treatment precipitates the Jarisch-Herxheimer reaction [15, 16].

Herpes simplex virus (HSV)

HSV is the most common ulcerative STI in the United States. **The seroprevalence of HSV is 17%** affecting approximately 880,000 pregnant women [17, 18]. Genital herpes can be caused by either serotypes 1 or 2 (HSV-1; HSV-2). Neonatal HSV infection can have devastating consequences but the effects of HSV on obstetrical outcome are unclear. HSV infection can be divided into primary infection, non-primary first episode, and recurrent infection based on urogenital and serum testing. **Both asymptomatic and symptomatic primary HSV infection [19] increase the risk of PTB** (57 pregnant women with asymptomatic shedding, rate of PTB<37 weeks 25%, median gestational age for primary infection 33 weeks) [20]. **Asymptomatic shedding due to reactivation and symptomatic recurrent infection, however, is not associated with PTB [20]**.

Prevention

Approximately 2.1% of women will acquire genital herpes during pregnancy [21]. As with other ulcerative diseases, latex condoms decrease the risk of transmission only when the ulcer is in a location that is covered.

Screening

Current guidelines do not recommend universal testing of pregnant women (Table 15.1). However, some experts suggest that all women be screened [21]. **Seventy percent of infections are asymptomatic, therefore the clinician should consider HSV in the differential diagnosis of women presenting with subtle vulvovaginal symptoms.** Diagnostic tests are shown in Table 15.1.

Treatment

There is no evidence that either treatment or suppression of genetal herpes prevents PTB. Women with PPROM complicated by activation of recurrent genital herpes can be managed expectantly if <34 weeks [22] (Chapter 19).

Other ulcerative diseases

Granuloma inguinale or Donovanosis *(Klebsiella granulomatis)*, **chancroid** *(Haemophilus ducreyi)* **and lymphogranuloma venereum** (*Chlamydia trachomatis* **serovars L1-3**) **are ulcerative diseases that primarily occur in tropical countries.** In the United States, hot spots of granuloma inguinale are found in southern states and in non-Caucasian urban populations [23]. Chancroid is still endemic in some areas of the United States. **There is no evidence that these infections are associated with an increased risk of PTB [24].** Recommended antibiotic regimens are listed in Table 15.2.

Gonorrhea (NG)

NG is caused by *Neisseria gonorrhea*, a Gram-negative diplococcus, and can infect the cervix and/or urethra. Cervical infection is frequently asymptomatic but may present as a mucopurulent cervical discharge. **At least five studies have demonstrated an association between NG and PTB** [2]; however, some of these studies failed to adjust for other risk factors [9], and therefore the exact risk is uncertain. **When NG is diagnosed, the RR of PTB is between 2.0 and 6.0 [1, 25, 26].**

Screening

There is no evidence that screening low risk women is beneficial [27]. Current guidelines recommend screening women with risk factors (Table 15.1). Repeat testing should be performed for those at continued risk [16]. Screening and diagnostic tests are shown in Table 15.1.

Treatment

Current treatment regimens are shown in Table 15.2. **Antibiotic resistance is an important consideration as resistance to penicillin and quinilones have been reported. Presumptive treatment for Chlamydia should be given unless co-infection has been ruled out. A test cure should be performed 4–6 weeks after treatment.**

Chlamydia (CT)

CT is caused by *Chlamydia trochomatis* serovars D–K. Like NG, infection can cause cervicitis and/or urethritis and is frequently asymptomatic. However, some women present with vaginal discharge or dysuria. There are approximately 100,000 new cases of CT each year in pregnant US women. The relationship between CT and PTB is less clear than for NG. CT infection is associated with a RR 2.0 for PTB [1, 2, 9, 28] but the risk may depend on serologic status (270 pregnant women with endocervical *CT* vs 270 controls, no significant difference in PTB; rate of PTB in IgM+ subset = 19% vs controls = 8% [*P* = 0.03] [29].

Screening

Recommendations for screening are shown in Table 15.1. **There is insufficient evidence that routine screening for Chlamydia will prevent the adverse pregnancy outcomes [16].** Screening and diagnostic tests are shown in Table 15.1.

Treatment

Current treatment regimens are shown in Table 15.2. **Treatment may decrease the incidence of PPROM and low birthweight [28] but the effect of treatment on the rate of PTB is unclear [2, 30].** A test of cure should be performed 4–6 weeks after treatment.

Pelvic inflammatory disease (PID)

PID is rare after the first trimester of pregnancy. However, because of the high risk for maternal morbidity and PTB, pregnant women who have suspected PID should be hospitalized and treated with parenteral antibiotics [16].

Trichomonas

Trichomonas is caused by the protozoa *Trichomonas vaginalis*. The prevalence of trichomonas during pregnancy is as high as 10–12.6% [2, 31]. **Trichomonas infection during pregnancy is associated with PTB and PPROM [32–34].** The largest study found that the odds ratio (OR) of PTB was 1.3 (95% CI 1.1–1.4) (13,914 women, prevalence of trichomonas 12.6%) [32].

Screening

Universal screening of pregnant women for trichomonas is not currently recommended. Despite this, in a survey, 27% of obstetricians reported that they routinely screen for trichomonas as an attempt to prevent PTB [35]. Diagnostic tests are shown in Table 15.1.

Treatment

Currently there is no data to support treatment of asymptomatic women with metronidazole to prevent PTB [36], and there is a potential harm. A trial of asymptomatic women between 16 and 23 weeks randomized to treatment with 4g of metronidazole or placebo was stopped early because of an 80% increase in PTB [37]. Proposed mechanisms for treatment with metronidazole causing PTB are that lysis of trichomonads elicits an inflammatory response and metronidazole may alter the balance of vaginal flora eradicating beneficial microorganisms. Despite this evidence, 98% of obstetricians would treat a trichomonas infection to prevent PTB [35]. **If treating trichomonas during pregnancy, no more than a single 2g dose should be used.**

Hepatitis C virus (HCV)

HCV, a single-stranded RNA virus, is the most common chronic bloodborne infection in the United States, occurring in 0.6–4.5% of pregnant women. HCV can be acquired by exposure to infected blood and, rarely, sexual contact or exposure to infected blood [38]. HCV infections can be divided into three categories: acute, chronic, and chronic active. In a study of opioid-dependent women, HCV positivity was not associated with an increased risk of PTB [39]. **However, studies controlling for type of infection have found an increased risk of PTB among women with chronic-active HCV (positive viral load and abnormal liver function tests) [40].**

Screening

Screening for HCV should be offered to women with risk factors (Table 15.1). Diagnostic tests are shown in Table 15.1.

Treatment

Treatment for HCV chronic infection with efficacious therapy (pegylated interferon-α and ribavirin) is recommended for non-pregnant adults but cannot be used during or immediately prior to pregnancy, because of the teratogenicity of ribavirin [38].

Human immunodeficiency virus (HIV)

The most devastating consequence of maternal HIV is vertical transmission. The risk of PTB is increased in women with HIV infection even after controlling for other risk factors including co-infection with other STIs [41]. Not all studies have confirmed this association [42], but **a systematic review of 31 prospective trials found an odds ratio of PTB of 1.83 (95%CI 1.63–2.06) [43]**.

Screening

HIV testing should be included in the routine panel of prenatal screening tests for all pregnant women. State law varies as to whether a separate written consent is required. Rescreening is recommended for all women living in areas with high rates of HIV infection. The screening test is shown in Table 15.1. A positive ELISA should be confirmed with a Western blot.

Treatment

Combination drug regimens are considered the standard of care for treatment of HIV infection during pregnancy and should be started according to standard criteria (available at www.aidsinfo.gov). Combination regimens are more effective than single drug regimens in reducing perinatal transmission. Several studies have found an increased risk of PTB among women treated with combination antiretroviral therapy during pregnancy (with and without a protease inhibitor). **However, two large meta-analyses did not find an increased risk of PTB associated with combination therapy compared with no treatment or treatment with one drug [44]**.

Presumptive treatment for vaginal infections (metronidazole and erythromycin vs placebo) did not reduce PTB among HIV positive women in Africa [45].

Human papillomavirus (HPV)

There are more than 40 types of HPV virus which cause anogenital diseases including genital warts, cervical dysplasia, and cervical cancer. More than half of sexually active men and women age 15–45 years old acquire HPV at some point in their lives. **There is no evidence that infection with HPV is directly associated with PTB.** Genital warts rarely can cause pregnancy complications by obstructing the birth canal or causing laryngeal warts in the neonate. **Surgical treatment of cervical dysplasia (cold-knife conization RR 1.99–2.59; large loop excision of the transformation zone RR 1.7; loop electrosurgical excision procedure RR 1.8) and invasive cancer (radical trachelectomy RR 2.0) is associated with an increased risk of PTB [46]**. HPV 16 and 18 account for 70% of cervical dysplasia. **In women who would have been**

treated for cervical intraepithelial neoplasia grade 2 or 3, it is estimated that vaccination with the quadrivalent vaccine (Guardisil®) could reduce PTB by 60% [47]. Women with cervical cancer diagnosed during pregnancy may need to be delivered prematurely to start treatment sooner.

Screening and treatment

The benefit of screening for STIs to reduce PTB has not been proven. Prior studies evaluated screening for common vaginal bacteria (*Gardnerella, Mycoplasma, Ureaplasma*) in addition to STIs. Presumptive treatment of STIs (metronidazole 2 g, cefixime 400 mg, azithromycin 1 g + penicillin if positive for syphilis) did not reduce PTB compared with screening among women in Uganda [48]. Current screening and treatment recommendations reflect maternal and neonatal health benefits. The necessity of performing a test of cure after treatment for STIs for prevention of PTB is insufficiently studied. Future research should also focus on prevention, including preconception, of STIs.

References

1 Goldenberg RL, Culhane JF, Iams JD, Romero R. Epidemiology and causes of preterm birth. Lancet 2008; 371: 75–84.
2 Romero R, Espinoza J, Chaiworapongsa T, Kalache K. Infection and prematurity and the role of preventive strategies. Semin Neonatol 2002; 7: 259–74.
3 Lettieri L, Vintzeleos AM, Rodis JF, Albini SM, Salafia CM. Does 'idiopathic' preterm labor resulting in preterm birth exist? Am J Obstet Gynecol 1993; 168: 1480–5.
4 Cram LF, Zapata MI, Toy EC, Baker B 3rd. Genitourinary infections and their association with preterm labor. Am Fam Physician 2002; 65: 241–8.
5 Swadpanich U, Lumbiganon P, Prasertcharoensook W, Laopaiboon M. Antenatal lower genital tract infection screening and treatment programs for preventing preterm delivery. Cochrane Database Syst Rev 2008; (2): CD006178.
6 Centers for Disease Control and Prevention (CDC). Trends in Reportable Sexually Transmitted Diseases in the United States, 2007. December 2008.
7 Schmid GP, Stoner BP, Hawkes S, Broutet N. The need and plan for global elimination of congenital syphilis. Sex Transm Dis 2007; 34(7 Suppl): s5–10.
8 Finelli L, Berman SM, Koumans EH, Levine WC. Congenital syphilis. Bull World Health Org 1998; 76 (suppl 2): 126–8.
9 Goldenberg RL, Culhane JF, Johnson DC. Maternal infection and adverse fetal and neonatal outcomes. Clin Perinatol 2005; 32: 523–59.
10 Watson-Jones D, Changalucha J, Gumodoka B, *et al.* Syphilis in pregnancy in Tanzania. I. Impact of maternal syphilis on outcome of pregnancy. J Infect Dis 2002; 186: 940–7.

11 Walker GJA, Walker DG. Congenital syphilis: a continuing but neglected problem. Semin Fetal Neonatal Med 2007; 12: 198–206.
12 Walker GJ. Antibiotics for syphilis diagnosed during pregnancy. Cochrane Database Syst Rev 2001; (3): CD001143.
13 Alexander JM, Sheffield JS, Sanchez PJ, *et al.* Efficacy of treatment for syphilis in pregnancy. Obstet Gynecol 1999; 93: 5–8.
14 Donders GGG, Desmyter J, Hooft P, *et al.* Apparent failure of one injection of benzathine penicillin G for syphilis during pregnancy in human immunodeficiency virus-negative African women. Sex Transm Dis 1997; 24: 96–101.
15 Donders GGG. Treatment of sexually transmitted bacterial diseases in pregnant women. Drugs 2000; 59: 477–85.
16 Workowski KA, Berman SM. Sexually Transmitted Disease Treatment Guidelines, 2006. Morbidity and Mortality Weekly Report, volume 55, RR11, August 4, 2006.
17 Xu F, Sternberg MR, Kottiri BJ, *et al.* Trends in Herpes Simplex Virus Type 1 and Type 2 seroprevalence in the United States. JAMA 2006; 8: 964–73.
18 Centers for Disease Control and Prevention. How common are STDs in Pregnant Women in the United States? http: //www.cdc.gov/std/STDFact-STDs&Pregnancy.htm#Common. Last accessed 3/29/09.
19 Brown ZA, Vontver LA, Bendetti J, *et al.* Effects of infants of a first episode of genital herpes during pregnancy. N Engl J Med 1987; 317: 1246–51.
20 Brown ZA, Benedetti J, Selke S, Ashley R, Watts H, Corey L. Asypmtomatic maternal shedding of herpes simplex virus at the onset of labor: relationship to preterm labor. Obstet Gynecol 1996; 87: 483–8.
21 Brown ZA, Gardella C, Wald A, Morrow RA, Corey L. Genital herpes complicating pregnancy. Obstet Gynecol 2005; 106: 845–56.
22 Major CA, Towers CV, Lewis DF, Garite TJ. Expectant management of preterm premature rupture of membranes complicated by active recurrent genital herpes. Am J Obstet Gynecol 2003; 188: 1551–4.
23 Baldwin HE. STD update: screening and therapeutic options. Int J Fertil Womens Med 2001; 2: 79–88.
24 Hoosen AA, Mphatsoe M, Kharsany AB, Moodley J, Bassa A, Bramdev A. Granuloma inguinale in association with pregnancy and HIV infection. Int J Gynaecol Obstet 1996; 53: 133–8.
25 Donders GGG, Desmyter J, De Wet GH, *et al.* The association of gonorrhoea and syphilis with premature birth and low birth weight. Genitourin Med 1993; 69: 98–101.
26 Elliott B, Brunham RC, Laga M, *et al.* Maternal gonococcal infection as a preventable risk factor for low birth weight. J Infect Dis 1990; 161: 531–6
27 O'Neill MA. Gonorrhea. In: Berghella V, ed. Maternal-Fetal Evidence Based Guidelines. London; Informa, 2007: 234–8.
28 O'Neill MA. Chlamydia. In: Berghella V, ed. Maternal-Fetal Evidence Based Guidelines. London; Informa, 2007: 239–4.
29 Sweet RL, Landers DV, Walker C, Schachter J. Chlamydia trachomatis infection and pregnancy outcome. Am J Obstet Gynecol 1987; 156: 824–33.
30 Martin DH, Eschenbach DA, Cotch MF, *et al.* Double-blind placebo-controlled treatment trial of *Chlamydia trachomatis* endocervical infections in pregnant women. Inf Dis Obstet Gynecol 1997; 5: 10–17.
31 Okun, N, Gronau KA, Hannah ME. Antibiotics for bacterial vaginosis or trichomonas vaginalis in pregnancy: a systematic review. Obstet Gynecol 2005; 105: 857–68.

32 Cotch MF, Pastorek JG, Nugent RP, *et al.* Trichomonas vaginalis associated with low birth weight and preterm delivery. The Vaginal Infections and Prematurity Study Group. Sex Transm Dis 1997; 24: 353–60.
33 Grice AC. Vaginal infection causing spontaneous rupture of the membranes and premature delivery. Aust NZ J Obstet Gynaecol 1974; 14: 156–8.
34 Minkoff H, Grunebaum AN, Schwarz RH, *et al.* Risk factor for prematurity and premature rupture of membranes: a prospective study of the vaginal flora in pregnancy. Am J Obstet Gynecol 1984; 150: 965–72.
35 Morgan M, Goldenberg RL, Schulkin J. Obstetrician-gynecologists' screening and management of preterm birth. Obstet Gynecol 2008; 112: 35–40.
36 Gülmezoglu AM. Interventions for treating trichomoniasis in women. Cochrane Database Syst Rev 2003; (2): CD000220.
37 Klebanoff MA, Carey JC, Hauth JC, *et al.* Failure of metronidazole to prevent preterm delivery among pregnant women with asymptomatic Trichomonas vaginalis infection. N Engl J Med 2001; 345: 487–93.
38 Airoldi J. Hepatitis C. In: Berghella V ed. Maternal-Fetal Evidence Based Guidelines. London; Informa: 2007; 219-22.
39 Berkley EM, Leslie KK, Arora S, Qualls C, Dunkelberg JC. Chronic hepatitis C in pregnancy. Obstet Gynecol 2008; 112(2 Pt 1): 304–10.
40 Simms J, Duff P. Viral hepatitis in pregnancy. Semin Perinatol 1993; 17(6): 384–93.
41 Leroy V, Ladner J, Nyiraziraje M, *et al.* Effect of HIV-1 infection on pregnancy outcome in women in Kigali, Rwanda, 1992–1994. Pregnancy and HIV Study Group. AIDS 1998; 12: 643–50.
42 Coley JL, Msamanga GI, Fawzi MC, *et al.* The association between maternal HIV-1 infection and pregnancy outcomes in Dar es Salaam, Tanzania. Br J Obstet Gynecol 2001; 108: 1125–33.
43 Brocklehurst P, French R. The association between maternal HIV infection and perinatal outcome: a systematic review of the literature and meta-analysis. Br J Obstet Gynaecol 1998; 105: 836–48.
44 Public Health Service Task Force. Recommendations for Use of Antiretroviral Drugs in Pregnant HIV-1-Infected Women for Maternal Health and Interventions to Reduce Perinatal HIV-1 Transmission in the United States, July 8, 2008.
45 Goldenberg RL, Mwatha A, Read JS, *et al.* The HPTN 024 Study: the efficacy of antibiotics to prevent chorioamnionitis and preterm birth. Am J Obstet Gynecol 2006; 194: 650–61.
46 Jolley JA, Wing DA. Pregnancy management after cervical surgery. Curr Opin Obstet Gynecol 2008; 20: 528–33.
47 Sjøborg KD, Eskild A. Vaccination against human papillomavirus–an impact on preterm delivery? Estimations based on literature review. Acta Obstet Gynecol Scand 2009; 88: 255–60
48 Gray RH, Wabwire-Mangen F, Kigozi G, *et al.* Randomized trial of presumptive sexually transmitted disease therapy during pregnancy in Rakai, Uganda. Am J Obstet Gynecol 2001; 185: 1209–17.
49 Brocklehurst P. Antibiotics for gonorrhoea in pregnancy. Cochrane Database Syst Rev 2002; (2): CD000098.
50 Brocklehurst P, Rooney G. Interventions for treating genital Chlamydia trachomatis infection in pregnancy. Cochrane Database Syst Rev 2000; (2): CD000054.

CHAPTER 16

Multiple Gestations: Preventing and Managing Preterm Birth

Edward J. Hayes[1] *& Suneet P. Chauhan*[2]

[1]Division of Maternal-Fetal Medicine, The Women's Center at Aurora Bay Care Medical Center and [2]Aurora Sinai Medical Center, Milwaukee, Wisconsin, USA

Key points

- The incidence of multiple gestations has increased over the past several decades.
- Preterm birth (PTB) is the primary reason for increased morbidity and mortality in multiples.
- Interventions which appear to be beneficial to decrease the incidence of PTB in multiples are:
  - Reduced embryo and blastocyst transfers
  - Reduction of higher order (≥ 3) multiples
- Interventions which have not been shown to decrease the incidence of PTB, and therefore should be abandoned, are:
  - Prophylactic tocolytics
  - Progesterone supplementation
  - Bed rest
  - Cerclage
  - Home uterine activity monitoring
  - Cervical length (CL) screening in asymptomatic patients
- Currently, the only proven effective approach to prevention of PTB in multiple gestations is avoidance of multiple gestations.
- Of twin gestations who present with symptoms of preterm labor only 20% will deliver within 7 days.
- Fetal fibronectin's negative predictive value is 97% for delivery in the next 14 days in multiples with symptoms of preterm labor.
- CL < 25 mm in women with multiple gestations between 24 and 36 weeks can be used as a threshold that distinguishes true from false labor.
- Tocolysis use has not been shown to decrease neonatal morbidity or mortality and is associated with an increased incidence of side effects in multiples.
- Antenatal corticosteroids should be given to woman diagnosed with preterm labor or preterm premature rupture of the membranes (PPROM) between 24 and 34 weeks gestation regardless of the number of fetuses.

Preterm Birth. Edited by Vincenzo Berghella. © 2010 Blackwell Publishing

Background

The recent increases in preterm birth (PTB) rates in the United States are attributable in part to increases in multiple gestations (Chapter 4). The incidence of multiple gestations has increased substantially over the past several decades due to assisted reproductive technology. The total rate for multiple gestations reported in the US in 2005 was 33.8 per 1000 live births [1]. Twins rates are stable at 32.2/1000 live births, while triplets and higher order multiples live births have declined 16% from the peak in 1998 of 193.5/100 00 to 161.8/100 000 [1].

Preterm birth is the primary reason for the increased morbidity and mortality associated with multiples. Interestingly, the gestational age of delivery with multiple gestations has decreased over the past 15 years. The percentage of twins delivered prior to 37 weeks has risen from 48 to 60% from 1990 to 2005. This trend toward earlier delivery has been mirrored in triplets with 50.2% delivering prior to 34 weeks in 2000 and then 64.1% in 2005 [1]. This trend toward increasing numbers of multiples and early gestational age at delivery has resulted in multiples accounting for 30% of very low birth infants and 20% of infant mortality [2]. Long-term morbidity can also be correlated based on the number of fetuses at the time of delivery. The cerebral palsy rate of 1.6 per 1000 for a singleton increases by several fold with each additional fetus to 7.3 per 1000 for twins and 28 per 1000 for triplets [3].

Prevention strategies for preterm birth in multiples (Table 16.1)

Asymptomatic women

Reduced IVF transfers

Understanding the adverse outcomes associated with higher order multiples, the practice Committee of the Society for Assisted Reproductive Technology and the Practice Committee of the American Society for Reproductive Medicine reported that one should view higher-order multiple pregnancy (three or more implanted embryos) as an undesirable consequence (outcome) of assisted reproductive technologies (ART). In order to decrease the likelihood of a higher order multiple, **recommendations were made for the number of embryo transfers at IVF** (Table 16.2) [4].

The clinical impact of these recommendations has already been observed. The percentage of pregnancies with three or more fetuses has declined consistently since the implementation of the guidelines, with the steepest decline in those pregnancies achieved with ART (20.8% decrease) between

Table 16.1 Strategies for prevention of preterm birth (PTB) related to multiple gestations.

Effective in preventing PTB
- Reduced embryo and blastocyst transfers
- Reduction of higher order (≥3) multiples

Not shown to be beneficial
- Prophylactic tocolytics
- Progesterone supplementation
- Bed rest
- Cervical length screening
- Fetal fibronectin screening
- Cerclage
- Home uterine activity monitoring

Table 16.2 Society for Assisted Reproductive Technology and American Society for Reproductive Medicine Recommendations for IVF (in-vitro fertilization) transfers. *Favorable prognosis is first cycle of IVF, good embryo quality, excess embryos available for cryopreservation, or previous successful IVF cycle.

Maternal age	Prognosis*	Transfers	
		Embryos	Blastocysts
<35 years	Favorable	1-2	1
	Others	2	2
35–37 years	Favorable	2	2
	Others	3	2
38–40 years	Favorable	3	2
	Others	4	3
>40 years	Favorable	5	3
	Others	5	3

1998 and 1999, after the publication in 1998 of the American Society for Reproductive Guidelines [5].

Reduction of higher order multiples

One strategy for reducing the rate of PTB in multiple gestations is **selective reduction**. Pregnancy reduction to twins has been associated with a reduction in pregnancy loss, antenatal complications, PTB < 36 weeks, low birth weight and neonatal death. The resulting conception outcomes are comparable to spontaneously conceived twins. It is important to consider that the evidence for this intervention is drawn from non-randomized trials, and therefore any results or conclusions must be interpreted with caution [6]. Although **the reduction from quadruplets or greater to twins has been endorsed**, selective reduction from triplets to twins has not been uniformly recommended due to whether the increased risk of pregnancy loss associated with selective reduction would be offset by the improved outcome. The largest cohort study examined the rate of pregnancy loss prior to 24 weeks in those electing embryo reduction (8.1% vs 4.4%; RR 1.83, 95% CI = 1.08–3.16), which was compared with the rate of PTB < 32 weeks (10.4% vs 26.7%; RR = 0.37, 95% CI 0.27–0.51). Seven (95% CI = 5–9) reductions needed to be performed to prevent one early PTB, while the number of reductions that will cause one miscarriage was 26 (95% CI 14–193) [7].

Prophylactic tocolytics

Several trials have examined the use of prophylactic oral betamimetics to delay delivery in twins. A meta-analysis which examined this intervention showed that it did not reduce PTB < 37 weeks (RR 0.85, 95% CI 0.65–1.10) or <34 weeks (RR 0.47, 95% CI 0.15–1.50). There was no change in low birth weight (RR 1.19, 95% CI 0.77–1.85) or neonatal mortality (RR 0.80, 95% CI 0.35–1.82). Therefore there is insufficient evidence to support prophylactic oral betamimetics in twins [8].

Progesterone

Progesterone has been shown to decrease the incidence of recurrent PTB in those with a singleton gestation [9]. The use of progesterone in multiples has **not been shown to decrease** the incidence of perinatal death (RR 1.95, 0.37–10.33), **PTB < 37 weeks** (RR 1.01, 0.92–1.12), birthweight < 2500 g (RR 0.94, 0.86–1.02), respiratory distress (RR 1.13, 0.86–1.48), intraventricular hemorrhage grade 3 or 4 (RR 1.20, 0.40–3.54), necrotizing enterocolitis (RR 0.77, 0.17–3.42)) or neonatal sepsis (RR 0.95, 0.55–1.63) [10].

Bed rest

Routine hospitalization for bed rest in multiple pregnancy **has not been proven to be beneficial** for a reduction in PTB or perinatal death. In fact, it is associated with an increase in PTB < 34 weeks in asymptomatic twin gestations [11].

Cervical length screening

A common practice today is to routinely perform cervical lengths (CL) in asymptomatic women with multiple gestations. In a recent retrospective analysis of this practice there was no difference in gestational age at delivery (34.8 weeks vs 35.3, $P = 0.35$), delivery less than 28 weeks (8.2% vs 3.9%, $P = 0.21$), but an increase in maternal antepartum length of stay (CL 34.5 days vs No CL 31.3 days [$P < 0.001$]) [12]. Moreover, cerclage for short cervix has not been shown to be beneficial (see below). Therefore this practice **can not be endorsed** (Chapter 12).

Fetal fibronectin (FFN) screening

Women with twin gestations with a CL ≥ 30 mm or FFN negative at 24 weeks have approximately a 5% incidence of PTB < 32 weeks. Nonetheless, there are **no trials evaluating FFN screening in multiple gestations**, and therefore this practice is not evidence-based, and should be discouraged (Chapter 13).

Cerclage

The use of cerclage in multiple gestations has been examined both as a prophylactic intervention and when a short cervix is noted on ultrasound. The use of **history-indicated** cerclage for twin gestations in a randomized trial was shown **not to prevent PTB** [13]. History-indicated cerclage did not show improvement in triplet gestations [14]. The use of cerclage for prevention of PTB in asymptomatic women with twins with a **short CL < 25 mm** on transvaginal ultrasound appears to **increase the risk of PTB < 35 weeks** (RR 2.15, CI 1.15–4.01) [15].

Home uterine activity monitoring

This practice has **not been shown to be beneficial** in the prevention of PTB in multiple gestations and should be abandoned [16].

Symptomatic women

Preterm labor

Diagnosis

Of twin gestations who present with symptoms of preterm labor (PTL), only 20% will deliver within 7 days [17].

- **FFN.** The utility of FFN in evaluation of twin gestations with symptoms of PTL is not related to its ability to predict who will deliver in the next 14 days (19% positive predictive value), but rather to the test ability to determine who is not going to deliver during this time frame (97% negative predictive value) [18]. FFN's high negative predictive value identifies low risk women, therefore avoiding hospitalization and unnecessary intervention (Chapters 13 and 18).
- **CL. A CL of 25 mm** in woman presenting with regular and painful uterine contractions between 24 and 36 weeks, **can be used as a threshold that distinguishes between true and false labor, again avoiding unnecessary interventions** (Chapters 12 and 18) [17].

Interventions

- **Tocolytics.** The use of tocolytics for the treatment of PTL in multiple gestations has **not been shown to decrease the incidence of delivery within 7 days** of treatment, perinatal or neonatal death, or the neonatal complications of respiratory distress syndrome, necrotizing enterocolitis or cerebral palsy [19]. This lack of proven efficacy and the amplification of side effects with these medications in multiples, lead the American College of Obstetrics and Gynecology to comment they should be used judiciously in this population [20].

- **Antenatal corticosteroids.** The use of antenatal corticosteroids has been shown to decrease the incidence of neonatal death (RR 0.69, 95% CI 0.58–0.81), respiratory distress syndrome (RR 0.66, 95% CI 0.43–0.69), cerebroventricular hemorrhage (RR 0.54, 95% CI 0.43–0.69), necrotizing enterocolitis (RR 0.46, 95% CI 0.29–0.74) and systemic infections within the first 48 hours of life (RR 0.56, 95% CI 0.38–0.58) in a large meta-analyses of trials involving mostly singleton gestations [21]. Although none of the studies specifically addressed use in multiples, the National Institutes of Health recommends that **all women in preterm labor between 24–34 weeks, regardless of the number of fetuses, should be given a course of antenatal corticosteroids [22]** (Chapter 20).

Preterm premature rupture of the membranes (PPROM)

There are **no interventions proven specifically in multiple gestations to decrease PTB once PPROM has occurred**. Management of PPROM in multiple gestations usually follows recommendations for singleton gestations (Chapter 19).

References

1 Martin JA, Hamilton BE, Sutton PD, *et al.* Births: Final data for 2005. National Vital Statistics Reports. Vol 56 #6.
2 Magee BD. Role of multiple births in very low birth weight and infant mortality. J Repro Med 2004; 49: 812–6
3 Peterson B, Nelson KB, Watson L, Stanly F. Twins, triplets and cerebral palsy in births in Western Australia in the 1980s. BMJ 1993; 307: 1239–43.
4 The Practice Committee of the Society for Assisted Reproductive Technology and the Practice Committee of the American Society for Reproductive Medicine. Guidelines on Number Of Embryos Transferred. Fertil Steril 2006; 86 (Suppl 4): S51–2.
5 Jain T, Missmer SA, Hornstein MD. Trends in embryo-transfer practice and in outcomes of the use of assisted reproductive technology in the United States. N Engl J Med 2004; 350: 1639–45.
6 Dodd JM, Crowther CA. Reduction of the number of fetuses for women with triplet and higher order multiple pregnancies. Cochrane Database Syst Rev 2003, Issue 2. Art. No.: CD003932. DOI: 10.1002/14651858.CD003932.
7 Papageorghiou AT, Avigidou K, Bakoulas V, Sebire NJ, Nicolaides KH. Risk of miscarriage and early preterm birth in trichorionic triplet pregnancies with embryo reduction versus expectant management: new data and systematic review. Hum Reprod 2006; 21: 912–7.
8 Yamasmit W, Chaithongwongwatthana S, Tolosa JE, Pereira L, Lumbiganon P. Prophylactic oral betamimetics for reducing preterm birth in woman with a twin

pregnancy. Cochrane Database Syst Rev 2005, Issue 3. Art. No.: CD004733. DOI: 10.1002/14651858.CD004733.pub2.
9 Meis PJ, Klebanoff M, Thom E, *et al.* Prevention of recurrent preterm delivery by 17 alpha-hydroxyprogesterone caproate. N Engl J Med 2003; 348: 2379–85.
10 Dodd JM, Flenady VJ, Concotta R, Crowther CA. Progesterone for the prevention of preterm birth a systematic review. Obstet Gynecol 2008; 112: 127–34.
11 Crowther CA. Hospitalisation and bed rest for multiple pregnancy. Cochrane Database Systematic Rev 2001, Issue 1. Art. No.: CD000110.DOI: 10.1002/14651858. CD000110.
12 Gyamfi C, Lerner V, Holzman I, Stone J. Routine cervical length in twins and perinatal outcomes. Am J Perinatol 2007; 24: 65–70.
13 Dor J, Shalev J. Mashiach S, *et al.* Elective cervical suture of twin pregnancies diagnosed ultrasonically in the first trimester following induced ovulation. Gynecol Obstet Invest 1982; 13: 55–60.
14 Rebarber A, Roman AS, Istwan N, Rhea D, Staziano G. Prophylactic cerclage in the management of triplet pregnancies. Am J Obstet Gynecol 2005; 193: 1193–6.
15 Berghella V, Obido A, To M, Rust O, Althuisius S. Cerclage for short cervix on ultrasound meta-analysis of trials using individual patient-level data. Obstet Gynecol 2005; 106: 181–9.
16 Colton T, Kayne H, Zhang Y. A meta-analysis of home uterine activity monitoring. Am J Obstet Gynecol 1995; 173: 1499–505.
17 Fuchs I, Tsoi E, Henrich W, Dudenhausen J, Nicolaides K. Sonographic measurement of cervical length in twin pregnancies in threatened preterm labor. Ultrasound Obstet Gynecol 2004; 23: 42–5.
18 Singer E, Pilpel S, Bsat F, Plevyak M, Healy A, Markenson, G. Accuracy of fetal fibronectin to predict preterm birth in twin gestations with symptoms of labor. Obstet Gynecol 2007; 109: 1083–7.
19 Anotayanonth S, Subhedar NV, Garner P, Neilson JP, Harigopal S. Betamimetics for inhibiting preterm labour. Cochrane Database Syst Rev 2004 Oct 18; (4) CD004352.
20 Multiple gestation: Complicated Twin, Triplet, and Higher-Order Multifetal Pregnancy. ACOG Practice Bulletin. Number 56, October 2004.
21 Roberts D, Dalziel S. Antenatal corticosteroids for accelerating fetal lung maturation for women at risk of preterm birth. Cochrane Database Syst Rev 2006; 3: CD004454.
22 Effect of corticosteroids for fetal maturation on perinatal outcomes. NIH Consensus Statement 1994; 12: 1–24.

CHAPTER 17

Asymptomatic Manual Cervical Changes

Leonardo Pereira
Division of Maternal-Fetal Medicine, Oregon Health and Science University, Oregon, USA

Key points

- In contrast to cervical shortening noted only on ultrasound, 90% of women with cervical dilation in the second trimester deliver preterm. Therefore clinical interventions should be considered in these women.
- In all women with asymptomatic manually-detected cervical changes, active labor, bleeding, ruptured membranes, and intra-amniotic infection (IAI) must be excluded before cerclage can be offered. An amniocentesis to rule-out IAI should be strongly considered.
- Placement of a physical exam-indicated cerclage should be considered for all women with a singleton gestation and premature manually-detected cervical dilation prior to 24 weeks gestation.
- Cerclage cannot be recommended at this time for women with multifetal gestations or uterine anomalies.
- There is insufficient evidence to recommend bed rest, progesterone, pessary, indomethacin or other therapies for the asymptomatic woman with manually-detected cervical changes in the second trimester.

Introduction

Asymptomatic cervical changes prior to 28 weeks gestation occur commonly and are associated with increased risk for preterm birth (PTB), intra-amniotic infection (IAI), and preterm premature rupture of the membranes (PPROM). The factors that determine which individuals with asymptomatic cervical changes will go on to deliver healthy term infants and which ones will develop adverse pregnancy outcomes are as yet unidentified and the focus of ongoing research. At present, individuals who display cervical changes in the second trimester and then suffer a miscarriage, early PTB or PPROM, are identified as having cervical insufficiency, a clinical diagnosis with a poorly defined phenotype (Chapter 6). The following chapter reviews the **identification and management of**

Preterm Birth. Edited by Vincenzo Berghella. © 2010 Blackwell Publishing

asymptomatic cervical changes detected by manual exam in the second trimester and suspicious for cervical insufficiency, highlighting the deficits in our knowledge base which limit the effectiveness of available treatments.

The changing cervix during pregnancy

Presentation and natural history

Unfortunately, cervical effacement and dilation are usually asymptomatic unless the process is advanced. In fact, the classic definition of cervical insufficiency is recurrent painless second trimester cervical dilation. Occasionally, cervical changes are accompanied by increased vaginal discharge or increased pelvic pressure, but these symptoms are not reliable enough to serve as sufficient screening questions. In one recent multicentered observational study, over 40% of patients with cervical dilation did not present until after amniotic membranes had prolapsed to the external cervical os, and 15% of women did not present until amniotic membranes or fetal parts had prolapsed into the vagina [1]. Typically, patients present with clinical symptoms only once they are in preterm labor (PTL) (Chapter 18) or have developed chorioamnionitis or PPROM (Chapter 19).

Assessing the cervix during pregnancy: manually-detected asymptomatic cervical changes

Spontaneous birth must occur through a dilated cervix. Therefore, assessing cervical status during pregnancy can predict, and perhaps help prevent PTB. Cervical status can be checked by ultrasound or manual (digital) exam. Cervical assessment by ultrasound for prevention of PTB was extensively reviewed in Chapter 12.

Ultrasound-detected cervical changes occur earlier than manually-detected changes. About 75% of women with a short cervical length (CL) on transvaginal ultrasound (TVU) (defined as < 25 mm) have no detectable changes on manual exam. That is, the cervix feels closed and long on digital exam [2]. Most low-risk women with a short CL before 24 weeks deliver at term (Chapter 12). Instead, **second trimester cervical dilation and/or effacement detected on manual exam are never normal** and should always be considered an ominous finding. This is because manual exam detects changes that, starting originally at the internal os and detectable first only on TVU CL, now have extended all the way to the external os, which is the part palpable on manual cervical exam. With regards to **infectious morbidity**, the prevalence of subclinical chorioamnionitis in this population is substantial, affecting at least 25% of women with premature cervical dilation [3] (Chapter 7). Furthermore, the risk for

PTB is extremely high. Without treatment, over 90% of women with premature cervical dilation deliver prior to 37 weeks gestation, and approximately 2/3 of them deliver prior to 28 weeks [1, 4–7]. This outcome appears to be independent of obstetric history. In a cohort of 73 women with second trimester cervical dilation who were expectantly managed, the risk of PTB prior to 28 weeks was 68% among women with a history of PTB and 67% in women with no prior PTB [1].

Work-up

When a woman with asymptomatic cervical changes detected by manual exam in the second trimester (before 28 weeks) is identified, a **detailed history** should be obtained (Chapter 4). The history should focus on obstetric outcomes, prior cervical surgeries, known gynecologic pathology, or uterine cavity malformations. Symptoms of increased discharge, bleeding, cramping or leaking need to be explored. Risk factors for cervical insufficiency include a history of prior PTBs (especially before 32 weeks gestation), previous midtrimester pregnancy losses, history of cervical conization or loop electrosurgical excision procedure, exposure to diethylstilbestrol, previous procedures requiring cervical dilation, or known uterine anomaly.

On physical exam, a sterile speculum examination should be performed first to exclude cervical–vaginal infections (Chapter 15), bleeding and ruptured membranes. A gentle digital examination should be performed to evaluate the degree of cervical dilation in centimeters, effacement recorded as centimeters of cervical length (more reliable than effacement reported as percentage), station, cervical position and cervical consistency. **Repeated manual cervical exams should be avoided**, as they may worsen the inflammation and infectious processes that may be already in process. An ultrasound should be performed to confirm gestational age, plurality, placentation and to exclude any congenital malformations. A **TVU CL should be considered**, as the risk of PTB can be better estimated by this test. In fact, a few women with a minimally-dilated cervix on manual exam have a reassuring CL > 25 mm on TVU, and can be reassured. A finding of a TVU CL ≤ 15 mm confirms high risk for PTB. **Tocodynanometry** should be considered to assess contraction frequency. Prior to any surgical interventions, **IAI should be excluded**. In the absence of reliable non-invasive tests to diagnosis IAI, the best available option is to **perform a transabdominal amniocentesis**. This procedure is safe in this setting [8]. Amniotic fluid evaluation should include amniotic fluid cultures (aerobic, anaerobic and ureaplasmas), microbial PCR if available, Gram stain, leukocyte count and glucose (Chapter 7).

Treatment options

For patients with asymptomatic cervical changes, treatment options, both surgical and non-surgical, should be based on at least three aspects: cervical assessment, gestational age, and history including review of all risk factors of PTB.

Bed rest

Bed rest is used in nearly one in five pregnancies to prevent or treat a wide variety of conditions, including threatened PTB [9]. However, there is **little evidence of effectiveness** [10]. Despite the assumption that bed rest is benign, the psychological and financial costs are considerable. For women with a dilated cervix, particularly in the setting of prolapsed or bulging amniotic membranes, bed rest appears to be universally prescribed, again without supportive evidence. Any decision to place a patient with asymptomatic cervical changes on bed rest should be made with respect to the emotional and financial consequences to the patient and disclosure that published data does not demonstrate efficacy.

Physical-exam indicated cervical cerclage

With the exception of patients with uterine anomalies or multifetal gestations, there appears to be a beneficial role for cervical cerclage in select women with asymptomatic cervical changes, particularly for those who are being followed serially during pregnancy and in whom progressive cervical changes during pregnancy are observed. In all cases, the benefits and risks of cerclage compared with noninvasive therapies must be discussed with the patient. **Contraindications** to cerclage includes labor, active bleeding, intra-amniotic infection and ruptured membranes. In addition, the fetus should be carefully evaluated preoperatively to exclude aneuploidy or any life threatening congenital anomalies that may impact a patient's decision about whether or not to undergo cerclage.

The clinical approach to women with an obstetric history suggestive of cervical insufficiency and the use of history-indicated cerclage (also referred to as prophylactic cerclage) typically performed at 11–15 weeks gestational age in the absence of any asymptomatic cervical changes are discussed further in Chapter 11. Ultrasound-indicated cerclage, performed for the finding of a short CL on ultrasound before 24 weeks, is discussed in Chapter 12.

Unlike women with asymptomatic cervical shortening, **all women with second trimester cervical dilation should be considered at increased risk of PTB**. Perhaps because cervical insufficiency is common among these patients, multiple studies suggest that physical examination-indicated cerclage is beneficial [1, 4–7]. However, only one of these trials was randomized [7]. That study, published by Althuisius in 2003, reported that among women with a history of cervical insufficiency who developed premature cervical dilation, 100% of those randomly assigned to bed rest delivered prior to 34 weeks gestation (10/10), compared with only 54% of women assigned to bed rest plus cerclage (7/13). These findings are consistent with the findings of two retrospective case series with controls, which included 37 [4] and 70 [5] women, and one prospective nonrandomized study of 46 women without a history of cervical insufficiency [6]. In our own observational cohort study of 225 women, placement of cerclage similarly resulted in a favorable outcome (reduced PTB, increased birth weight, increased neonatal survival), once labor, bleeding, PPROM and chorioamnionitis were ruled out [1]. These observed benefits persisted after controlling for cervical dilation and gestational age, and appeared beneficial even in the subgroup of women with no prior PTB who were considered low risk for cervical insufficiency at the start of the pregnancy.

Among women with multifetal gestations who develop premature cervical dilation, data on cerclage efficacy is lacking. Since there is evidence that ultrasound-indicated cerclage is not beneficial in this population [11–13], physical examination-indicated cerclage in the face of cervical dilation cannot be recommended for women with multifetal gestations.

Excluding women with uterine anomalies, **a physical-exam indicated cerclage should be offered to all women with a singleton gestation and premature cervical dilation prior to 24 weeks** as long as contraindications (labor, bleeding, ruptured membranes, intra-amniotic infection) have been excluded. Although supporting data is lacking, cerclage after 24 weeks gestation may be a reasonable option in settings where clinical care for extremely preterm neonates is unavailable and delivery prior to 26 weeks gestation is likely.

Once the decision to perform a cerclage has been made, **many techniques and surgical variations have been described**. One option is the McDonald cerclage, which involves placing a continuous purse string suture around the base of the cervix. Alternate techniques, including the Shirodkar (without or without posterior vaginal dissection) and the Wurm techniques are also employed, although less commonly. Additional clinical adjuncts, such as the use of perioperative antibiotics, anti-inflammatory medication, activity restriction, and tocolytic therapy are commonly employed despite lack of evidence supporting their efficacy. Direct comparisons between methods and other surgical considerations, such as selection of suture material, need further study before specific recommendations can be made.

Cerclage placement, especially in the setting of advanced cervical dilation, can be technically difficult. The reported rate of intraoperative membrane rupture with physical examination-indicated cerclage is between 4 and 19% [14–16] and is likely even higher when amniotic membranes have prolapsed into the vagina. Multiple techniques to reduce amniotic membrane prolapse have been published including amnioreduction [17], use of a Foley catheter balloon or covered sponge stick to push the membranes up into the lower uterine segment [18], and Trendelenberg positioning. None of these strategies has been definitively shown to improve cerclage success, and implementation of these techniques should be left to individual operator judgment and experience.

Pessary

Theoretically, placement of a vaginal pessary may prolong pregnancy by altering gravitational force vectors that promote cervical dilation among women with cervical insufficiency. **No trial comparing pessary with no pessary for prevention of PTB has been published**. To date, one prospective randomized study has been performed comparing pessary with cerclage, and concluded that pessary and cerclage were of equal efficacy [19]. In this study, published by Forster in 1986, 250 patients thought to have cervical insufficiency were enrolled: 112 patients received inpatient cerclage, 130 patients received outpatient pessary, and eight patients received bed rest alone (however, these eight were subsequently dropped from the analysis). Limitations of this study, in addition to post-enrollment exclusion of subjects, include no mention of the type of pessary used, vague inclusion criteria, and late initiation of therapy (mean gestational age of 27 weeks), calling into question whether the study population had true cervical insufficiency. A review article, published in 2000, concluded that pessaries should not replace cerclage in women with cervical insufficiency because of the poor nature of most studies (the majority are retrospective case reviews) [20]. At this time, **pessaries should not be offered as first line therapy for women with cervical insufficiency**. However, in light of the safety benefits of non-surgical treatment options and recent observational studies in which pessary use compared favorably to bed rest and cerclage [21–23], the potential role of pessaries for prevention of PTB among women with suspected cervical insufficiency merits further study.

Progesterone

There is **no randomized trial** on the effectiveness of progesterone, of any kind, to prevent PTB in women with asymptomatic manually-detected cervical changes in the second trimester. Based on current data, women with a short cervix (<15 mm) prior to 24 weeks gestation can be counseled regarding one positive trial showing benefit with micronized vaginal progesterone supplementation from time of diagnosis of short TVU CL until 37 weeks gestation [24] (Chapter 12).

Indomethacin

Given that premature cervical changes in the second trimester have been associated with severe inflammation, anti-inflammatory therapy has been proposed as an intervention for women with such changes. Women with asymptomatic cervical changes also often have contractions, so a tocolytic agent could be postulated to help. Indomethacin is both an anti-inflammatory agent and an effective tocolytic (Chapter 18). There are **no randomized trials** to assess its efficacy in women with asymptomatic cervical changes in the second trimester. In a prospective cohort, indomethacin therapy in women with a dilated cervix at 14–25 weeks had no significant effects on pregnancy outcomes [25]. Given trends for benefit, further study is warranted.

References

1 Pereira L, Cotter A, Gómez R, *et al.* Expectant management compared with physical examination-indicated cerclage (EM-PEC) in selected women with a dilated cervix at 14(0/7)-25(6/7) weeks: results from the EM-PEC international cohort study. Am J Obstet Gynecol 2007; 197: 483 e1–8.

2 Berghella V, Tolosa JE, Kuhlman K, Weiner S, Bolognese RJ, Wapner RJ. Cervical ultrasonography compared with manual examination as a predictor of preterm delivery. Am J Obstet Gynecol 1997; 177: 723–30.

3 Gomez R, Romero R, Nien JK, *et al.* A short cervix in women with preterm labor and intact membranes: a risk factor for microbial invasion of the amniotic cavity. Am J Obstet Gynecol 2005; 192: 678–89.

4 Novy MJ, Gupta A, Wothe DD, Gupta S, Kennedy KA, Gravett MG. Cervical cerclage in the second trimester of pregnancy: a historical cohort study. Am J Obstet Gynecol 2001; 184: 1447–54; discussion 1454–6.

5 Olatunbosun OA, al-Nuaim L, Turnell RW. Emergency cerclage compared with bed rest for advanced cervical dilatation in pregnancy. Int Surg 1995; 80: 170–4.

6 Daskalakis G, Papantoniou N, Mesogitis S, Antsaklis A. Management of cervical insufficiency and bulging fetal membranes. Obstet Gynecol 2006; 107(2 Pt 1): 221–6.

7 Althuisius SM, Dekker GA, Hummel P, van Geijn HP. Cervical incompetence prevention randomized cerclage trial: emergency cerclage with bed rest versus bed rest alone. Am J Obstet Gynecol 2003; 189: 907–10.

8 Airoldi J, Pereira L, Cotter A *et al.* Amniocentesis prior to physical exam-indicated cerclage in women with midtrimester cervical dilation: results from the expectant management compared to Physical Exam-indicated Cerclage international cohort study. Am J Perinatol 2009; 26: 63–8.

9 Goldenberg RL, Cliver SP, Bronstein J, Cutter GR, Andrews WW, Mennemeyer ST. Bed rest in pregnancy. Obstet Gynecol 1994; 84: 131–6.

10 Sosa C, Althabe F, Belizán J, Bergel E. Bed rest in singleton pregnancies for preventing preterm birth. Cochrane Database Syst Rev 2004(1): p. CD003581.
11 Roman AS, Rebarber A, Pereira L, Sfakianaki AK, Mulholland J, Berghella V. The efficacy of sonographically indicated cerclage in multiple gestations. J Ultrasound Med 2005; 24: 763–8; quiz 770–1.
12 Rebarber A, Roman AS, Istwan N, Rhea D, Stanziano G. Prophylactic cerclage in the management of triplet pregnancies. Am J Obstet Gynecol 2005; 193: 1193–6.
13 Berghella V, Odibo AO, To MS, Rust OA, Althuisius SM. Cerclage for short cervix on ultrasonography: meta-analysis of trials using individual patient-level data. Obstet Gynecol 2005; 106: 181–9.
14 Higuchi M, Hirano H, Maki M. Emergency cervical cerclage using a metreurynter in patients with bulging membranes. Acta Obstet Gynecol Scand 1992; 71: 34–8.
15 Wong GP, Farquharson DF, Dansereau J. Emergency cervical cerclage: a retrospective review of 51 cases. Am J Perinatol 1993; 10: 341–7.
16 Barth WH, Jr, Yeomans ER, Hankins GD. Emergent cerclage. Surg Gynecol Obstet 1990; 170: 323–6.
17 Locatelli A, Vergani P, Bellini P, Strobelt N, Arreghini A, Ghidini A. Amnioreduction in emergency cerclage with prolapsed membranes: comparison of two methods for reducing the membranes. Am J Perinatol 1999; 16: 73–7.
18 Holman MR. An aid for cervical cerclage. Obstet Gynecol 1973; 42: 68–9.
19 Förster F, During R, Schwarzlos G. Therapy of cervix insufficiency-cerclage or support pessary?. Zentralbl Gynaekol 1986; 108: 230–7.
20 Newcomer J. Pessaries for the treatment of incompetent cervix and premature delivery. Obstet Gynecol Surv 2000; 55: 443–8.
21 Acharya G, Eschler B, Grønberg M, Hentemann M, Ottersen T, Maltau JM. Noninvasive cerclage for the management of cervical incompetence: a prospective study. Arch Gynecol Obstet 2006; 273: 283–7.
22 Antczak-Judycka A, Sawicki W, Spiewankiewicz B, Cendrowski K, Stelmachów J. [Comparison of cerclage and cerclage pessary in the treatment of pregnant women with incompetent cervix and threatened preterm delivery]. Ginekol Pol 2003; 74: 1029–36.
23 Arabin B, Halbesma JR, Vork F, Hübener M, van Eyck J. Is treatment with vaginal pessaries an option in patients with a sonographically detected short cervix? J Perinat Med 2003; 31: 122–33.
24 Fonseca EB, Celik E, Parra M, Singh M, Nicolaides KH. Fetal Medicine Foundation Second Trimester Screening Group. Progesterone and the risk of preterm birth among women with a short cervix. N Engl J Med 2007; 357: 462–9.
25 Berghella V, Prasertcharoensuk W, Cotter A, *et al.* Does indomethacin prevent preterm birth in women with cervical dilatation in the second trimester? Am J Perinatol 2009; 26: 13–9.

CHAPTER 18

Preterm Labor

Amen Ness, Yair Blumenfeld & Joyce F. Sung

Division of Maternal-Fetal Medicine, Department of Obstetrics and Gynecology, Stanford University Medical Center, CA, USA

Key points

- Preterm labor (PTL) is responsible for about half of all preterm births (PTB).
- Treatment of symptomatic women with PTL has not reduced the rate of PTB.
- PTL must be considered and ruled out in any pregnant woman after 16–20 weeks with abdominal or pelvic symptoms (e.g. persistent pelvic pressure, increasing vaginal discharge, backache and menstrual-like cramps), but treatment should only be initiated once the diagnosis is made.
- Early in pregnancy, especially the late second and early third trimester, symptoms may be subtle and easily confused with common pregnancy symptoms.
- Digital examination in women less than 3 cm dilated is subjective and imprecise, yet, most women being evaluated for PTL are less than 3 cm dilated.
- Women without cervical change or with advanced dilation should not be treated with tocolytics.
- Pooled data suggests a transvaginal ultrasound (TVU) cervical length (CL) of >30 mm has a negative predictive value of 80–100% for PTB < 34–37 weeks and >95% for delivery within 7 days. On the other hand, women with CL < 15–20 mm have a 20–50% risk for PTB within 7 days and a >60% chance of PTB < 35 weeks. Management of PTL based on knowledge of TVU CL (in association with fetal fibronectin) has been shown to be associated with a lower incidence of PTB.
- Appropriate management of PTL depends on what the anticipated neonatal morbidity/mortality would be if the fetus delivered.
- Overt clinical signs of intramniotic infection and contraindications to tocolysis should be identified.
- Transport of mothers with PTL to the appropriate level of facilities for their gestational age is an important means to reduce neonatal mortality and morbidity. Use of tocolytics may allow for this transport.
- The goals of tocolysis are to prevent imminent PTB in order to have sufficient time to administer corticosteroids, and (if needed) allow for maternal *in utero* transfer to a hospital with appropriate neonatal care.

(Continued)

Preterm Birth. Edited by Vincenzo Berghella.

- Given their safety profiles and effectiveness at delaying delivery for both 48 hours and 7 days, nifedipine (as usual first line) and indomethacin (for ≤48 hours) are the primary tocolyics we mostly use clinically.
- There is no evidence to support the use of maintenance tocolysis after successful arrest of PTL.
- All women being treated for PTL between 24 and 34 weeks should be given antenatal steroids (ACS). Use of ACS is recommended between 24 and 34 weeks gestation. In earlier or later gestational ages, use of ACS is still experimental.
- Weekly dosing of ACS is not recommended. Recent evidence suggests that a single 'rescue' course of ACS may safe for short-term outcomes and effective at reducing respiratory complications.

Introduction

Preterm labor (PTL) is the final phenotypic pathway associated with about half of all preterm births (PTBs). In this chapter we will discuss evaluation, management, and follow-up of women with PTL (Table 18.1).

Diagnosis of PTL

Whenever a pregnant woman presents with abdominal or pelvic symptoms (e.g. persistent pelvic pressure, increasing vaginal discharge, backache and menstrual-like cramps) after 16–20 weeks of pregnancy and before 37 weeks, PTL must be considered and ruled out. **Treatment should be initiated only once the diagnosis is made**. Early in pregnancy, especially the late second and early third trimester, symptoms may be subtle and easily confused with common pregnancy symptoms.

Table 18.1 Major issues in management of preterm labour (PTL).

1 Making an accurate diagnosis (Table 18.2)
2 Attempt to determine the underlying causes of PTL or co-morbidities that may alter management (see assessment)
3 Confirming the gestational age (see assessment)
4 Assessing obstetrical and neonatal resources and evaluating options for maternal transport and/or availability of adequately trained personnel (see maternal transport)
5 Deciding whether to treat with tocolytics and which drug to choose (see tocolytics)
6 Antenatal steroids (see steroids)
7 Should antibiotics be given? (see antibiotics)

Table 18.2 Diagnosis of preterm labour (at 23–36 6/7 weeks).

Traditional
1 Persistent uterine contractions with dilatation and/or effacement of the cervix
2 These criteria are most accurate with:
- Contractions ≥6 /hour
- Cervical dilatation ≥3 cm and/or effacement ≥80%
- Vaginal bleeding
- Documented change in the cervical exam.

Modern
1 Persistent uterine contractions (≥6 /hour), *and*
2 Transvaginal ultrasound (TVU) cervical length ≤20 mm, *or* TVU 20–30 mm and positive fetal fibronectin

Traditional **criteria for the diagnosis of PTL are listed in Table 18.2**. Using less stringent criteria to diagnose PTL results in about a 40% false positive diagnosis but does not increase sensitivity (does not identify more women who would deliver preterm) [1]. Digital examination in women less than 3 cm dilated is subjective and imprecise [2]; yet, most women being evaluated for PTL are less than 3 cm dilated. Women without cervical change or advanced dilation should not be treated with tocolytics. Using these criteria, about 40–70% of women diagnosed with PTL deliver at term, and less than 10% deliver within 1 week [1, 2]. **Transvaginal ultrasound cervical length** (TVU CL) and cervicovaginal **fetal fibronectin** (FFN) have been used to **improve the diagnostic accuracy for PTL** and assess the likelihood of PTB.

Many studies of TVU CL and FFN use PTB before 37 or 35 weeks as the outcome of interest, but more relevant and important to the management of symptomatic women is the risk for imminent delivery — delivery within 48 hours to 7 days, since it is this interval for which tocolytics have shown clear benefits and for which steroids are effective. Pooled data suggests a **TVU CL > 30 mm has a negative predictive value of 80–100% for PTB < 34–37 weeks and >95% for delivery within 7 days**. On the other hand, **women with CL < 15–20 mm have a 20–50% risk for PTB within 7 days and a >60% chance of PTB < 35 weeks** [3]. A negative FFN is also associated with a low risk for delivery within 7 days (6%) and delivery ≤35 weeks (8%) but its use in combination with CL is much more predictive. This is especially true in women with CL between 16 and 30 mm [4–6].

Conclusion

Based on this data, **the diagnosis of PTL should be based on the presence of contractions, but also results of TVU CL and FFN tests**

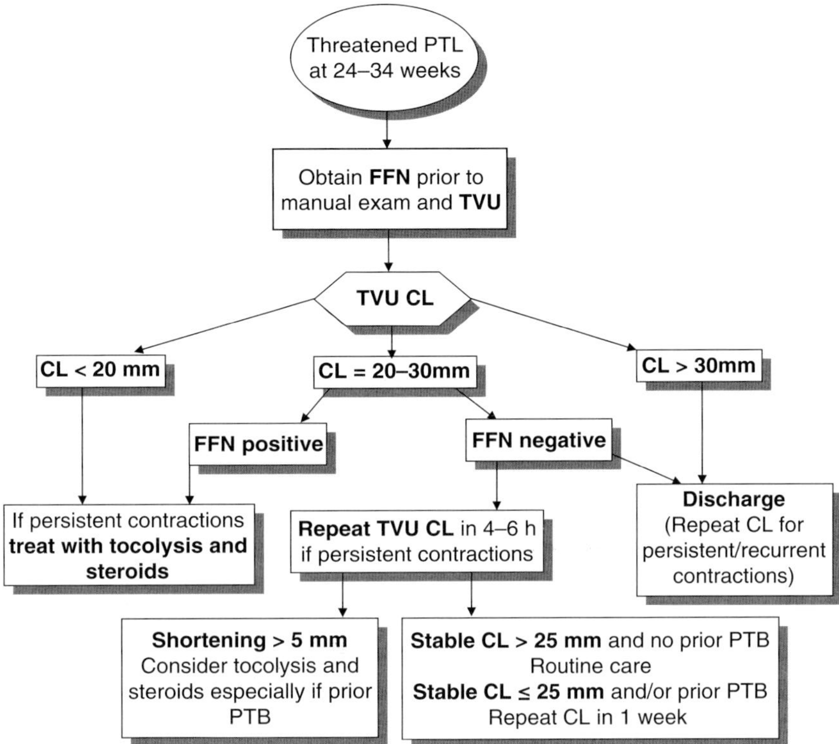

Figure 18.1 Preterm labor management algorithm.

(Table 18.2). Symptomatic women with a CL < 20 mm are at high enough risk for delivery within 7–14 days to justify treatment. If the TVU CL is between 20 and 30 mm, management can be based on the results of a FFN. **Since over half of women presenting with threatened PTL have CL > 30 mm, a majority of symptomatic women do not have true PTL, can be more rapidly triaged, and avoid unnecessary interventions [7] (Figure 18.1)**.

Assessment (Table 18.3)

The **history** should ask about symptoms of PTL such as cramping, 'tightening', menstrual- like symptoms, backache and pelvic pressure as well as bleeding, leakage and fever. Risk factors for PTB should be evaluated (see Table 4.1). An assessment should be made for intercurrent illness or exacerbation of chronic medical conditions. Women should be assessed for acute maternal conditions such as preeclampsia, urinary tract infections, pyelonephritis, trauma, abruption, chorioamnionitis as well as exacerba-

Table 18.3 Assessment of women with suspected preterm labor.

1 History
- Symptoms-cramping, bleeding, leakage etc.
- Risk factors for preterm birth
- Pregnancy history
- Medical history

2 Maternal vital signs

3 Monitor fetal heart rate and contractions

4 Physical exam
- Uterine tone and tenderness
- Sterile speculum for fetal fibronectin, rule out rupture of membranes (ROM) and assess cervix
- GBS culture
- Manual cervical exam if no ROM

5 Ultrasound
- Gestational age, growth and fluid
- Transvaginal cervical length

6 Additional labs
- Urine analysis and culture
- Complete blood count
- Gonorrhea/Chlamydia if suspected

tions of chronic maternal medical problems such as poorly controlled diabetes, asthma or hypertension. Fetal conditions such as fetal growth restriction, oligohydramnios, or nonreassuring fetal status should be identified.

- **Physical examination** should include vital signs, uterine size, tone, and tenderness, fetal heart rate monitoring, and cervical speculum exam. **Specimens** for evaluation for rupture of membranes (PPROM), FFN, group B streptococcus should be obtained and cultures for sexually transmitted infections considered in high risk patients. Once PPROM is excluded, a manual examination of the cervix should be done on women with suspected PTL. Significant bleeding should prompt evaluation for placental previa or abruption. **Ultrasound** should be performed to assess for gestational age, presentation, growth, amniotic fluid, fetal anomalies, placental location and demise. Transvaginal ultrasound cervical length is recommended if available.
- Overt clinical signs of **intramniotic infection** (IAI) and contraindications to tocolysis should be identified. Clinical IAI is diagnosed if there are ≥2 of the following: uterine tenderness, fever ≥38 °C (100.4 °F), maternal and fetal tachycardia in the absence of other sources of infection. About 15–20% of women with PTL have IAI (Chapter 7). The diagnosis of IAI should prompt delivery. Amniocentesis can be per-

formed to evaluate for IAI in equivocal cases and to determine fetal lung maturity (especially beyond 33 weeks).

- Appropriate management of PTL depends on what the anticipated neonatal morbidity/mortality would be if the fetus delivered. Knowledge of the **gestational age** allows for an informed decision regarding the need for intervention and how aggressive that intervention should be. Accurate neonatal outcome statistics should be part of the discussion with the woman to justify whatever management is chosen. **Neonatal consultation** should be obtained if available (Chapter 22).

Transfer to tertiary care centers

The availability of necessary equipment and trained personnel should be considered in light of the gestational age of the potential neonate. If resources at the presenting hospital are inadequate to care for the mother or neonate, prompt arrangements should be made with the nearest center capable of providing appropriate care. Regionalization of perinatal care developed in the 1970s as part of an effort to reduce infant mortality. An important aspect of regionalization is identification of high-risk pregnancies for maternal transport. **Maternal (*in utero*) transport has been shown to improve outcomes over neonatal transport**, with decreases in neonatal mortality and morbidity, including severe intraventricular hemorrhage (IVH), respiratory distress syndrome (RDS), patent ductus arteriosus and nosocomial infection [8–10].

Conclusion

Transport of mothers with PTL to the appropriate level of facilities for their gestational age is an important means to reduce neonatal mortality and morbidity. Use of tocolytics may allow for this transport.

Treatment

The current goals of tocolysis are to prevent imminent PTB in order to have sufficient time to administer antenatal corticosteroids (ACS) (Chapter 20), allow for maternal *in utero* transfer to a hospital with appropriate neonatal care, and in some women, to interrupt transitory causes for PTL in order to delay delivery to a later gestational age. Tocolysis and other interventions such as corticosteroids should be limited to women with TVU CL < 20 mm or TVU 20–30 mm and positive FFN (Figure 18.1).

Table 18.4 Effectiveness of tocolytics *against placebo or no tocolysis* for primary tocolysis based on level 1 evidence. +, yes (beneficial effect in prevention). –, no effect. NA, not available, i.e. not studied. *Most data is pre-steroids. †One trial only. ‡Includes respiratory distress disorder, intraventricular hemorrhage, necrotizing enterocolitis. RCT, randomized controlled trial.

Tocolytic	<48h	<7 days	<34–37weeks	Perinatal mortality	Perinatal morbidity‡
Betamimetics	+	+	–	–*	–*
Magnesium	–	–	–	–	–
Calcium channel blockers (CCB)	No RCT	No RCT	No RCT	No RCT	No RCT
Cyclooxygenase inhibitors (COX)	+	+	+	–	–
Oxytocin receptor antagonists (ORA)	–	–	–	–	–
Nitric oxide donors (NOD)	–	NA	NA	–	+†

Tocolytics (Tables 18.4 and 18.5)

Betamimetics

Ritodrine and terbutaline have been studied in multiple randomized controlled trials (RCTs). Ritodrine remains the first and only tocolytic agent FDA-approved for the treatment of PTL. Despite this initial approval and acceptance by the medical community, the introduction of newer tocolytics, and the potential for significant maternal side effects, limit their use.

- *Mechanism.* Bind to beta-2 adrenergic receptors on the myometrial cell membrane, which increase the levels of intracellular cyclic AMP and inactivate myosin light-chain kinase.
- *Effectiveness.* A Cochrane review including 11 randomized, placebo-controlled trials found that betamimetics significantly **decrease the rate of PTB within 48 hours** by 37% (RR 0.63, 95% CI 0.53–0.75) and showed a **trend toward decreased PTB within 7 days** of 33% (RR 0.67, 95% CI 0.48–1.01) [11]. A trend towards lower rates of RDS (RR 0.87, 95% CI 0.71–1.08), but no effect on the neonatal death rate (RR 1.00, 95% CI 0.48–2.09) was noted. The findings of this review are limited because **many of the trials included did not routinely use ACS**.
- *Side effects.*
  - *Maternal.* Nausea, headaches, nasal stuffiness; hypokalemia (K < 3 mEq/L in 50%); increased in serum glucose levels (20–50%); nervousness, tremors, tachycardia and palpitations, chest pain (5–

Table 18.5 Comparisons among tocolytics for primary treatment based on level 1 evidence. Tocolytics listed inside the table are significantly beneficial in the comparison. –, no effect. NA, not available in report of studies. CCB, calcium channel blockers. Mg, magnesium sulfate. COX, cyclo-oxygenase (COX) inhibitors. ORA, oxytocin receptor antagonists. NOD, nitric oxide donors.

Tocolytic	<48h	<7 days	<34–37 weeks	Perinatal mortality	Perinatal morbidity
CCB vs betamimetics	CCB	CCB	CCB	–	CCB
CCB vs Mg	–	NA	–	–	–
CCB vs COX	No RCT	No RCT	No RCT	No RCT	No RCT
CCB vs ORA	No RCT	No RCT	No RCT	No RCT	No RCT
CCB vs NOD	No RCT	No RCT	No RCT	No RCT	No RCT
COX vs betamimetics	COX	–	–	–	–
COX vs Mg	–	NA	COX	–	–
COX vs ORA	No RCT	No RCT	No RCT	No RCT	No RCT
COX vs NOD	No RCT	No RCT	No RCT	No RCT	No RCT
ORA vs betamimetics	–	–	–	–	–
ORA vs Mg	No RCT	No RCT	No RCT	No RCT	No RCT
ORA vs NOD	No RCT	No RCT	No RCT	No RCT	No RCT
Mg vs betamimetics	–	NA	–	–	–
Mg vs NOD	NA	NA	NA	NA	NA
NOD vs betamimetics	–	–	NOD	–	–

10%), shortness of breath (10%), arrhythmia (3%); ECG changes (2–3%), pulmonary edema (<5%) and rarely myocardial ischemia.
 - *Fetal/neonatal.* Tachycardia, hypoglycemia, hypocalcemia, hyperbilirubinemia, hypotension, and possibly IVH.
- *Contraindications.* Significant cardiac disease, arrhythmia, difficult or poorly controlled diabetes, thyroid disease. Use with caution in women with risk for massive hemorrhage.
- *Dose.* Ritodrine: Begin with 50–100 μg/min IV then increase 50 μg/min every 10 minutes (maximum 350 μg/min). Terbutaline: 0.25 mg subcutaneously every 20–30 minutes up to four doses then every 3–4 hours or 2.5–5.0 mg for 24 hours orally every 2–4 hours; OR IV infusion 2.5–5 μg/min then increase by 2.5–5.0 μg/min every 20–30 minutes to a maximum of 25 μg/min until contractions controlled. Then decrease to lowest dose for uterine quiescence. (Hold dose or reduce if maternal heart rate ≥120 b.p.m.)
- *Conclusion.* **Due to the significance and high frequency of side effects, we never use these medications as treatment for PTL.**

Magnesium sulfate

Magnesium sulfate remains the number one tocolytic used in the United States. A survey of over 700 general obstetrician-gynecologists revealed that 94% use magnesium sulfate as their primary tocolytic [12]. A similar survey of 827 maternal-fetal medicine specialists found magnesium sulfate to be the most common first-line tocolytic for acute PTL (45%) and repeat acute PTL (41%) [13].

- *Mechanism.* Inhibits voltage independent calcium channels at the myometrial cell surface, and likely has an intracellular mechanism of action as well. Extracellular magnesium suppresses calcium influx across the cell membrane, whereas intracellular magnesium competes with calcium, thereby inhibiting myosin light-chain kinase activity.
- *Effectiveness.* A Cochrane review **failed to prove any benefit in delaying birth or preventing PTB** compared with placebo or no therapy [14] (Table 18.4). Comparative data between magnesium sulfate and beta-agonsists did not demonstrate any difference in efficacy [15, 16]. Despite this data, a recent meta-analysis of all tocolytics found magnesium sulfate to be superior to placebo in delaying delivery for 48 hours [17].
- *Side effects.*
  - *Maternal.* Flushing, nausea, visual disturbances, and headache, while rare complications include pulmonary edema and cardiac arrest [18]. Toxicity is related to serum concentration. Loss of deep tendon reflexes occurs at about 10–12 mg/dl (4.0–5.0 mmol/l) and respiratory arrest at 12–18 µg/l (5–7.5 mmol/l). Prolonged use of magnesium sulfate has been reported [19]; however, such use may also carry a risk of osteopenia [20]. Toxicity is treated by discontinuation of the infusion, and for life threatening symptoms, administration of calcium gluconate (1 g IV over 5 minutes).
  - *Fetal.* Early reports described increased adverse neurological outcomes [21] and pediatric mortality [22]. Recent data suggests short exposure may be neuroprotective. A large randomized controlled trial (RCT) of over 2200 women described reduced rates of moderate or severe cerebral palsy in the magnesium sulfate group (1.9% vs 3.5%) [23]. This protective effect was also described in a follow-up Cochrane review of five trials (6,145 babies) [24].
- *Contraindications.* Myasthenia gravis, cardiac compromise, cardiac conduction defects. Caution with impaired renal function.
- *Dose.* 4–6 g IV over 20 minutes, then continuous infusion of 2 g/hour. The serum magnesium level may continue to rise over time, therefore the rate should be adjusted to lowest dose based on clinical response and maternal toxicity. With impaired renal function (serum creatinine ≥1 mg/dl [88.4 mmol/l]), give the usual loading dose and reduce

the maintenance dose to 1 g/hour or hold the maintenance infusion until a magnesium level is obtained in 4–6 hours. Close monitoring of patellar reflexes and urine output should be performed in all women receiving magnesium.

- *Conclusion.* **Because of side effects, the need for an intravenous infusion, and limited data of proven benefit, many have called for the discontinuation of its use as a first-line tocolytic agent** [25]. **We tend to agree with this recommendation**.

Calcium channel blockers

The most commonly studied calcium channel blocker (CCB) for PTL is nifedipine, which can be administered orally or sublingually.

- *Mechanism.* Inhibits calcium re-uptake by voltage dependent calcium channels on the myometrial cell wall.
- *Efficacy.* There are **no studies comparing CCB with placebo to prevent PTB**, but the **overall data of nifedipine as a tocolytic appears favorable**. Early studies comparing nifedipine to magnesium sulfate found similar efficacy with fewer side effects in the nifedipine group [26]. A Cochrane review showed CCB to be superior to betamimetics, reducing PTB within 7 days by 24% and before 34 weeks by 17% [27]. It also reduced the frequency of RDS by 37%, necrotizing enterocolitis (NEC) by 79%, and IVH by 41%. Of considerable importance, CCB reduced the need to discontinue treatment because of adverse side effects by 86%. A recent RCT comparing magnesium sulfate with nifedipine showed similar rates of delay of delivery, gestational age at delivery and neonatal outcomes [28]; however, nifedipine was associated with fewer maternal side effects. A recent meta-analysis found nifedipine to be superior to all other tocolytics in delaying delivery until after 37 weeks, though this difference was not statistically significant [29].
- *Side effects.*
  - *Maternal.* Hypotension, tachycardia, flushing and dizziness.
  - *Fetal.* None.
- *Contraindications.* Left ventricular dysfunction or congestive heart failure. Due to largely theoretical concerns regarding synergistic suppression of muscle contractility, the use of magnesium sulfate with CCB is not recommended.
- *Dose.* There is no agreement on the optimal dosing of nifedipine. Typical initial dosing is 20 mg orally repeated in 90 minutes, or alternatively we often use 10–20 mg orally every 20 minutes up to three doses. We then continue with 10–20 mg every 4–6 hours.
- *Conclusion.* Because of its overall favorable profile, **nifedipine is the most commonly utilized tocolytic in our practice**.

Prostaglandin (cyclooxygenase) inhibitors

The main prostaglandin inhibitor used for PTL is indomethacin, a non-selective cyclooxygenase (COX) inhibitor.

- *Mechanism.* Inhibits prostaglandin production by inhibiting COX, the enzyme which converts arachidonic acid to prostaglandin.
- *Efficacy.* The Cochrane review included 13 trials (10 used indomethacin). Only three trials totalling 106 women (two included women up to 35 weeks and allowed rescue tocolysis within 2 hours) compared indomethacin with placebo. Compared with placebo, indomethacin **reduced PTB < 37 weeks**, increased birth weight, and showed **trends towards reducing delivery within 48 hours and 7 days**. There were no improvements in neonatal mortality or morbidity [30].
- Compared with other tocolytics (mainly beta-mimetics), COX inhibitors significantly reduced the risk for delivery <37 weeks (RR 0.53; 95% CI 0.31–0.94) and low rates of discontinuation of medication due to side effects (RR 0.07; 95% CI 0.02–0.29). Trends toward reduction in delivery within 48 hours (RR 59; 95% CI 0.34–1.02) were noted. No differences were found between deliveries <7 days or for any fetal or neonatal outcome. Several inhibitors (e.g. celcoxib and rofecoxib) of cyclooxygenase-2 (COX-2), the enzyme required to produce the prostaglandins most likely involved in PTL, have been described and compared with magnesium sulfate. No differences were found in the efficacy of these medications and magnesium sulfate in arresting PTL. A recent decision analysis and meta-analysis of all tocolytics (after 28 weeks) demonstrated that prostaglandin inhibitors provided the best combination of tolerance and delayed delivery for both 48 hours and 7 days [17].
- *Side effects.*
  - *Maternal.* Nausea, reflux and gastritis seen in about 4% of women.
  - *Fetal.* Premature constriction of the ductus arteriosis, fetal oliguria and oligohydramnios. Indomethacin has also been associated with NEC and periventricular leukomalacia (PVL) but a recent meta-analysis did not confirm these findings [31]. The best evidence from RCTs and meta-analyses regarding the risks for ductal constriction and oligohydramnios is reassuring, when COX inhibitors are used for ≤48 hours, and before 32 weeks [32]. A review of 61 patients exposed to a 48 hour course of indomethacin faied to show significant amniotic fluid changes [33]. Less commonly utilized prostaglandin inhibitors studied for acute tocolysis include sulindac and nimesulide. Both have similar adverse effects seen with antenatal indomethacin exposure. Data regarding their efficacy is limited.
- *Contraindications.* Platelet dysfunction, bleeding disorder, hepatic dysfunction, ulcer disease, asthma with hypersensitivity to aspirin.

- *Dose.* We begin with 50–100 mg by the vaginal, rectal or oral route, followed by 25 mg every 6 hours **for up to 48 hours up to 32 weeks**.
- *Conclusion.* In light of newer evidence, some have suggested that indomethacin should be considered as a first line agent, especially for PTL before 30 weeks, and if **used for only ≤48 hours before 32 weeks**.

Oxytocin-receptor antagonists

Atosiban is a selective oxytocin receptor antagonist commonly used in Europe, but not approved for use in the United States.

- *Mechanism.* Competes with oxytocin for binding to receptors in the myometrium and decidua.
- *Efficacy.* Data regarding atosiban, are mixed. A large unblinded study of atosiban compared with 'usual care' which included beta-agonists, calcium channel blockers, or magnesium sulfate, showed similar rates of women undelivered after 48 hours. However, fewer women in the atosiban group required additional tocolysis and maternal and fetal safety was superior [34]. On the other hand, a recent Cochrane review of oxytocin-receptor antagonists for PTL **failed to demonstrate the superiority of atosiban over betamimetics or placebo in terms of tocolytic efficacy or infant outcomes** [35]. Use of atosiban showed nonsignificant trends toward increased rates of birth at 48 hours, <28 weeks and <37 weeks and an increase in fetal deaths in one placebo-controlled trial. Yet this review also found atosiban as effective as betamimetics for preventing PTB within 48 hours and 7 days.
- *Side effects.*
  - *Maternal.* Hypersensitivity and injection site reactions. Overall fewer reported side effects than any other tocolytic.
  - *Fetal.* Concerns from one trial regarding higher rates of fetal-neonatal death and infection in infants delivered <28 weeks. This effect may have been due to a greater number of very preterm (<26 weeks) infants in the atosiban arm of that trial [35].
- *Dose.* Loading dose of 6.75 mg intravenously followed by 300 μg/minute infusion over 3 hours, followed by 100 μg/hour for up to 45 hours.
- *Contraindications.* None. Some avoid use for pregnancies <28 weeks.
- *Conclusion.* Because of this limited and contradictory data as well as its unavailability in the US, **we do not use atosiban in our management paradigm for PTL**.

Nitric oxide donors (NOD)

Nitroglycerine is the only NOD used in trials of PTL.

- *Mechanism.* Relaxes uterine muscle.

- *Efficacy.* In a Cochrane meta-analysis including 466 women in five trials, nitroglycerine **did not prevent prematurity** related outcomes compared with placebo or no treatment (Table 18.4) [36].
- *Dose.* Transdermal nitroglycerine patch 0.4 mg/h.
- *Conclusion.* Currently there is insufficient evidence to support the use of NOD as tocolytics.

Duration of tocolyis

Tocolysis is usually continued **for 48 hours until the completion of corticosteroid therapy**. Because each day gained *in utero* between 24 and 28 weeks increases survival by about 3%, tocolysis is prolonged or restarted beyond 48 hours in some practices in these women if needed, but there are **no studies proving effectiveness of extended tocolysis**.

Refractory PTL (failure of primary agent)

Treatment may be more aggressive when there is a risk of extreme prematurity and there is evidence of progressive cervical change despite tocolysis. A change to a second agent may be considered after reevaluation for possible chorioamnionitis or abruption. Occasionally a second agent may be added but the risks of side effects are increased. **There is little or no evidence to support any specific approach**. Some studies of magnesium sulfate in addition to ritodrine showed unacceptable maternal side effects, namely chest pain, and ECG changes suggestive of ischemia [37]. We would use indomethacin if primary tocolysis with nifedipine fails before 30 weeks.

Maintenance tocolysis

There is limited data regarding the efficacy of maintenance tocolysis following arrested acute PTL. The studied medications have been terbutaline, nifedipine, and magnesium. Despite early studies suggesting a benefit to oral betamimetics for maintanence tocolysis. A Cochrane review of oral betamimetics for maintenance therapy after threatened PTL **failed to support their use** [38]. Studies evaluating the role of **terbutaline pumps failed to show prolonged gestations** in women successfully treated for suspected PTL [39]. Multiple studies evaluating the use of nifedipine for maintenance therapy **failed to show any benefit [40. 41]**.A Cochrane review of magnesium maintenance therapy ($n = 303$) **did not show benefit** when compared with placebo or other tocolytics [42]. One trial of over 500 patients showed maintenance therapy with atosiban delayed the next episode of labor after successful treatment with atosiban of an acute episode of PTL, but **did not prevent PTB** or adverse neonatal outcomes [43].

Conclusions

We currently **never administer maintenance tocolysis**, which has no scientific basis for its use.

Contraindications to tocolysis

Most contraindications are relative [32]. When there is a high risk of gestational age related neonatal mortality or significant morbidity, tocolysis is usually justified even when there is some additional risk to the mother such as with diabetes, placenta previa with mild bleeding, and chronic hypertension [44].

Conclusion: putting it all together

The decision regarding which tocolytic to choose for a given clinical situation requires a thorough understanding of patient past medical history, gestational age and clinical assessment. A cost decision analysis of four tocolytics [45] analyzed 19 trials. The probability of adverse events was 57.9% for terbutaline, 22% for magnesium sulfate, 27.2% for nifedipine and 11.4% for indomethacin. When factoring the cost of medications and monitoring, both **nifedipine and indomethacin** appeared superior to terbutaline and magnesium sulfate. A 2009 metaanalysis and decision analysis of 58 trials showed that all tocolytics were better than placebo or control groups at delaying delivery for both 48 hours (75–93% versus 53%) and 7 days (61–78% versus 39 %) [22]. No differences in neonatal outcomes were noted. **Prostaglandin inhibitors and calcium channel blockers** had the best combination of tolerance and delayed delivery.

Therefore, unless contraindicated because of either prior sensitivity or hypotension, our first-line treatment for acute tocolysis is usually **nifedipine**. In patients who do not tolerate nifedipine well we usually switch to **indomethacin when gestational age is <32 weeks**. We administer tocolytics, especially indomethacin, **for 48 hours only**. If we achieve uterine quiescence we stop the medication and continue to observe the patient for at least 24 hours. We find that this paradigm allows for maximal benefit with the fewest maternal and neonatal risks.

Other interventions

Antenatal corticosteroids

A course of antenatal corticosteroids **should be given to all women with true PTL, or at high risk for PTB within the next 7 days when between 24 and 34 6/7 weeks**. See Chapter 20 for details.

Hydration

Although data is limited, two trials including 228 women showed **no benefit** was seen when hydration was compared with bed rest alone, even during the period of evaluation for PTL [46, 47]. The risks for delivery before 32, 34 and 37 weeks were similar in both groups.

Bed rest

There is no trial which evaluates the effectiveness of activity modification at the time of PTL. There was **no benefit** for bed rest in one trial that studied singletons hospitalized for bed rest after arrested PTL [48]. Both groups were advised to decrease activity but this was not enforced. In twins with cervical dilatation hospitalization did not decrease PTB.

Antibiotics

The Cochrane review evaluating prophylactic antibiotics in conjunction with tocolysis for PTL < 36 weeks in over 7,400 women with intact membranes in 11 trials **failed to show any overall benefit** on prolongation of pregnancy or neonatal outcomes, with a trend toward increased neonatal mortality in the antibiotics group [49]. There was a significant reduction in maternal infection. This review is dominated by the ORACLE II trial which included over 1400 women. In this trial, the risk of cerebral palsy was increased in children (about 7 years old) of women who received either co-amoxiclac or (especially) erythromycin compared with placebo [50]. A more recent meta-analysis limited to pregnancies <34 weeks, showed that aside from a reduction in clinically diagnosed infection, there was no increased latency or overall improvement in neonatal outcomes [51].

Conclusion

We currently **do not administer antibiotics in the setting of PTL with intact membranes** in order to prolong the latency period. We administer antibiotics for group B streptococcal (GBS) coverage in cases where delivery is felt to be imminent and the GBS status of the patient is unknown.

Progesterone

There are no trials of progesterone therapy used as primary tocolysis. Use of progesterone in addition to other tocolytics or as maintenance tocolysis has not been studied sufficiently to recommend use.

Magnesium for neuroprotection

Magnesium sulfate has been shown in five trials enrolling over 6,100 women to significantly **decrease cerebral palsy** from 5.3% in placebo controls to 4.1% [24]. Substantial motor dysfunction is decreased, while perinatal mortality and other outcomes are not significantly altered. The number needed to treat for the effect on cerebral palsy is 63.

Follow up

After successful arrest of PTL most women can be sent home after a period of 1–2 days of observation. There is **no evidence to support hospitalization after arrested PTL** [52]. Outpatient manual cervical exams, bed rest, as well as avoidance of intercourse, exercise and other strenuous activities have not been studies in trials. Some women may return to work if they remain stable, are less than 3 cm dilated and have sedentary occupations.

References

1 Iams JD, Romero R, Creasy RK. PTL and birth. In Creasy RK, Resnik R, Iams JD, Lockwood CJ, Moore TR, eds. *Maternal Fetal Medicine*, 6th edn. Philadelphia: Saunders, 2009: 545–82.

2 Iams JD, Romero R. Preterm birth. In Gabbe SG, Niebyl JR, Simpson JL, eds. *Obstetrics: Normal and Problem Pregnancies*, 5th edn. Philadelphia: Churchill Livingstone, 2007: 668–712.

3 Berghella V, Ness A, Bega G, Berghella M. Cervical sonography in women with symptoms of PTL. Obstet Gynecol Clin N Am 2005; 32: 383–96.

4 Tsoi E, Fuchs IB, Rane S, *et al.* Sonographic measurement of cervical length in threatened PTL in singleton pregnancies with intact membranes. Ultrasound Obstet Gynecol 2005; 25: 353–6.

5 Tsoi E, Akmal S, Geerts L, *et al.* Sonographic measurement of cervical length and fetal fibronectin testing in threatened PTL. Ultrasound Obstet Gynecol 2006; 27: 368–72.

6 Gomez R, Romero R, Medina L. Cervicovaginal fibronectin improves the prediction of preterm delivery based on sonographic cervical length in patients with preterm uterine contractions and intact membranes. Am J Obstet Gynecol 2005; 192: 350–9.

7 Ness A, Visintine J, Ricci E, Berghella V. Does knowledge of cervical length and fetal fibronectin affect management of women with threatened preterm labor? A randomized trial. Am J Obstet Gynecol 2007; 197: 426e1–426e7.

8 Kollee LA, Brand R, Schreuder AM, Ens-Dokkum MH, Veen S, Verloove-Vanhorick SP. Five-year outcome of preterm and very low birth weight infants: a comparison between maternal and neonatal transport. Obstet Gynecol 1992; 80: 635–8.

9 Shlossman PA, Manley JS, Sciscione AC, Colmorgen GH. An analysis of neonatal morbidity and mortality in maternal (in utero) and neonatal transports at 24–34 weeks' gestation. Am J Perinatol 1997; 14: 449–56.

10 Modanlou HD, Dorchester WL, Thorosian A, Freeman RK. Antenatal versus neonatal transport to a regional perinatal center: a comparison between matched pairs. Ob Gyn 1979; 53: 725–9.

11 Anotayanonth S, Subhedar NV, Neilson JP, Harigopal S. Betamimetics for inhibiting preterm labour. Cochrane Database Syst Rev 2009; CD 004352.

12 Morgan MA, Goldenberg RL, Schulkin J. Obstetrician-gynecologists' screening and management of preterm birth. Obstet Gynecol 2008; 112: 35–41.

13 Fox NS, Gelber SE, Kalish RB, Chasen ST. Contemporary practice patterns and beliefs regarding tocolysis among US Maternal-fetal medicine specialists. Obstet Gynecol 2008; 112: 42–7.

14 Crowther CA, Hiller JE, Doyle LW. Magnesium sulphate for preventing preterm birth in threatened preterm labour. Cochrane Database Syst Rev 2002: CD001060.

15 Cotton DB, Strassner HT, Hill LM, Schifrin BS, Paul RH. Comparison of magnesium sulfate, terbutaline and a placebo for inhibition of preterm labor. A randomized study. J Reprod Med 1984; 29: 92–7.

16 Macones GA, Sehdev HM, Berlin M, Morgan MA, Berlin JA. Evidence for magnesium sulfate as a tocolytic agent. Obstet Gynecol Surv 1997; 52: 652–8.

17 Haas DM, Imperiale TF, Kirkpatrick PR, Klein RW, Zollinger TW, Golichowski AM. Tocolytic therapy: a meta-analysis and decision analysis. Obstet Gynecol 2009; 13: 585–94.

18 Terrone DA, Rinehart BK, Kimmel ES, May WL, Larmon JE, Morrison JC. A prospective, randomized, controlled trial of high and low maintenance doses of magnesium sulfate for acute tocolysis. Am J Obstet Gynecol 2000; 182: 1477–82.

19 Wilkins IA, Goldberg JD, Phillips RN, Bacall CJ, Chervenak FA, Berkowitz RL. Long-term use of magnesium sulfate as a tocolytic agent. Obstet Gynecol 1986; 67: 38S–40S.

20 Hung JW, Tsai MY, Yang BY, Chen JF. Maternal osteoporosis after prolonged magnesium sulfate tocolysis therapy: a case report. Arch Phys Med Rehabil 2005; 86: 146–9.

21 Mittendorf R, Dambrosia J, Pryde PG, *et al.* Association between the use of antenatal magnesium sulfate in PTL and adverse health outcomes in infants. Am J Obstet Gynecol 2002; 186: 1111–8.

22 Scudiero R, Khoshnood B, Pryde PG, Lee KS, Wall S, Mitterndorf R. Perinatal death and tocolytic magnesium sulfate. Am J Obstet Gynecol 2000; 96: 178–82.

23 Rouse DJ, Hirtz DG, Thom E, *et al.* A randomized, controlled trial of magnesium sulfate for the prevention of cerebral palsy. N Engl J Med 2008; 359: 895–905.

24 Doyle LW, Crowther CA, Middleton P, Marret S, Rouse D. Magnesium sulphate for women at risk of preterm birth for neuroprotection of the fetus. Cochrane Database Syst Rev 2009: CD004661.

25 Grimes DA, Nanda K. Magnesium sulfate tocolysis: time to quit. Obstet Gynecol 2006; 108: 986–9.

26 Haghighi L. Prevention of preterm delivery: nifedipine or magnesium sulfate. Int J Gynaecol Obstet 1999; 66: 297–8.

27 King JF, Flenady VJ, Papatsonis DN, Dekker GA, Carbonne B. Calcium channel blockers for inhibiting preterm labour. Cochrane Database Syst Rev 2003: CD002255.

28 Lyell DJ, Pullen K, Campbell L, *et al.* Magnesium sulfate compared with nifedipine for acute tocolysis of PTL: a randomized controlled trial. Obstet Gynecol 2007; 110: 61–7.

29 Haas DM, Imperiale TF, Kirkpatrick PR, Klein RW, Zollinger TW, Golichowski AM. Tocolytic therapy: a meta-analysis and decision analysis. Obstet Gynecol 2009; 113: 585–94.

30 King J, Flenady V, Cole S, Thornton S. Cyclo-oxygenase (COX) inhibitors for treating preterm labour. Cochrane Database Syst Rev 2005: CD001992.

31 Loe SM, Sanchez-Ramos L, Kaunitz AM. Assessing the neonatal safety of indomethacin tocolysis: a systematic review with meta-analysis. Obstet Gynecol 2005; 106: 173–9.

32 Berghella V. Prevention of prematurity. In: Berghella V, ed. *Obstetric Evidence Based Guidelines*. London: Informa Healthcare, 2007.

33 Sandruck JC, Grobman WA, Gerber SE. The effect of short-term indomethacin therapy on amniotic fluid volume. Am J Obstet Gynecol 2005; 192: 1443–5.

34 Husslein P, Cabero Roura L, Dudenhausen JW, *et al.* Atosiban versus usual care for the management of PTL. J Perinat Med 2007; 35: 305–13.

35 Papatsonis D, Flenady V, Cole S, Liley H. Oxytocin receptor antagonists for inhibiting preterm labour. Cochrane Database Syst Rev 2005: CD004452.

36 Duckitt K, Thornton S . Nitric oxide donors for the treatment of preterm labour. Cochrane Database Syst Rev 2009.

37 Ferguson JE, 2nd, Hensleigh PA, Kredenster D. Adjunctive use of magnesium sulfate with ritodrine for PTL tocolysis. Am J Obstet Gynecol 1984; 148: 166–71.

38 Dodd JM, Crowther CA, Dare MR, Middleton P. Oral betamimetics for maintenance therapy after threatened preterm labour. Cochrane Database Syst Rev 2006: CD003927.

39 Guinn DA, Goepfert AR, Owen J, Wenstrom KD, Hauth JC. Terbutaline pump maintenance therapy for prevention of preterm delivery: a double-blind trial. Am J Obstet Gynecol 1998; 179: 874–8.

40 Carr DB, Clark AL, Kernek K, Spinnato JA. Maintenance oral nifedipine for PTL: a randomized clinical trial. Am J Obstet Gynecol 1999; 181: 822–7.

41 Lyell DJ, Pullen KM, Mannan J, *et al.* Maintenance nifedipine tocolysis compared with placebo: a randomized controlled trial. Obstet Gynecol 2008; 112: 1221–6.

42 Crowther C, Moore V. Magnesium maintenance therapy for preventing preterm birth after threatened preterm labour. Cochrane Database Syst Rev, 2000; CD000940.

43 Valenzuela G, Sanchez-Ramos L, Romero R, *et al.* Maintenance treatment of preterm labor with the oxytocin antagonist atosiban. The Atosiban PTL-098 Study Group. Am J Obstet Gynecol 2000; 182: 1184–90.

44 Berghella V. Prevention of preterm birth. In Berghella V, ed. *Obstetric Evidence Based Guidelines*. London: Informa Healthcare, 2007: 116–37.

45 Hayes E, Moroz L, Pizzi L, Baxter J. A cost decision analysis of four tocolytic drugs. Am J Obstet Gynecol 2007; 197: 383 e1–6.

46 Yost NP, Bloom SL, McIntire DD, Leveno KJ. Hospitalization for women with arrested preterm labor: a randomized trial. Am J Obstet Gynecol 2005; 106: 14.

47 Stan C, Boulvain M, Pfister R, Hirsbrunner-Almagbaly P. Hydration for the treatment of preterm labour. Cochrane Database Syst Rev 2002; (2): CD003096.

48 Yost NP, Bloom SL, McIntire DD, Leveno KJ. Hospitalization for women with arrested preterm labor: a randomized trial. Obstet Gynecol 2005; 106: 14–8.

49 King J, Flenady V. Prophylactic antibiotics for inhibiting preterm labour with intact membranes. Cochrane Database Syst Rev 2002; CD000246.

50 Kenyon S, Pike K, Jones DR, Brocklehurst P, Marlow N, Taylor DJ. Childhood outcomes after prescription of antibiotics to pregnant women with spontaneous labour: 7-year follow-up of the ORACLE II trial. Lancet 2008; 372: 1319–27.
51 Hutzal CE, Boyle EM, Kenyon SL, *et al.* Use of antibiotics for the treatment of preterm parturition and prevention of neonatal morbidity: a metaanalysis. Am J Obstet Gynecol 2008; 199: 620e1–8.
52 Yost NP, Bloom SL, McIntire DD, Leveno KJ. Hospitalization for women with arrested preterm labor. Obstet Gynecol 2005; 106: 14–18.

CHAPTER 19

Preterm Premature Rupture of the Membranes

Brian M. Mercer
Reproductive Biology, Case Western Reserve University and Department of Obstetrics and Gynecology, MetroHealth Medical Center, Ohio, USA

Key points

- The hallmarks of preterm premature rupture of the membranes (PPROM) are brief latency, intrauterine infection, placental abruption, and umbilical cord compression.
- Neonatal complications after PPROM vary directly with the gestational age at membrane rupture and delivery.
- Advanced labor, intrauterine infection, significant uterine bleeding, and non-reassuring fetal testing are indications for delivery at any gestational age.
- Antenatal corticosteroid treatment after PPROM results in less frequent respiratory distress syndrome, intraventricular hemorrhage and necrotizing enterocolitis without increasing perinatal or maternal infections.
- Broad spectrum antibiotic therapy during conservative management of PPROM can improve latency and reduce neonatal morbidities. Ampicillin-clavulanic acid should not be given for this indication.
- If pulmonary maturity is evident after PROM at 32–33 weeks' gestation, there is little to be gained from conservative management and delivery is encouraged. At ≥34 0/7 weeks, delivery is usually recommended.
- Weekly intramuscular 17 hydroxyprogesterone caproate or daily vaginal progesterone suppositories may prevent recurrent preterm birth due to preterm labor or PROM.

Introduction

Preterm premature rupture of membranes (PROM) occurs in 3% of pregnancies and results in approximately one third of all preterm births (PTB) [1]. While the incidence of PTB in the United States continues to increase, **PTB due to spontaneous labor and PROM appears to have declined in singleton gestations** among both Caucasian and African-American women [2]. Preterm PROM (PPROM) can be separated into three general groups to guide evaluation and treatment.

Preterm Birth. Edited by Vincenzo Berghella. © 2010 Blackwell Publishing

(1) PPROM before the limit of viability (currently 23 weeks' gestation)
(2) PPROM remote from term (23–31 weeks' gestation)
(3) PPROM near term (32–36 weeks' gestation).

With PROM occurring before the limit of viability, immediate delivery results in neonatal death. Conservative management can end in previable or periviable birth, and less likely with delivery at an advanced gestational age. However, lethal pulmonary hypoplasia can occur despite extended latency. Midtrimester PROM (occurring at ~16–26 weeks' gestation) is no longer a relevant delineation as it crosses the limit of viability. With PPROM remote from term, perinatal morbidities and mortality are common with immediate delivery. These can decrease progressively with each week gained before delivery. When PROM occurs at 32 weeks or later, there is a high likelihood of survival and a low risk of long-term morbidities. Further, severe short term morbidities are unlikely if pulmonary maturity is present. Though late PTB is associated with more infant complications than delivery at term, PPROM can lead to fetal death, intrauterine infection and cord compression. Delivery under this circumstance should be undertaken when the risks of conservative management outweigh the potential benefits.

Risk factors and etiology

Risk factors for PPROM include prior PTB, low socioeconomic status, low body mass index, cervical conization or cerclage, and current pregnancy preterm labor (PTL) or contractions, urinary tract infection, sexually transmitted diseases, uterine over-distention (e.g. twins or polyhydramnios), amniocentesis, vaginal bleeding and cigarette smoking (Chapter 4). These can result in membrane degradation with decreased strength, chorio–decidual inflammation, and/or decreased maternal resistance to ascending bacterial colonization.

Near term, physiologic weakening with apoptosis (programmed cell death) and dissolution of the membrane extracellular matrix exacerbated by contraction-induced shearing forces is likely the most prevalent cause of PROM. Ascending bacterial colonization, inflammation and infection initiate a cytokine cascade resulting in apoptosis, protease production and dissolution of the extra-cellular matrix, and is more prevalent remote from term. Abruptio placentae can result in decidual thrombin expression, triggering thrombin–thrombin receptor interactions to increase local protease production. Mechanical stretch may increase protease production via cytokine expression. However, the inciting cause of PROM is often not evident (Chapters 2, 7 and 8).

Clinical course, maternal and fetal/neonatal risks

The hallmarks of PPROM are **brief latency, intrauterine infection, placental abruption, and umbilical cord compression** which can result in non-reassuring fetal testing (NRFT) or death. Though not guaranteed after PROM, each is more common in this setting. Spontaneous sealing of the membranes with cessation of leakage and restoration of intrauterine fluid rarely occurs (<5%), with the exception of PPROM occurring after amniocentesis.

The **latency** from membrane rupture to delivery increases with decreasing gestational age at rupture. With PROM before 34 weeks', 93% overall and 50–60% of those conservatively managed will deliver within 1 week [3]. Median latency is between 6 and 13 days [4]. A recent study found 38% will deliver within 1 week and 69% within 5 weeks after PROM near the limit of viability [5].

Chorioamnionitis is the most common maternal complication after PPROM and this risk is increased with membrane rupture remote from term. Conservative management increases this risk further. Intra-amniotic infection complicates 13–60% of conservatively managed pregnancies, and endometritis is not uncommon (2–13%). The frequency of **abruptio placentae** related to PPROM is 4–12%. Retained placenta and postpartum hemorrhage necessitating uterine curettage, maternal sepsis, and death are uncommon but serious complications of conservatively managed PROM near or before the limit of viability.

The frequencies of **fetal and neonatal complications** after PROM are potentially increased with intrauterine infection, placental abruption and umbilical cord compression. **Respiratory distress syndrome** is the most common serious complication, regardless of gestational age at delivery. **Necrotizing enterocolitis**, **intraventricular hemorrhage** and **sepsis**, are common with early PTB, but do not frequently occur with near term delivery. Neonatal sepsis is twofold more common after PROM than after PTL and PTB. With delivery remote from term, serious acute morbidities can lead to death or long-term sequelae. Membrane rupture at the critical phase before 20 weeks' gestation can result in lethal **pulmonary hypoplasia** from arrested alveolar development. With PROM closer to the limit of viability, nonlethal pulmonary hypoplasia can result in complications due to poor pulmonary compliance and high ventilatory pressures (e.g. pneumothorax, pneumo-mediastinum). Restriction deformities can occur with prolonged oligohydramnios but are not life threatening. Although specific survival and morbidity curves are not available for infants delivering after PPROM, care-givers should be aware of gestational age specific curves and incorporate these into their decision making and counseling [6]. A recently published web-based calculator for infant outcomes delivering near the limit of viability and adjusting for infant gender, and antenatal corticosteroid administration, is available for easy access [7] **(http://www.nichd.nih.gov/about/org/cdbpm/pp/prog_epbo/)** (Chapter 22).

Accumulating data have linked perinatal infection to infant neurologic complications. **Cerebral palsy** and **cystic periventricular leukomalacia** have been linked to chorioamnionitis [8, 9]. Elevated amniotic fluid cytokines and fetal systemic inflammation have been associated with PPROM, periventricular leukomalacia, and cerebral palsy [10, 11]. However, it has not been demonstrated that immediate delivery after PPROM will avert these complications. In some cases, these may actually result from the inciting cause of membrane rupture rather than to complications after PROM.

Diagnosis

PROM occurs when the fetal membranes rupture before the onset of symptomatic uterine contractions, regardless of whether labor subsequently ensues before or after admission. Pragmatically, the diagnosis is optimally confirmed soon after symptoms occur.

Membrane rupture can usually be confirmed clinically, based on history, physical examination and laboratory evaluation. When PPROM is suspected, a **sterile speculum examination** should be performed to confirm the diagnosis, inspect for cervicitis, assess cervical dilatation and effacement, and to obtain samples for culture or DNA testing for *Neisseria gonorrhoeae* and *Chlamydia trachomatis*. Urine leakage, increased vaginal discharge with cervical dilatation or membrane prolapse, cervicitis, cervical mucous discharge, and semen or vaginal douching can also cause increased vaginal discharge. **Digital examination should be avoided** when membrane rupture is suspected unless imminent delivery is anticipated, because this can shorten latency and has been shown to increase the risk of infection in some studies [12–14].

If **amniotic fluid** is not seen **passing from the cervix** on speculum examination, vaginal sidewall or pooled vaginal fluid pH can be evaluated. Amniotic fluid is generally neutral (pH 7.1–7.3) while secretions are more acidic (pH in the 4.5–6.0 range). **Nitrazine™** paper will turn blue with a pH above 6.0–6.5 9. Blood, semen, alkaline antiseptics and bacterial vaginosis can result in a false positive Nitrazine™ result. Prolonged membrane rupture with low residual fluid can result in a false negative test. Microscopic evaluation for arborized crystals (**ferning** test) in an air-dried sample from the vaginal sidewalls or pooled vaginal fluid can be performed if the diagnosis remains unclear. Cervical mucus can also display a ferning pattern as can heavy blood contamination, but the test is unaffected by meconium and pH [15, 16]. If the diagnosis continues to be suspected but testing is negative or equivocal, options include re-examination after prolonged recumbency and/or amniocentesis with instillation of indigo carmine dye (1 ml in 9 ml of sterile normal saline) followed by observation for blue fluid passing onto a perineal pad. Those with suspicious history but negative testing should be encouraged to return if symptoms persist or recur.

Ancillary confirmatory testing with **alternative cervico-vaginal markers** (e.g. placental alpha microglobulin-1 [PAMG-1], insulin-like growth factor-binding protein-1 [IGFBP-1], fetal fibronectin, alpha-fetoprotein, diamino-oxydase, human chorionic gonadotropin, prolactin) has been studied by several investigators [17–19]. These have generally been evaluated when the diagnosis of PROM was clear and ancillary testing was not needed. In a recent study, Lee *et al.* found cervicovaginal PAMG-1 to confirm PROM in 99% cases of known PROM, and to be positive in some equivocal cases. It is unknown if all of these actually had membrane rupture as amnioinfusion was not routinely performed [17]. This group subsequently found a rapid test for PAMG-1 (Amnisure®) to be positive in 31% of laboring and 5% of non-laboring women in whom membrane rupture was not suspected, raising question regarding the test's utility [20].

Assessment and management (Figure 19.1)

Advanced labor, intrauterine infection, significant uterine bleeding, and non-reassuring fetal testing are indications for delivery regardless of the gestational age. If needed, the mother should be **transferred** before delivery where possible to a facility with the resources needed to care for the premature neonate. **If chorioamnionitis is suspected but the diagnosis is unclear**, an amniocentesis sample revealing a glucose value <16–20 mg/dl or a positive Gram stain can support the diagnosis. Aerobic and anaerobic amniotic fluid cultures can be performed, but results are typically unavailable until after management has been decided. Though not specific, a maternal white blood cell count above 18 000/mm^3 is also supportive of infection if antenatal corticosteroids have not recently been given, especially if the count is rising. Intrapartum broad spectrum antibiotics are indicated if chorioamnionitis is suspected. Intrapartum narrow-spectrum intrapartum **group B streptococcus prophylaxis** is indicated unless a recent anovaginal culture was negative [21]. Vaginal **bleeding** that has resolved before PROM is not necessarily an indication for delivery. However, heavy vaginal bleeding is an indica-

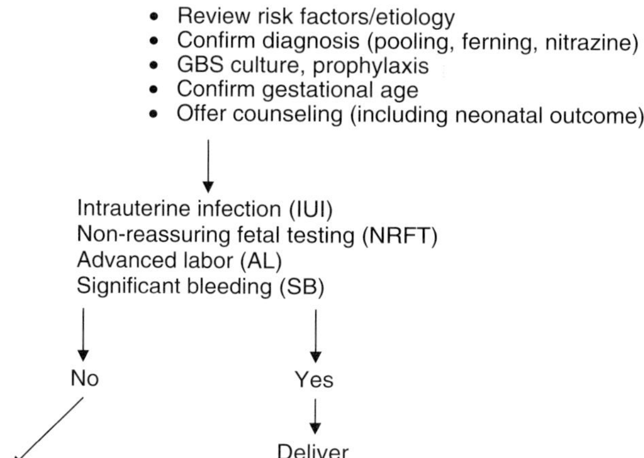

- GA < 23 weeks
  - Often delivery vs expectant management
- GA 23–31 weeks
  - Conservative management
  - Hospitalization
  - Corticosteroids for fetal maturity
  - Broad spectrum antibiotics (e.g. erythromycin and ampicillin)
  - Delivery for IUI, NRFT, AL, SB or attainment of fetal maturity or ≥ 34 weeks
- GA 32–33 weeks
  - Consider evaluation of fetal maturity. If mature, deliver.
  - Consider delivery after antenatal corticosteroid benefit achieved or at 34 weeks
  - Treat as per GA 23–31 weeks if managed conservatively
- GA ≥ 34 weeks
  - Deliver

Figure 19.1 Management of preterm premature rupture of the membranes. GA, gestational age. GBS, group B streptococcus.

tion for delivery at any gestational age. Delivery is generally indicated for any ongoing or new onset bleeding from suspected placental abruption unless the risk of neonatal death is high with delivery. Similarly, the fetus at risk for imminent asphyxia or death because of recurrent moderate–severe variable or late **decelerations** is best delivered. Mild variable decelerations with an otherwise reassuring heart rate pattern may be amenable to conservative management, but evaluation for fetal malpresentation and umbilical cord prolapse should be considered. Extended fetal heart rate monitoring and/or delivery may be appropriate after completion of antenatal corticosteroid administration if decelerations persist.

After initial assessment, targeted treatment of women with PPROM amenable to conservative management is adjusted based on gestational age at membrane rupture. Anovaginal **group B streptococcus cultures** should be obtained if conservative management is undertaken, if not recently performed. **Hospitalization** is indicated once viability is reached.

Only 18% of women with PPROM are eligible for outpatient management, and home management removes the patient from the opportunity for emergency intervention for labor, infection, bleeding or umbilical cord prolapsed [22].

PROM before the limit of viability (<23 weeks' gestation)

If the woman does not desire conservative management after detailed counseling, **delivery** can be accomplished by dilatation and evacuation or by labor induction with oxytocin infusion or prostaglandins (PgE2 or PgE1 unless contra-indicated). There is no evidence to guide inpatient versus outpatient **conservative management** after initial assessment. It is unclear whether broad spectrum antibiotics (see below) will enhance latency sufficiently to accrue neonatal benefits in this setting, but initial treatment may be appropriate. A detailed ultrasound study should be performed to evaluate for fetal anomalies, and serial evaluation of fetal lung growth can be performed. Direct (lung length, volume) and indirect markers (e.g. chest circumference, chest–abdomen circumference ratio, chest circumference–femur length ratio) have a high positive predictive value for lethal pulmonary hypoplasia [23, 24]. Based on this information, some women will proceed to delivery. Experimental measures to reseal the membranes after PROM have been explored but cannot be recommended [25–27]. Typically, women with previable PROM are re-admitted to hospital when the limit of viability is reached, and they are subsequently treated similarly to those with PROM remote from term. Antenatal corticosteroids can be administered at this time. However, administration of broad spectrum antibiotics to prolong pregnancy will not likely be beneficial at this point if extended latency has already occurred.

PROM remote from term (23–31 weeks' gestation)

After initial assessment, daily **evaluation of the fetal heart rate** pattern is advised. Continuous monitoring or reconsideration of delivery is recommended if abnormalities are evident. Fetal well-being can be assessed by nonstress test, biophysical profile, or both. Neither has high sensitivity for predicting infectious complications [28]. Fetal heart rate monitoring allows assessment for asymptomatic uterine contractions and the fetal response to these. Bed rest increases the risk of deep venous thrombophlebitis, and **prophylactic leg exercises, [intermittent] compression stockings and/or prophylactic subcutaneous heparin** should be considered. For those few women with extended latency, **delivery is generally undertaken at ~34 weeks' gestation**.

Antenatal corticosteroids should be administered to reduce neonatal complications during conservative management of PROM remote from term. A 2006 Cochrane meta-analysis found antenatal corticosteroid treatment led to less frequent neonatal death, respiratory distress syndrome, chronic lung disease, intraventricular hemorrhage and necrotizing enterocolitis, with no evident increase in perinatal or maternal infections [29] (Chapter 20).

Broad spectrum antibiotic therapy has also been explored in at least 22 randomized trials, including over 6000 women with PPROM. Taken together, these have shown improved latency at 48 hours and 7 days, less frequent chorioamnionitis, and reductions in neonatal morbidities including intraventricular hemorrhage, infections and the need for oxygen therapy [30]. In one of the two largest studies, aggressive therapy with ampicillin/amoxicillin and erythromycin (2 days intravenous and 5 days oral therapy) improved latency up to 3 weeks after initiation of treatment and reduced gestational age dependent morbidities including respiratory distress and the composite primary outcome [31]. The largest multicenter trial found that ampicillin-clavulanic acid treatment increased neonatal necrotizing enterocolitis, but that **erythromycin** alone prolonged pregnancy and reduced the incidences of death or major cerebral abnormality and chronic neonatal lung disease [32]. Seven year follow-up of these infants revealed no benefits or risks from antibiotic treatment [33]. While transcervical or transabdominal amnioinfusion of antibiotics has been a subject of interest, rapid penetration of antibiotics into the amniotic cavity is generally achieved with systemic administration and amnioinfusion is unneeded [34–37].

While it has been speculated that tocolytic treatment might extend latency and allow time for corticosteroid therapy, this benefit has not been proven. Parenteral tocolysis with betamimetic agents may prolong pregnancy briefly, but neither this nor other tocolytic treatments have been shown to improve infant outcomes. The potential benefits and risks of tocolytic therapy remain unclear for those treated concurrently with broad spectrum antibiotics in this setting.

Prevention of cerebral palsy and other neurologic complications with antenatal **magnesium sulfate** administration before PTB has been studied in several trials [38]. In one of these, more than 90% of included patients were enrolled because of PPROM before 32 weeks' gestation [39]. Treatment reduced cerebral palsy without an increase in fetal/infant death. Because none of the currently published studies demonstrated a reduction in the primary outcome with magnesium sulfate administration, its final place in practice for this indication has not been decided. Readers are encouraged to watch for new information.

PROM near term (32–36 weeks' gestation)

If PROM occurs at **34 weeks 0 days or after, delivery is generally recommended** because the risk of major neonatal morbidities is low and latency can be anticipated to be too brief to reduce morbidity and mortality, and because the risks of intrauterine infection and umbilical cord compression are increased if conservative management is pursued [40].

With PPROM **at 32–33 weeks' gestation, fetal pulmonary maturity can be evaluated** from a vaginal pool or amniocentesis specimen. If pulmonary maturity is evident, little is to be gained from conservative management as latency will likely be brief and the risk of chorioamnionitis increases with delayed delivery [41]. For those with evident pulmonary immaturity, or if fluid is not available for testing, antenatal corticosteroids can be administered. During this time, it is prudent to administer broad spectrum antibiotics to reduce the risk of infection. With PROM at 33 weeks 0 days or more, it is reasonable to proceed to delivery after antenatal corticosteroids have been administered as delivery would typically be induced within ~1 week. Conservative management after antenatal corticosteroids is acceptable for PROM at 32 weeks' gestation.

Special circumstances

Multiple gestations

Several studies have evaluated PPROM in twin pregnancies. The vast majority of these result from rupture of the presenting sac. This complication occurs more frequently in twins than singletons (7.4 versus 3.7%, $P < 0.001$) [42]. In published studies, latency is either similar or shorter in twin pregnancies, with 50–74% delivering within 48 hours and 78–91% delivering within 7 days [42–44]. As in singleton gestations, latency is longer with membrane rupture before 30 weeks' gestation, but median latencies remain less than 2 days [42–45]. Other than an increased risk for Cesarean delivery in twin gestations, maternal and neonatal outcomes are similar to singletons when matched for gestational age. The incidence of PROM involving the non-presenting sac is unknown but this has been documented in one case which was managed conservatively and resealed to ultimately deliver after recurrent PPROM at 32 weeks [46].

Management of twin pregnancies complicated by PPROM is generally similar to that for singletons. Because the non-presenting twin appears to have more frequent hyaline membrane disease (21 versus 7.1 %; $P < 0.01$) and oxygen requirement (44 versus 23%; $P < 0.003$) [42] it may be preferable to sample the non-presenting gestational sac when amniocentesis is performed to evaluate fetal pulmonary maturity after PROM in twins (Chapter 16).

Herpes simplex virus (HSV) infection

Neonatal HSV infection usually results from vertical transmission in labor. Neonatal infection occurs in up to 34–80% of infants delivered with primary maternal infection versus 1–5% with secondary infection. Based on small case series, it has been believed that membrane rupture for more than 4–6 hours is associated with increased neonatal infection [47, 48]. However, in a series of 29 pregnancies managed conservatively with PROM and active recurrent herpes infection before 32 weeks gestation, Major *et al.* found no cases on neonatal infection after latencies ranging from 1to35 days [49]. These data suggest that PROM complicated by recurrent maternal herpes infection can be managed conservatively when the risk of death and long term complications is high with immediate delivery. Prophylactic treatment with antiviral agents (e.g. acyclovir) has not been studied specifically after PROM, but is likely appropriate. When PROM occurs near term, abdominal delivery should be undertaken expeditiously.

Cervical cerclage

PROM complicates approximately one of four pregnancies with a cervical cerclage, and half of those after physical-exam cerclage placement. Retrospective studies suggest that cerclage removal after PPROM results in similar outcomes to PROM without cerclage. Studies of cerclage retention versus removal after PROM have yielded conflicting results but none has found a significant reduction in infant morbidities with cerclage retention [50, 51]. Each found insignificant trends toward increased maternal infection with this practice, and one study found increased infant mortality and death from sepsis with retained cerclage despite brief pregnancy prolongation. One study found improved pregnancy prolongation with cerclage retention, but this may have reflected differences in patient populations or practices at the two institutions that were compared [52]. Given potential risk without evident neonatal benefit, **the cerclage should generally be removed when PPROM occurs**. Short-term cerclage retention (≤48 hours) during antenatal corticosteroid administration has not been studied.

Prevention of PPROM

Prior PTB, especially that due to PROM, is associated with subsequent PPROM, and this risk increases with decreasing gestational age at PTB.

Women with a prior history are at 3.3-fold increased risk for PTB due to PROM (13.5 versus 4.1%, $P < 0.01$) and have a 13.5-fold increased risk for PPROM before 28 weeks of gestation (1.8 versus 0.13%, $P < 0.01$) [53]. Multiparas with a history of PPROM, a short cervix, and a positive fetal fibronectin at 22–24 weeks gestation have a 25% risk of recurrence before 35 weeks' gestation (a 31-fold increased risk, $P = 0.001$), while nulliparas with similar findings have a 16.7% risk of preterm birth due to PROM. Only a fraction of those destined to deliver preterm are identified by these expensive technologies, and an effective intervention has not yet been identified. Because of this, routine screening is not recommended.

Given a history of prior PTB due to PTL or PROM, guidance is directed to limit factors associated with an increased risk (**adequate nutrition, smoking cessation, avoid heavy lifting, limit prolonged standing without breaks**) (Chapter 9). **Weekly 17-hydroxyprogesterone caproate** therapy can reduce the risk of recurrent PTB due to PTL or PROM [54]. While vaginal progesterone suppositories (100 mg daily) have also resulted in a reduction in PTB (13.8 versus 28.5%, $P < 0.05$) [55], daily treatment with 90 mg progesterone vaginal gel resulted in no benefit [56].

Though vitamin C deficiency has been linked to PPROM, supplementation with this vitamin may has not been found to prevent this complication [57]. In a placebo controlled trial, Spinnato *et al.* found treatment with vitamin C (1000 mg) and E (400 IU) supplements starting at 12–19 weeks' gestation to increase the risks of PROM (10.6 versus 5.5%, $P = 0.015$), and PPROM (4.6 versus 1.7%, $P = 0.025$) [58].

References

1 Ventura SJ, Martin JA, Taffel SM, Mathews TJ, Clarke SC. Advance report of final natality statistics, 1993. Monthly Vital Statistics Report from the Centers For Disease Control and Prevention 1995; 44(3S): 1–88.

2 Ananth CV, Joseph KS, Oyelese Y, Demissie K, Vintzileos AM. Trends in preterm birth and perinatal mortality among singletons: United States, 1989 through 2000. Obstet Gynecol 2005; 105: 1084–91.

3 Mercer BM, Arheart KL. Antimicrobial therapy in expectant management of preterm premature rupture of the membranes. Lancet 1995; 346: 1271–9.

4 Waters TP, Mercer BM. The management of preterm premature rupture of the membranes near the limit of fetal viability. Am J Obstet Gynecol 2009; 201: 230–40.

5 Muris C, Girard B, Creveuil C, *et al.* Management of premature rupture of membranes before 25 weeks. Eur J Obstet Gynecol Reprod Biol 2007; 131: 163–8.

6 Mercer BM. Preterm premature rupture of the membranes. Obstet Gynecol 2003; 101: 178–93.
7 Tyson JE, Parikh NA, Langer J, Green C, Higgins RD. Intensive care for extreme prematurity: moving beyond gestational age. N Engl J Med 2008; 358: 1672–81.
8 Locatelli A, Ghidini A, Paterlini G, *et al.* Gestational age at preterm premature rupture of membranes: a risk factor for neonatal white matter damage. Am J Obstet Gynecol 2005; 193: 947–51.
9 Wu YW, Colford JM Jr. Chorioamnionitis as a risk factor for cerebral palsy: a meta-analysis. JAMA 2000; 284: 1417–24.
10 Yoon BH, Jun JK, Romero R, *et al.* Amniotic fluid inflammatory cytokines (interleukin-6, interleukin-1 beta, and tumor necrosis factor-alpha), neonatal brain white matter lesions, and cerebral palsy. Am J Obstet Gynecol 1997; 177: 19–26.
11 Yoon BH, Romero R, Yang SH, *et al.* Interleukin-6 concentrations in umbilical cord plasma are elevated in neonates with white matter lesions associated with periventricular leukomalacia. Am J Obstet Gynecol 1996; 174: 1433–40.
12 Alexander JM, Mercer BM, Miodovnik M, *et al.* The impact of digital cervical examination on expectantly managed preterm rupture of membranes. Am J Obstet Gynecol 2000; 183: 1003–7.
13 Lewis DF, Major CA, Towers CV, *et al.* Effects of digital vaginal examinations on latency period in preterm premature rupture of membranes. Obstet Gynecol 1992; 80: 630–4.
14 Imseis HM, Trout WC, Gabbe SG. The microbiologic effect of digital cervical examination. Am J Obstet Gynecol 1999; 180: 578–80.
15 Reece EA, Chervenak FA, Moya FR, Hobbins JC. Amniotic fluid arborization: effect of blood, meconium, and pH alterations. Obstet Gynecol 1984; 64: 248–50.
16 Rosemond RL, Lombardi SJ, Boehm FH. Ferning of amniotic fluid contaminated with blood. Obstet Gynecol 1990; 75: 338–40.
17 Lee SE, Park JS, Norwitz ER, Kim KW, Park HS, Jun JK. Measurement of placental alpha-microglobulin-1 in cervicovaginal discharge to diagnose rupture of membranes. Obstet Gynecol 2007; 109: 634–40.
18 Lockwood CJ, Wein R, Chien D, *et al.* Fetal membrane rupture is associated with the presence of insulin-like growth factor-binding protein-1 in vaginal secretions. Am J Obstet Gynecol 1994; 171: 146–50.
19 Gaucherand P, Guibaud S, Awada A, Rudigoz RC. Comparative study of three amniotic fluid markers in premature rupture of membranes: fetal fibronectin, alpha-fetoprotein, diamino-oxydase. Acta Obstet Gynecol Scand 1995; 74: 118–21.
20 Lee SM, Lee J, Seong HS, *et al.* The clinical significance of a positive Amnisure test in women with term labor with intact membranes. J Matern Fetal Neonatal Med 2009; 22: 305–10.
21 Prevention of early-onset group B streptococcal disease in newborns. ACOG Committee Opinion No. 279. American College of Obstetricians and Gynecologists. Obstet Gynecol 2002; 100: 1405–12.
22. Carlan SJ, O'Brien WF, Parsons MT, Lense JJ. Preterm premature rupture of membranes: a randomized study of home vs hospital management. Obstet Gynecol 1993: 81: 61–4.
23 Laudy JA, Tibboel D, Robben SG, *et al.* Prenatal prediction of pulmonary hypoplasia: clinical, biometric, and Doppler velocity correlates. Pediatrics 2002; 109: 250–8.

24 Rizzo G, Capponi A, Angelini E, Mazzoleni A, Romanini C. Blood flow velocity waveforms from fetal peripheral pulmonary arteries in pregnancies with preterm premature rupture of the membranes: relationship with pulmonary hypoplasia. Ultrasound Obstet Gynecol 2000; 15: 98–103.
25 Sciscione AC, Manley JS, Pollock M, *et al.* Intracervical fibrin sealants: a potential treatment for early preterm premature rupture of the membranes. Am J Obstet Gynecol 2001; 184: 368–73.
26 Quintero RA, Morales WJ, Bornick PW, Allen M, Garabelis N. Surgical treatment of spontaneous rupture of membranes: the amniograft- first experience. Am J Obstet Gynecol 2002; 186: 155–7.
27 O'Brien JM, Barton JR, Milligan DA. An aggressive interventional protocol for early midtrimester premature rupture of the membranes using gelatin sponge for cervical plugging. Am J Obstet Gynecol 2002; 187: 1143–6.
28 Lewis DF, Adair CD, Weeks JW, Barrilleaux PS, Edwards MS, Garite TJ. A randomized clinical trial of daily nonstress testing versus biophysical profile in the management of preterm premature rupture of membranes. Am J Obstet Gynecol 1999; 181: 1495–9.
29 Roberts D, Dalziel SR. Antenatal corticosteroids for accelerating fetal lung maturation for women at risk of preterm birth. Cochrane Database Syst Rev 2006, Issue 3. Art. No.: CD004454. DOI:10.1002/14651858.CD004454.pub2.
30 Kenyon S, Boulvain M, Neilson JP. Antibiotics for preterm rupture of membranes. Cochrane Database Syst Rev 2003, Issue 2. Art. No.: CD001058. DOI: 10.1002/14651858.CD001058
31 Mercer BM, Miodovnik M, Thurnau G *et al.* Antibiotic therapy for reduction of infant morbidity after preterm premature rupture of the membranes. A randomized controlled trial. JAMA 1997; 278: 989–95.
32 Kenyon SL, Taylor DJ, Tarnow-Mordi W; Oracle Collaborative Group. Broad spectrum antibiotics for preterm, prelabor rupture of fetal membranes: the ORACLE I Randomized trial. Lancet 2001; 357: 979–88.
33 Kenyon S, Pike K, Jones DR *et al.* Childhood outcomes after prescription of antibiotics to pregnant women with preterm rupture of the membranes: 7-year follow-up of the ORACLE I trial. Lancet 2008; 372: 1310–8.
34 Fortunato SJ, Bottom BW, Don RE, Welt SI, Swan KS. Study state cord and amniotic fluid Ceftizoxime levels continuously surpass maternal levels. Am J Obstet Gynecol 1988; 159: 570–3.
35 De Leeuw JW, Roumen FJME, Bouckaert PXJM, Cremers HMHG, Vree TB. Achievement of therapeutic concentrations of Cephuroxime in early preterm gestations with premature rupture of the membranes. Obstet Gynecol 1993; 81: 255–60.
36 Philpson A. Pharmacokinetics of antibiotics in pregnancy and labour. Clin Pharmacokinet 1979; 4: 297–307.
37 Bloom SL, Cox SM, Bawdon RE, Gilstrap LC. Ampicillin for neonatal group B streptococcal prophylaxis: how rapidly can bactericidal concentrations be achieved? Am J Obstet Gynecol 1996; 175: 974–6.
38 Doyle LW, Crowther CA, Middleton P, Marret S, Rouse D. Magnesium sulphate for women at risk of preterm birth for neuroprotection of the fetus. Cochrane Database Syst Rev 2009, Issue 1. Art. No.: CD004661. DOI:10.1002/14651858.CD004661.pub3.
39 Rouse DJ, Hirtz DG, Thom E *et al.* A randomized, controlled trial of magnesium sulfate for the prevention of cerebral palsy. N Engl J Med 2008; 359: 895–905.

40 Naef RW 3rd, Allbert JR, Ross EL *et al.* Premature rupture of membranes at 34 to 37 weeks' gestation: aggressive versus conservative management. Am J Obstet Gynecol 1998; 178: 126–30.
41 Mercer BM, Crocker L, Boe N, Sibai B. Induction vs expectant management in PROM with mature amniotic fluid at 32-36 weeks: a randomized trial. Am J Obstet Gynecol 1993; 82: 775–82.
42 Mercer BM, Crocker LG, Pierce WF, Sibai BM. Clinical characteristics and outcome of twin gestation complicated by preterm premature rupture of the membranes. Am J Obstet Gynecol 1993; 168: 1467–73.
43 Trentacoste SV, Jean-Pierre C, Baergen R, Chasen ST. Outcomes of preterm premature rupture of membranes in twin pregnancies. J Matern Fetal Neonatal Med 2008; 21: 555–7.
44 Hsieh YY, Chang CC, Tsai HD *et al.* Twin vs singleton pregnancy. Clinical characteristics and latency periods in preterm premature rupture of membranes. J Reprod Med 1999; 44: 616–20.
45 Bianco AT, Stone J, Lapinski R, Lockwood C, Lynch L, Berkowitz RL. The clinical outcome of preterm premature rupture of membranes in twin versus singleton pregnancies. Am J Perinatol 1996; 13: 135–8.
46 Borenstein R, Shoham Z. Premature rupture of the membranes in a single twin gestational sac: a case report. J Reprod Med 1990; 35: 270.
47 Amstey MS. Management of pregnancy complicated by genital herpes virus infection. Obstet Gynecol 1971; 37: 515–20.
48 Nahmias AJ, Josey WE, Naib ZM, Freeman MG, Fernandez RJ, Wheeler JH. Perinatal risk associated with maternal genital herpes simplex virus infection. Am J Obstet Gynecol 1971; 110: 825–37.
49 Major CA, Towers CV, Lewis DF, Garite TJ. Expectant management of preterm premature rupture of membranes complicated by active recurrent genital herpes. Am J Obstet Gynecol 2003; 188: 1551–5.
50 Ludmir J, Bader T, Chen L, Lindenbaum C, Wong G. Poor perinatal outcome associated with retained cerclage in patients with premature rupture of membranes. Obstet Gynecol 1994; 84: 823–6.
51 Jenkins TM, Berghella V, Shlossman PA *et al.* Timing of cerclage removal after preterm premature rupture of membranes: maternal and neonatal outcomes. Am J Obstet Gynecol 2000; 183: 847–52.
52 McElrath TF, Norwitz ER, Lieberman ES, Heffner LJ. Perinatal outcome after preterm premature rupture of membranes with in situ cervical cerclage. Am J Obstet Gynecol 2002; 187: 1147–52.
53 Mercer BM, Goldenberg RL, Meis PJ, *et al.* The Preterm Prediction Study: prediction of preterm premature rupture of the membranes through clinical findings and ancillary testing. Am J Obstet Gynecol 2000; 183: 738–45.
54 Meis PJ, Klebanoff M, Thom E *et al.* Prevention of recurrent preterm delivery by 17 alpha-hydroxyprogesterone caproate. N Engl J Med 2003; 348: 2379–85.
55 da Fonseca EB, Bittar RE, Carvalho MH, Zugaib M. Prophylactic administration of progesterone by vaginal suppository to reduce the incidence of spontaneous preterm birth in women at increased risk: a randomized placebo-controlled double-blind study. Am J Obstet Gynecol 2003; 188: 419–24.
56 O'Brien JM, Adair CD, Lewis DF *et al.* Progesterone vaginal gel for the reduction of recurrent preterm birth: primary results from a randomized, double-blind, placebo-controlled trial. Ultrasound Obstet Gynecol 2007; 30: 687–96.

57 Casanueva E, Ripoll C, Tolentino M *et al.* Vitamin C supplementation to prevent premature rupture of the chorioamniotic membranes: a randomized trial. Am J Clin Nutr 2005; 81: 859–63.

58 Spinnato JA 2nd, Freire S, Pinto e Silva JL *et al.* Antioxidant supplementation and premature rupture of the membranes: a planned secondary analysis. Am J Obstet Gynecol 2008; 199: 433.e1–8.

CHAPTER 20

Promotion of Fetal Maturation

Kellie E. Murphy
University of Toronto, Mount Sinai Hospital, Toronto, Ontario, Canada

Key points

- All pregnant women between 24 and 34 weeks at risk of preterm birth (PTB) should be offered treatment with a single course of antenatal corticosteroids (ACS).
- This single course of ACS consists of two doses of 12 mg of betamethasone given intramuscularly 24 hours apart; or four doses of 6 mg of dexamethasone given intramuscularly 12 hours apart.
- A single course of ACS administered to women at increased risk of PTB between 24 and 34 weeks reduces morbidity (respiratory distress syndrome, intraventricular hemorrhage (IVH), necrotizing enterocolitis, newborn intensive care unit admission, etc.) and mortality in infants.
- There is equipoise regarding the effects of betamethasone vs dexamethasone, with meta-analysis data showing a lower incidence of IVH with betamethasone.
- The benefits of a single course of ACS are proven for women with preterm premature rupture of the membranes, while evidence is limited for those with multiple gestations.
- The current benefit and risk data are insufficient to support routine use of repeat or rescue courses of ACS in clinical practice. Repeat courses of antenatal corticosteroids, including rescue therapy, should be reserved for patients enrolled in clinical trials.

Introduction

Preterm birth (PTB) is associated with increased morbidity and mortality for the neonate born too soon [1]. Morbidity includes several complications (Chapter 22). Respiratory distress syndrome (RDS) is one of the most common. A single course of antenatal corticosteroids (ACS) to the mother to promote fetal maturation and decrease neonatal morbidity and mortality is a rare example of a treatment that yields both a cost saving and an improved health outcome. The objectives of this chapter are to review this therapy: its history; fetal lung development; pharmacology and physiology

Preterm Birth. Edited by Vincenzo Berghella. © 2010 Blackwell Publishing

of ACS therapy; the use of ACS in clinical practice, including the controversy that exists today regarding the use of rescue and multiple courses of ACS.

History of antenatal corticosteroids

The effect of steroids in relationship to accelerated organ maturation in animals has been known for more than 50 years. **Liggins and Howie**, while studying parturition in pregnant sheep, noted that fetal lambs when exposed to ACS appeared viable at an earlier age. Furthermore, he and colleagues hypothesized that antenatal steroids could be given to humans to accelerate fetal lung development. In **1972**, his team performed the **first randomized controlled trial** (RCT) of ACS in women at risk of PTB [2]. In this hallmark study, a single course of ACS not only reduced the risk of RDS (from 25.8 to 9%), but also was associated with a decrease in neonatal mortality (15–3.2%) [2].

Over the next 18 years, several investigators conducted randomized controlled trials of ACS in women at risk of PTB. Like Liggins, many found that ACS were associated with benefits, including a decrease in RDS and neonatal mortality, while other investigators reported no benefits. During this time, the use of ACS was a controversial and passionately debated topic in the medical literature. Antenatal therapy was challenged with criticism as there were concerns that exposure to steroids would be detrimental, leading to sequelae such as maternal and fetal immune suppression. In addition, animal studies provided concerns that steroids would alter neuronal development and force cell differentiation at the expense of cell multiplication, while others argued that the benefits of ACS outweighed the potential risks and argued for the universal adoption of this practice.

In **1990 Patricia Crowley** summarized the results of the first 12 RCTs. Incorporating the results of over 3000 participants, this analysis clearly demonstrated that ACS were beneficial and highly effective in reducing rates of RDS and neonatal mortality [3]. Despite this convincing summary, many clinicians were slow to adopt this life-saving antenatal therapy.

Four years later, the **National Institutes of Child Health and Infant Development** held a consensus conference which reviewed the evidence and summarized the risks and benefits of a single course of ACS in women at increased risk of PTB. The consensus panel concluded that ACS led to a **reduction in neonatal mortality, RDS and intraventricular hemorrhage (IVH)**. Furthermore, they concluded that these benefits extended over a wide range of gestational age (**24–34 weeks**) and were **not limited by gender or race** [4].

Table 20.1 Phases of lung development.

Phase	Duration
1 Pseudoglandular	Embryonic period—17 weeks
2 Canalicular	13–25 weeks
3 Terminal-sac	24 weeks—birth
4 Alveolar	29 weeks—postnatal life

Lung development

To understand fetal maturation and effect of ACS therapy, its important to review the four phases of lung development [5] (Table 20.1).

The **pseudoglandular phase** begins in the embryonic period and extends until approximately 17 weeks gestation. The lung begins as an epithelial tree. The branches become bronchi and bronchioles and by the end of this phase the number of bronchi and bronchioles are complete. Columnar epithelium line the proximal part of the tree, whereas cuboidal epithelium line the distal part of the tree. The cuboidal epithelium is composed of the precursor or immature type 2 alveolar cells or pneumonocytes [5].

The **canalicular phase** extends from approximately 13 to 25 weeks gestational age. This phase is characterized by 'canalisation' or invasion of the cuboidal epithelium by capillaries and by the formation of the respiratory units called acini. The acinar tubules are lined by type 2 alveolar cells. The end of this stage is the beginning of current fetal viability [5].

The **terminal-sac phase** extends from 24 weeks until birth. This phase is characterized by the development of saccules. Saccules end the respiratory tree. These thin-walled saccules are lined by flat epithelium. This epithelial lining is composed of type 1 and type 2 alveolar cells. Postnatally, saccules become alveolar ducts. At birth the saccules give rise to alveoli.

Type 2 alveolar cells synthesize and secrete pulmonary surfactant. Surfactant production begins before birth and is composed primarily of lecithin. Surfactant reduces the surface air-liquid interface in the neonatal lung and is essential in the transition to air-breathing. Surfactant production increases with pulmonary maturation [5].

The **alveolar phase** begins at approximately 29 weeks gestational age and extends into postnatal life. This phase is characterized by the development of alveoli. One third or more of the 300 million alveoli of the adult are present at term birth. Following birth and during the first two years of life, the alveoli increase in number. The alveoli then grow at a slower rate up to approximately 8 years of life. Subsequently, the lungs simply grow in size [5].

Pharmacology and physiology of antenatal corticosteroids

Endogenous cortisol is derived from cholesterol, following several enzymatically controlled metabolic steps. Corticosteroids act by controlling the rate of production of various proteins. This is accomplished when corticosteroids bind with the cytoplasmic receptors of cells and form steroid–receptor complexes. These complexes move into the cell nucleus and bind to DNA regulating the production of specific proteins.

Corticosteroids have a wide variety of pharmacological effects. These pharmacological effects include direct and indirect effects on skeletal muscle, cardiovascular, renal and nervous systems. In the inflammatory response and the immune system, corticosteroids modulate various enzymatic pathways. Additionally, corticosteroids inhibit cell division in a variety of tissues and participate in regulation of electrolyte balance. Corticosteroids influence carbohydrate, lipid and protein metabolism. Finally, corticosteroids are known to accelerate maturation of developmentally regulated proteins and to stimulate cytodifferentiation in numerous cells, including type II pneumocytes [6].

Dexamethasone and betamethasone are the preferred corticosteroids for antenatal fetal maturation. There are several reasons why these corticosteroids are preferred: (1) readily cross the placenta in their biologically active forms; (2) are weak in immunosuppressive activity and are devoid of mineralocorticoid activity and (3) have a longer duration of action than cortisol [7]. The bioavailability of corticosteroids to the fetus is reduced secondary to placental metabolism. The umbilical vein concentrations of betamethasone are approximately 25–30% of maternal venous concentrations. In addition, the corticosteroids do not remain in the fetal circulation for long. In one study, when the levels of betamethasone, administered prior to birth, were assayed in cord blood, the drug was undetectable 40 hours following the injection [8].

Risks and benefits of a single course of antenatal corticosteroids

A **single course** of ACS is defined as either **betamethasone 12 mg intramuscularly (IM) every 24 hours for two doses**, or **dexamethasone 6 mg IM every 12 hours for four doses**. The benefits of a single course of ACS for fetuses at increased risk of PTB are shown in **Table 20.2**, as summarized in the most recent Cochrane meta-analysis, which includes 21 trials in 3885 women and 4269 infants [9]. Infants exposed

Table 20.2 Effects to infants and children of a single course of corticosteroids for women at risk for preterm birth[9].

	RR	95% CI	*n* (infants)
Neonatal death	0.69	0.58–0.81	3956
Respiratory distress syndrome	0.66	0.59–0.73	4038
Cerebroventricular hemorrhage	0.54	0.43–0.69	2872
Necrotizing enterocolitis	0.46	0.29–0.74	1675
Intensive care admission	0.80	0.65–0.99	277
Systemic infections in first 48 hours of life	0.56	0.38–0.85	1319
Developmental delay in childhood (~3 y.o.)	0.49	0.24–1.00	518
Cerebral palsy (~6 y.o.)	0.60	0.34–1.03	904

to ACS also have improved circulatory stability, and require less oxygen and ventilatory support [10]. To date, follow up studies of infants enrolled in RCTs have not demonstrated any long-term adverse effects following a single course of ACS. The most recent of these studies followed children to 30 years of age [11]. A meta-analysis of over 1400 women with preterm premature rupture of membranes (**PPROM**) shows that a single course of ACS was associated with a decrease in RDS (RR 0.56:CI 0.46–0.70), IVH (RR 0.47: CI 0.31–0.70) and necrotizing enterocolitis (RR 0.21: CI 0.05–0.82) [12]. **ACS are beneficial** for the fetus/infant/child, and safe for the mother. The **frequency of maternal infection is similar** between women who received and those who did not receive a single course of ACS [9]. The only significant maternal side effect is a **transient (<7 days) increase in glucose intolerance** [9]. Effect and dosing in multiple pregnancy deserves further study. Betamethasone is associated with a greater reduction in RDS and less puerperal sepsis than dexamethasone in a meta-analysis [9], but a recent trial showed no difference in RDS and death [13]. The most recent Cochrane meta-analysis of 10 trials and over 1100 infants reported a **56% lower incidence of IVH with betamethasone compared with dexamethasone** [14]. Gestational age of proven effectiveness is from **24 to 34 6/7 weeks** [9]. **Limited data shows benefit also at 23 weeks** [15], while limited data is available for efficacy at 35–36 weeks.

Risks and benefits of repeated courses of ACS

There is uncertainty as to how long ACS treatment should continue to be effective if the woman remains undelivered ≥7 days following a single

Table 20.3 Randomized controlled trials of single vs repeated doses of antenatal corticosteroids (ACS).

Study group	Sample size	Intervention (after one single course of ACS)	Primary outcome	Primary outcome findings percent ACS vs placebo OR/RR (CI)	Respiratory distress syndrome OR/RR (CI)
USA (Chicago) Guinn *et al.* [18]	502	Betametasone 12 mg or placebo q 24 h × 2 doses q 7 days until 34 weeks	Death or adverse neonatal outcome	No difference between groups 22.5% vs 28%, 0.80 (0.59–1.10) $P = 0.16$	Severe 15.3% vs 24.1%, 0.63 (0.44–0.91) $P = 0.01$
ACTORDS [20]	982	11.4 mg Celestone Chronodose or placebo × 1 dose q 7 days until 32 weeks	Neonatal lung disease	12% vs 20%, 0.60 (0.46–0.79) $P = 0.0003$	33% vs 41%, 0.82 (0.71–0.95) $P = 0.01$
NICHD [19]	495	Betametasone 12 mg or placebo q 24 h × 2 doses q 7 days until 33 weeks	Death or adverse neonatal outcome	No difference between groups 8.0% vs 9.1%, 0.88 (0.49–1.57) $P = 0.67$	Severe 2.4% vs 4.1%, 0.58 (0.21–1.57) $P = 0.28$
MACS (Canadian) [22]	1858	Betametasone 12 mg or placebo q 24 h × 2 doses q 14 days until 33 weeks	Death or adverse neonatal outcome	No difference between groups 12.9% vs 12.5%, 1.04 (0.77–1.39) $P = 0.83$	Severe 7.8% vs 7.0%, 1.14 (0.80–1.58) $P = 0.51$

course of treatment. Repeated doses in animals were first associated with adverse effects including growth restriction and alterations in neuronal maturation [16]. There are now **several RCTs which have investigated the short term benefits and risks of repeated courses of ACS in humans** (**Table 20.3**).

Overall, smaller RCTs investigating single vs weekly courses of ACS demonstrated no benefit from repeated courses of ACS [17, 18]. However, the National Institutes of Child Health and Human Development (NICHD) Maternal Fetal Medicine Units Network trial found a trend toward improved composite outcome for infants born at less than 32 weeks gestational age (23.3% ACS vs 38.5% placebo, $P = 0.08$) [19]. A larger trial which enrolled 982 women, the Australasian Collaborative Trial of Repeat

Doses of Steroids (ACTORDS), demonstrated benefit overall [20]. Fewer infants in the ACS group had RDS (33% vs 41%; RR 0.82 [95% CI 0.71–0.95], $P = 0.01$) and severe lung disease (12% vs 20%; RR 0.60 [95% CI 0.46–0.79], $P = 0.0003$). The Cochrane systematic review, incorporating the results of these trials, suggests that weekly courses of ACS are associated with a reduction in occurrence (RR 0.82 [95% CI 0.72–0.93]) and severity (RR 0.60 [95% CI 0.48–0.75]) of neonatal lung disease and a reduction in serious infant morbidity (RR 0.79 [95% CI 0.67–0.93]) [21].

The 'Multiple courses of Antenatal Corticosteroids for preterm birth Study' (MACS), which enrolled 1858 women, found no difference in the primary composite outcome (perinatal or neonatal mortality, severe RDS, bronchopulmonary dysplasia, IVH [Grade III or IV], periventricular leukomalacia or necrotizing entercolitis) between the ACS and placebo groups (12.9% vs 12.5% [OR 1.04 (CI 0.77–1.39);($P = 0.83$)] respectively). However, compared with placebo, infants who received multiple courses of ACS weighed less (2216 g [SE 28.3] vs 2330 g [SE 28.7], $P = 0.0026$), were shorter (44.5 cm [SE 0.2] vs 45.4 cm [SE 0.2], $P < 0.001$) and had a smaller head circumference (31.1 cm [SE 0.1] vs 31.7 cm [SE 0.1], $P < 0.001$) (Table 20.3) [22]. The results of MACS have not yet been incorporated into the current Cochrane meta-analysis on repeated courses of antenatal corticosteroids [21].

Risks and benefits of rescue courses of ACS in humans

'Rescue coursing' is another type of prescribing pattern for ACS which has gained popularity. For women who remain at risk of PTB, a **rescue course (a second and final course [or partial course, one injection]) is given ≥7 days following an initial course of ACS (between 25 and 33 weeks gestational age) prior to anticipated delivery**.

To date, **two RCTs** have reported discrepant results in regards to the efficacy of rescue course therapy. The first randomized 249 women to a single repeat dose of betamethasone vs placebo, 7 or more days following a single course of betamethasone. No difference was seen in the primary outcome (intact survival without RDS; OR 0.84, CI 0.55–1.30) or in RDS (OR 1.16, CI 0.75–1.79) between the two groups [23].

A second RCT randomized 437 women to a rescue course of ACS (12 mg betamethasone × 2 doses, 24 hours apart) vs placebo 14 or more days after an initial course of ACS. This study reported a decreased risk of composite morbidity for infants who received a rescue course of ACS vs placebo (32.1% vs 42.6%; OR 0.65, CI 0.44–0.97) [24].

Long-term risks and benefits of repeated courses of ACS

Infants in the MACS study **weighed less** and had a **smaller head circumference** at birth. The clinical importance of decreased fetal size is not clear, thus long-term follow-up of these infants is important. Children of the NICHD study were followed to 2–3 years of age. Physical and neurocognitive measures did not differ between groups but there was a non-significant increased risk of cerebral palsy in those exposed to weekly courses of ACS (2.9% ACS vs 0.5% placebo) [25]. In ACTORDS, the rate of survival free of major disability was similar between the two groups at 2 years of age. However, the children exposed to weekly courses of ACS were more likely to warrant an assessment for attention problems than were controls ($P = 0.04$) [26]. It is important to note that the majority of participants in ACTORDS (66%) received one or two courses of study treatment (11.4 mg Celestone Chronodose × 1 dose, every 7 days vs placebo) [20]. **These results are concerning and caution against the use of repeated or rescue courses of ACS at this time**. The 18–24 month follow-up assessments for the children in MACS and five year follow-up assessments for the children in MACS [27] and ACTORDS [28] are ongoing.

Other interventions

Prenatal thyrotropin-releasing hormones, in addition to ACS, given to women at risk of very PTB do not improve infant outcomes and can cause maternal side-effects, based on a meta-analysis of 13 trials involving over 4600 women [29]. Similarly, phenobarbital [30] and vitamin K [31] have not been shown to be efficacious.

Conclusion

A single course of ACS has substantial and immediate benefits for preterm infants and is indicated in most women at risk of PTB between 24 and 34 6/7 weeks. However, the evidence in regards to risks and benefits from repeated, or rescue courses, of ACS is unclear. Therefore, **the practice of administering repeated or rescue courses of ACS should be postponed** until additional trials (rescue coursing) are performed and the existing long-term follow-up studies assessing growth and neurodevelopment are published [32, 33].

References

1 Joseph KS, Kramer MS, Marcoux S, *et al.* Determinants of preterm birth rates in Canada from 1981 through 1983 and from 1992 through 1994. N Engl J Med 1998: 339: 1434–9.
2 Liggins GC, Howie RN. A controlled trial of antepartum glucocorticoid treatment for prevention of the respiratory distress syndrome in premature infants. Pediatrics 1972: 50; 515–25.
3 Crowley P, Chalmers I, Keirse MJ. The effects of corticosteroid administration before preterm delivery: an overview of the evidence from controlled trials. Br J Obstet Gynaecol 1990; 97: 11–25.
4 The effect of antenatal steroids for fetal maturation on perinatal outcomes. NIH Consensus Statement 1994; 12: 1–24
5 O'Rahilly R. Human Embryology and Teratology. New York: Wiley-Liss, Inc., 1992.
6 Ballard PL. Hormonal regulation of pulmonary surfactant. Endocr Rev 1989; 10: 165–81.
7 Goodman LS, Gilman A, Rall TW. The Pharmacological Basis of Therapeutics. Oxford: Pergamon, 1990.
8 Ballard PL, Granberg P, Ballard RA. Glucocorticoid levels in maternal and cord serum after prenatal betamethasone therapy to prevent respiratory distress syndrome. J Clin Invest 1975; 56: 1548–54.
9 Roberts D, Dalziel S. Antenatal corticosteroids for accelerating fetal lung maturation for women at risk of preterm birth. Cochrane Database Syst Rev 2006, Issue 3. Art. No.: CD004454. DOI: 10.1002/14651858.CD004454.pub2
10 Moise AA, Wearden ME, Kozinetz CA, Gest AL, Welty SE, Hansen TN *et al.* Antenatal steroids are associated with less need for blood pressure support in extremely premature infants. Pediatrics 1995; 95: 845–50.
11 Dalziel SR, Walker NK, Parag V, *et al.* Cardiovascular risk factors after antenatal exposure to betamethasone: 30-year follow-up of a randomised controlled trial. Lancet 2005; 365(9474): 1856–62.
12 Collaborative Group on Antenatal Steroid Therapy. Effect of antenatal dexamethasone administration on the prevention of respiratory distress syndrome. Am J Obstet Gynecol 1981; 141: 276–87.
13 Elimian A, Garry D, Figueroa R, Spitzer A, Wiencek V, Quirk JG. Antenatal betamethasone compared with dexamethasone (Betacode trial): a randomized controlled trial. Obstet Gynecol 2007; 110: 26–30.
14 Brownfoot FC, Crowther CA, Middleton P. Different corticosteroids and regimens for accelerating fetal lung maturation for women at risk of preterm birth. Cochrane Library 2008, vol. 4: CD006764.
15 Hayes J, Paul DA, Stahl GE, *et al.* Effect of antenatal corticosteroids on survival for neonates born at 23 weeks of gestation. Obstet Gynecol 2008; 111: 921–6.
16 Aghajafari F, Murphy K, Matthews S, Ohlsson A, Amankwah K, Hannah M. Repeated doses of antenatal corticosteroids in animals: a systematic review. Am J Obstet Gynecol 2002; 186: 843–9.
17 Aghajafari F, Murphy K, Willan A, *et al.* Multiple courses of antenatal corticosteroids: a systematic review and meta-analysis. Am J Obstet Gynecol 2001; 185: 1073–80.
18 Guinn DA, Atkinson MW, Sullivan L *et al.* Single vs weekly courses of antenatal corticosteroids for women at risk of preterm delivery: a randomized controlled trial. JAMA 2001; 286: 1581–7.

19 Wapner RJ, Sorokin Y, Thom EA, *et al.* Single versus weekly courses of antenatal corticosteroids: evaluation of safety and efficacy. Am J Obstet Gynecol 2006; 195: 633–42.
20 Crowther CA, Haslam RR, Hiller JE, Doyle LW, Robinson JS; Australasian Collaborative Trial of Repeat Doses of Steroids (ACTORDS) Study Group. Neonatal respiratory distress syndrome after repeat exposure to antenatal corticosteroids: a randomised controlled trial. Lancet 2006; 367: 1913–9.
21 Crowther CA, Harding JE. Repeat doses of prenatal corticosteroids for women at risk of preterm birth for preventing neonatal respiratory disease. Cochrane Review, 2008, vol. 4.
22 Murphy KE, Hannah ME, Willan AR, *et al.* Multiple courses of antenatal corticosteroids for preterm birth (MACS): a randomised controlled trial. Lancet 2008; 372: 2143–51.
23 Peltoniemi OM, Kari MA, Tammela O,*et al.* Randomized trial of a single repeat dose of prenatal betamethasone treatment in imminent preterm birth. Pediatrics 2007; 119: 290–8.
24 Garite TJ, Sorokin Y, Mele L, *et al.* Impact of a 'rescue course' of antenatal corticosteroids: a multicenter randomized placebo-controlled trial. Am J Obstet Gynecol 2009; 200: 248 e1–9.
25 Wapner RJ, Sorokin Y, Mele L, *et al.* Long-term outcomes after repeat doses of antenatal corticosteroids. N Engl J Med 2007; 357: 1190–8.
26 Crowther CA, Doyle LW, Haslam RR, *et al.* Outcomes at 2 years of age after repeat doses of antenatal corticosteroids. N Engl J Med 2007; 357: 1179–89.
27 www.utoronto.ca/macs
28 actords@medicine.adelaide.edu.au
29 Crowther CA, Alfirevic Z, Haslam RR. Thyrotropin-releasing hormone added to corticosteroids for women at risk of preterm birth for preventing neonatal respiratory disease. Cochrane Library, 2009, vol. 1.
30 Crowther CA, Crosby DD, Henderson-Smart DJ. Phenobarbital prior to preterm birth for preventing neonatal periventricular haemorrhage. Cochrane Database Syst Rev 1, 2009.
31 Crowther CA, Crosby DD, Henderson-Smart DJ. Vitamin K prior to preterm birth for preventing neonatal periventricular haemorrhage. Cochrane Database Syst Rev 1, 2009.
32 American College of Obstetrics and Gynecology. Antenatal corticosteroid therapy for fetal maturation. ACOG Committee Opinion No. 402. Obstet Gynecol 2008; 111: 805–6.
33 NIH Consensus Development Conference Statement. Antenatal corticosteroids revisited: repeat courses. August 2000.

CHAPTER 21

Location, Mode of Delivery and Intrapartum Issues for the Preterm Gestation

Dana Figueroa & Dwight J. Rouse
Division of Maternal-Fetal Medicine and Center for Women's Reproductive Health, The University of Alabama at Birmingham, Alabama, USA

Key points

- Women at risk of delivering a very low birth weight (<1500 g) infant should be transferred antenatally to a hospital with a Level III Neonatal Intensive Care Unit with adequate volume.
- Parents should be counseled that infants delivered before 24 weeks gestation are less likely to survive and have approximately a 50% risk of significant morbidity.
- Detecting abnormal fetal heart rate patterns early, whether on auscultation or electronic fetal monitoring, and acting promptly (with Cesarean delivery if indicated) is important for improved neonatal outcomes.
- Regional anesthesia provides the best pain control with least risk for the preterm fetus.
- Routine episiotomy, forceps, or elective Cesarean delivery does not provide proven protection to the preterm fetus.
- Cesarean delivery should be considered for the breech preterm fetus, especially if in footling breech presentation.
- Delaying cord clamping by 30 to 120 seconds, rather than early clamping, seems to be associated with less need for transfusion and less intraventricular haemorrhage in preterm infants.

Introduction

Despite the best efforts to prevent preterm birth (PTB) and manage preterm labor (PTL), many antepartum patients have progressive PTL leading to PTB. Thus, it is important to discuss the appropriate management, location, and mode of delivery for the preterm gestation.

Preterm Birth. Edited by Vincenzo Berghella. © 2010 Blackwell Publishing

Location of delivery

Level of neonatal care

The level of neonatal intensive care and experience of the preterm infant's birth hospital play an important role in neonatal outcomes. Consideration should be given to transporting the antepartum woman based on the level of neonatal care available for delivery of a preterm infant. The Sixth Edition of Guidelines for Perinatal Care defines an expanded system of classification for levels of neonatal care. Level 1 provides basic newborn nursery care. Level IIA provides specialty care in an intermediate care nursery. Level IIB has the additional capability to provide positive airway pressure or mechanical ventilation for up to 24 hours. Level IIIA can provide comprehensive care for infants born at more than 28 weeks and greater than 1000 g, provide sustained mechanical ventilation, but not more advanced life support, and can perform minor surgeries, such as placement of central vein catheters and inguinal hernia repairs. Level IIIB provides comprehensive care for infants born at less than 28 weeks of life and less than 1000 g; advanced respiratory support, such as high frequency ventilation and inhaled nitric oxide; advanced imaging; prompt on-site access to a full range of pediatric subspecialists, including anesthesiology and pediatric surgical subspecialists who can perform major surgeries. Level IIIC has the additional ability to provide extracorporeal life support and open heart surgery for repair of complex, congenital cardiac malformations [1].

Mortality was examined in almost 14 000 low birth weight infants (501–2250 g) born in three differing level hospitals in New York City between 1976 and 1978. **Level III care was associated with a lower mortality rate** of 129/1000 live births versus Level II (168/1000) or Level I (163/1000) care. Adjustment for social or demographic status, receipt of prenatal care, or medical complications of pregnancy did not alter their findings [2].

Volume of neonatal care

The volume, in addition to level of neonatal intensive care, was analyzed in over 53 000 newborns in California in 1990. Infants born in a hospital with a level III neonatal intensive care unit (NICU) and an average census of ≥15 patients per day had significantly lower risk-adjusted neonatal mortality (OR, 0.62; 95% CI, 0.47–0.82, P = 0.002). In contrast, risk-adjusted neonatal mortality for infants born in smaller level III NICUs and level II NICUs, regardless of average census, was not significantly different than infants born in hospitals with Level I NICUs and was significantly higher than Level III NICUs [3]. Later 48 000 very low birth weight infants (VLBW), <1500 g, born in California from 1991 to 2000 were reviewed.

This study was performed after the introduction of surfactant replacement therapy in 1990 and the recommendation for antenatal corticosteroid therapy by the NICHD in 1994 [4]. **Neonatal mortality decreased as patient volume increased** within each level of care. VLBW infants born in high volume (>100 VLBW infants/year) level IIIB or higher nurseries had a lower mortality rate (18.1%) than those born in lower level and lower volume hospitals. The worst mortality rate (34.2%) was for Level I nurseries that cared for <10 VLBW infants per year [5].

Antenatal transport

Preterm neonates born in specialized centers to women transported during the antepartum period have better survival rates and decreased risks of long term sequelae than neonates transferred after birth. The American Academy of Pediatrics in conjunction with the American College of Obstetricians and Gynecologists **recommend antenatal transport of women with a VLBW fetus to a regional medical center that can provide Level III newborn care** [1]. The decision to transfer must be individualized to the patient's clinical status. Although sometimes not avoidable, caution must be taken to not transfer patients who may deliver en route. Tocolytics, antibiotics, and corticosteroids may be considered for transport. The recent trend has been towards a de-regionalization of neonatal care due to an increasing number of level II NICUs. Thus, **fewer than 25% of VLBW infants deliver in Level III NICUs** [6]. Even so, efforts must be made to transport women at risk of PTB to hospitals with the appropriate NICU care.

Intrapartum management

Diagnosis of PTL or preterm, premature rupture of the membranes (PPROM) should be confirmed, and medical management with corticosteroids, group B Streptococcus prophylaxis, and tocolytics should be considered as discussed in Chapters 18, 19 and 20. These medications, intrapartum management, the mode of delivery, and neonatal resuscitation should be reviewed with the parents in the context of age-specific morbidity and mortality.

Age-specific counseling considerations

It is important to determine the best estimated gestational age and estimated fetal weight (EFW) for preterm gestations. These estimates guide counseling on the neonate's risk for short-term and long-term morbidity and mortality and help lead discussions of intrapartum care and neonatal resuscitation. This is of particular concern for gestations at the limit of viability. Obstetric gestational age is based on a combination of last menstrual period, ultrasound measurements, or clinical data. Gestational age can also be determined by the newborn Ballard score. Studies on neonatal survival have used either the best obstetric gestational age, estimated gestational age from Ballard score, or newborn weight. Studies using Ballard estimated gestational age alone can be inaccurate, as age determined by the Ballard score consistently overestimates gestational age by approximately 10 days for infants born before 28 weeks [7]. Estimation of survival using weight is confounded by infants with growth restriction [8]. By itself, **obstetric gestational age is the most reliable antenatal predictor of neonatal survival** [9, 10]. However, combining obstetric age, weight, and gender provides the best information on neonatal survival and morbidity.

The NICHD Neonatal Research Network's prospective trial of 4633 infants weighing between 400 g and 1500 g concluded that survival increases for each completed week of gestation. These infants had 0% survival at 21 weeks estimated obstetric age and 75% survival at 25 weeks. Survival also increased with increasing weight with a survival of 11% at 401–500 g, 54% at 501–750 g, 86% at 751–1000 g, 94% at 1001–1250 g, and 97% at 1251–1500 g. When obstetric gestational age, weight and gender are combined it is clear that lower weight infants and males have higher rates of mortality than their same gestational age counterparts [11]. Tyson *et al.* prospectively studied 4446 VLBW infants to determine risk factors assessable at or before birth that were associated with likelihood of survival, survival with profound neurodevelopmental impairment, and survival without profound neurodevelopmental impairment. They found four **factors in addition to gestational age that increase the likelihood of a favorable outcome: female gender, exposure to antenatal steroids, whether singleton vs multiple birth, and higher birth weight for any given gestational age** [12].

Morbidity of surviving VLBW infants is significant. Chronic lung disease occurs in 23%, proven necrotizing enterocolitis in 7%, and severe grade III or IV intraventricular hemorrhage (IVH) occurs in 11%. Almost all (99%) of VLBW infants will have poor postnatal growth [11]. Approximately half of extremely premature infants born at 25 weeks or less will manifest disability in mental and psychomotor development, neuromotor function, or sensory and communication function based on assessment at a median age of 30 months, corrected for gestational age, and 25% will have severe neurologic disability. Male infants have lower psychomotor scores and are more likely to have cerebral palsy than females [13] (Chapter 22).

Parents should be counseled that in general infants delivered before 24 weeks are less likely to survive and those who do survive have a 50% risk of significant morbidity. Survival increases with increasing gestational age and weight. In general, females have a better prognosis than males. The health care team should be consistent with parents on their assessment, prognosis, and recommendations for care [14] (Chapter 23).

Intrapartum fetal monitoring

Mean fetal heart rate at 22 weeks is 160 b.p.m. and drops to 140 b.p.m. at term. Fetal heart rate variability is reassuring for a preterm infant as for a term infant. Deviations from expected baseline fetal heart rate and variability should be addressed and may be of greater clinical significance in the preterm fetus. Acidemia in the preterm neonate is associated with increased mortality relative to matched preterm infants without acidosis (23 vs 7%) [15]. Metabolic acidosis is also associated with severe respiratory disease [16]. Fetal tachycardia may indicate infection or sepsis. **Continuous fetal heart monitoring of the preterm fetus during labor has been associated with a reduction in neonatal mortality in fetuses weighing less than 1500 g** [17]. In a study of 61 VLBW infants, ominous periodic changes or diminished variability on continuous fetal monitoring reliably predicted neonatal acidosis at delivery but did not predict central nervous system hemorrhage or survival. Seventy-five percent of fetuses with ominous fetal heart rate tracings were promptly delivered, which may explain the low number of neonatal deaths (1.5%) for this group in the study. This suggests that **fetal heart rate patterns can be useful in identifying the preterm fetus who should be promptly delivered** [18].

In contrast, another study did not find continuous electronic fetal monitoring to be effective in lowering the rate of perinatal mortality [19]. A later study by the same group found that electronic fetal monitoring allowed more accurate predictions about 5-minute Apgar scores and arterial cord pH, suggesting that electronic fetal monitoring provided better information about fetal well-being than does periodic auscultation [20]. It was reported elsewhere that electronic fetal monitoring did not result in improved neurologic development in preterm neonates. Of note, the time to delivery when an ominous fetal heart rate was present on electronic fetal monitoring was longer than auscultation (104 vs 60 minutes) [21]. Whatever the case, for preterm fetuses **detecting ominous fetal heart rate patterns early (by whatever method) and acting promptly on them (by willingness to perform a Cesarean) is important for improved neonatal outcomes.**

Anesthesia/analgesia

Pain management of the preterm parturient should be provided for medical indications and on maternal request [22]. The goal is to provide pain relief while minimizing central nervous system depression of the preterm fetus and avoiding fetal acidosis. Various methods are available to laboring women including regional, parenteral, local, and general anesthesia. Numerous studies indicate that **epidural anesthesia** provides the most effective pain relief compared with parenteral agents [23, 24]. The most common side effect from regional anesthesia is hypotension that can lead to fetal compromise and bradycardia [25]. This can be reduced with a 500–1000 ml infusion of crystalloid prior to placement of the regional anesthesia. Large parenteral doses of narcotics are required to achieve adequate pain control in labor and they mostly achieve their effect through sedation [26]. Careful monitoring of toxicity in the mother is required to avoid respiratory depression or aspiration. Parenteral agents can cause fetal and neonatal depression and decreased fetal heart rate variability [27]. Caution should be taken if the fetus has diminished fetal heart rate variability. Parental agents given to the mother have long neonatal half lives and can result in respiratory depression of the infant or may result in neonatal neurobehavioral depression up to day 3 of life [21, 27–29]. It is best to avoid these agents in the preterm gestation as the time to delivery is unpredictable and often occurs quickly [30].

Local agents last approximately 20–40 minutes and can be used for pudendal and local blocks. Local anesthesia is useful for operative vaginal deliveries, episiotomies, or laceration repairs but have little benefit for labor anesthesia. Paracervical blocks provide poor pain control in labor and can lead to bradycardia and these should also be avoided in the preterm gestation [31]. Inhaled anesthetics easily cross the placenta and may lead to neonatal depression within 8 minutes of induction [32]. General anesthesia should be reserved for emergency Cesarean delivery or for those women with contraindications to regional anesthesia who require Cesarean delivery. In general, induction of general anesthesia to delivery time should be minimized [21].

Delivery

As metabolic acidosis and birth trauma increase neonatal morbidity and mortality in the preterm infant, second stage interventions that reduce these risks have been sought. A retrospective analysis on the effect of type of delivery on neonatal outcomes in 118 VLBW singletons reported that routine **episiotomy** in a PTB **does not improve** neonatal outcomes. They also reviewed protection from birth trauma with the use of low forceps. There was **no benefit to forceps delivery** in the preterm fetus [33]. Standard use of forceps for obstetric indications is advised. **Vacuum should never be used before 34 weeks**, as it is associated with increased neonatal morbidity, in particular high rates of subgaleal hemorrhage [34].

There is not enough evidence concerning the use of intrapartum amnioinfusion for preterm rupture of membranes [35].

The approach to obstetric management significantly influences the outcome of extremely low-birth-weight infants. Above 26 weeks the obstetrician should be willing to perform Cesarean delivery for fetal indications. **Between 22 and 25 weeks willingness to intervene results in greater likelihood of both intact survival and survival with serious morbidity** [36]. In these cases women, families and physicians should be aware of the impact of the approach to obstetric management and consider the likelihood of serious morbidity and mortality when formulating plans for delivery.

Several trials have also considered **elective Cesarean delivery** for the preterm infant. The six randomized trials that studied vaginal vs Cesarean delivery in 122 preterm infants between 24 and 36 weeks were summarized in a Cochrane meta-analysis, which noted less respiratory distress syndrome, higher incidence of low cord pH, less neonatal seizures and fewer deaths with Cesarean delivery. However, this was based on limited numbers, and maternal morbidity was significantly increased in the elective Cesarean section group [37]. All these trials had recruitment difficulties. A review of 1765 neonates with birth weights of less than 1500 g found that there was no benefit in mortality or IVH with Cesarean delivery [38]. Based on these data, **vaginal delivery is preferred for cephalic-presenting preterm fetuses**.

The risk of neonatal mortality for the preterm infant with a vaginal **breech** delivery has been more controversial, with no specific randomized study aimed at this population. Several retrospective studies support Cesarean delivery for preterm breech presentation [39, 40]. In another study, Cesarean delivery for early preterm breech presentation was not associated with increased survival without disability or handicap, but footling breech negatively influenced survival in preterm breech deliveries [41]. There is also insufficient data to determine if external cephalic version of the preterm breech is safe. One study examined mode of delivery for high risk VLBW preterm fetuses (e.g. preeclampsia, non-reassuring fetal heart rate tracings, or bleeding) vs low risk VLBW preterm fetuses (e.g. preterm labor, PPROM) and found no benefit from Cesarean delivery for the low risk group but significantly decreased mortality for the high risk group [42]. It may be that in a high risk VLBW fetus with poor Bishop's score Cesarean delivery would be of benefit over a prolonged and possibly morbid induction of labor. If Cesarean section is undertaken for the preterm fetus **caution must be taken to avoid trauma**. **Low vertical or classical uterine incisions should be considered depending on the fetal presentation and development of the lower uterine segment.**

Delaying cord clamping by 30–120 seconds, rather than early clamping, seems to be associated with less need for transfusion and less IVH in preterm infants. There are no clear differences in other outcomes [43].

References

1 American Academy of Pediatrics, The American College of Obstetricians and Gynecologists. Guidelines for Perinatal Care, 6th Edn. October 2007.

2 Paneth N, Kiely JL, Wallenstein S, Marcus M, Pakter J, Susser M. Newborn intensive care and neonatal mortality in low-birth weight infants. N Engl J Med 1982; 307: 149–55.

3 Phibbs CS, Bronstein JM, Buxton E, Phibbs RH. The effects of patient volume and level of care at the hospital of birth on neonatal mortality. JAMA 1996; 276; 1054–9.

4 NIH Consensus Development Panel on the Effect of Corticosteroids for Fetal Maturation on Perinatal Outcomes. Effect of corticosteroids for fetal maturation on perinatal outcomes. JAMA 1995; 273: 413–8.

5 Phibbs CS, Baker LC, Caughey AB, Danielsen B, Schmitt SK, Phibbs RH. Level and volume of neonatal intensive care and mortality in very-low-birth-weight infants. N Engl J Med 2007; 356: 2165–75.

6 Haberland C, Phibbs CS, Baker LC. Effect of opening midlevel neonatal intensive care units on the location of low birth weight births in California. Pediatrics 2006; 118: 1667–79.

7 Donovan EF, Tyson JE, Ehrenkranz RA, *et al.* Inaccuracy of Ballard scores before 28 weeks' gestation. J Pediatr 1999; 135: 147–52.

8 Arnold CC, Kramer MS, Hobbs CA, McLean FH, Usher RH. Very low birth weight: a problematic cohort for epidemiologic studies of very small or immature neonates. Am J Epidemiol 1991; 134: 604–13.

9 Bahado-Singh RO, Dashe J, Deren O, Daftary G, Copel JA, Ehrenkranz RA. Prenatal prediction of neonatal outcome in the extremely low birth weight infant. Am J Obstet Gynecol 1998; 178: 462–8.

10 Bottoms SF, Paul RH, Mercer BM, *et al.* Obstetric determinants of neonatal survival: antenatal predictors of neonatal survival and morbidity in extremely low birth weight infants. Am J Obstet Gynecol 1999; 180: 665–9.

11 Lemons JA, Bauer CR, Oh W, *et al.* Very low birth weight outcomes of the National Institute of Child Health and Human Development Neonatal Research Network, January 1995 through December 1996. NICHD Neonatal Research Network. Pediatrics 2001; 107: E1.

12 Tyson JE, Parikh NA, Langer J, Green C, Higgins RD. For the National Institute of Child Health and Human Development Neonatal Research Network. Intensive Care for Extreme Prematurity — Moving Beyond Gestational Age. N Engl J Med 2008; 358: 1672–81.

13 Wood NS, Marlow N, Costeloe K, Gibson AT, Wilkinson AR. Neurologic and developmental disability after extremely preterm birth. EPICure Study Group. N Engl J Med 2000; 343: 378–84.

14 American College of Obstetricians and Gynecologists Practice Bulletin. Prenatal care at the threshold of viability. September 2002. No 38.

15 Low JA, Panagiotopoulos C, Derrick EJ. Newborn complications after intrapartum asphyxia with metabolic acidosis in the preterm fetus. J Obstet Gynecol 1995; 172: 805–10.

16 Kimberlin DF, Hauth JC, Goldenberg RL, *et al.* Relationship of acid-base status and neonatal morbidity in 1000g infants. Am J Obstet Gynecol 2006; 174: 382.

17 Paul RH, Hon EH. Clinical fetal monitoring: V. Effect on perinatal outcome. Am J Obstet Gynecol 1974; 118: 529–33.

18 Bowes WA, Gabbe SG, Bowes C. Fetal heart rate monitoring in premature infants weighing 1,00 grams or less. Am J Obstet Gynecol 1980; 137: 791–6.

19 Luthy DA, Shy KK, van Belle G, *et al.* A randomized trial of electronic fetal monitoring in preterm labor. Obstet Gynecol 1987; 69: 687–95.

20 Larson EB, van Belle G, Hsy KK, Luthy DA, Strickland D, Hughes JP. Fetal monitoring and predictions by clinicians: observations during a randomized clinical trial in very low birth weight infants. Obstet Gynecol 1989; 74: 584–9.

21 Shy KK, Luthy DA, Bennett FC, *et al.* Effects of electronic fetal-heart-rate monitoring, as compared with periodic auscultation, on the neurologic development of premature infants. N Engl J Med 1990; 322: 588–93.

22 American College of Obstetricians and Gynecologists Practice Bulletin. Obstetric analgesia and anesthesia. July 2002. No 36.

23 Ramin SM, Gambling DR, Lucas MJ, Sharma SK, Sidawi JE, Leveno KJ. Randomized trial of epidural versus intravenous analgesia during labor. Obstet Gynecol 1995; 86: 783–9 (Level I).

24 Thorp JA, Hu DH, Albin RM, *et al.* The effect of intrapartum epidural analgesia on nulliparous labor: a randomized, controlled, prospective trial. Am J Obstet Gynecol 1993; 169: 851–8 (Level I).

25 Brizgys RV, Dailey PA, Shnider SM, Kotelko DM, Levinson G. The incidence and neonatal effects of maternal hypotension during epidural anesthesia for Cesarean section. Anesthesiology 1987; 67: 782–6 (Level II-2).

26 Olofsson C, Ekblom A, Ekman-Ordeberg G, Hjelm A, Irestedg L. Lack of analgesic effect systemically administered morphine or pethidine on labour pain. Br J Obstet Gynaecol 1996; 103: 968–72 (Level II-1).

27 Halpern SH, Leighton BL, Ohlsson A, Barrett JF, Rice A. Effect of epidural vs parenteral opioid analgesia on the progress of labor: a meta-analysis. JAMA 1998; 280: 2105–10 (Meta-analysis).

28 Kuhnert BR, Kuhnert PM, Philipson EH, Syracuse CD. Disposition of meperidine and normeperidine following multiple doses in labor. II. Fetus and neonate. Am J Obstet Gynecol 1985; 151: 410–15 (Level III).

29 Kuhnert BR, Linn PL, Kennard MJ, Kuhnert PM. Effects of low doses of meperidine on neonatal behavior. Anesth Analg 1985; 64: 335–42 (Level II-2).

30 Gabbe SF, Niebyl JR, Leigh Simpson J, Eds. Obstetrics: Normal and Problem Pregnancies, 2002. 4th Edn. Churchill Livingstone.

31 LeFevre ML. Fetal heart rate pattern and postparacervical fetal bradycardia. Obstet Gynecol 1984; 64: 343–6 (Level II-2).

32 Datta S, Ostheimer GW, Weiss JB, Brown WU Jr, Alper MH. Neonatal effect of prolonged anesthetic induction for Cesarean section. Obstet Gynecol 1981; 58: 331–5 (Level II-3).

33 Barrett JM, Boehm FH, Vaughn WK. The effect of type of delivery on neonatal outcome in singleton infants of birth weight of 1,000g or less. JAMA 1983; 250: 625–9.

34 Miksovsky P, Watson WJ. Obstetric vacuum extraction: state of the art in the new millennium. Obstet Gynecol Surv 2001; 56: 736–51.

35 Nageotte MP, Freeman RK, Garite TJ, Dorchester W. Prophylactic intrapartum amnioinfusion in patients with preterm premature rupture of membranes. Am J Obstet Gynecol 1985; 153: 557–62.
36 Bottoms SF, Paul RH, Iams JD, *et al.* Obstetric determinants of neonatal survival: influence of willingness to perform Cesarean delivery on survival of extremely low-birth-weight infants. Am J Obstet Gynecol 1997; 176: 960–6.
37 Malloy MH, Onstad L, Wright E, National Institute of Child Health and Human Development Neonatal Research Network. The effect of Cesarean delivery on birth outcome in very low birth weight infants. Obstet Gynecol 1991; 77: 498–503.
38 Grant A, Penn ZJ, Steer PJ. Elective or selective caesarean delivery of the small baby? A systematic review of the controlled trials. Br J Obstet Gynaecol 1996; 103: 1197–200.
39 Lee KS, Khoshnook B, Sriram S, Hsieh HL, Singh J, Mittendorf R. Relationship of Cesarean delivery to lower birth weight-specific neonatal mortality in singleton breech infants in the United States. Obstet Gynecol 1998; 92: 769–74.
40 Effer SB, Moutquin JM, Farine D, *et al.* Neonatal survival rates in 860 singleton live births at 24 and 25 weeks gestational age. A Canadian multicentre study. Br J Obstet Gynaecol 2002; 109: 740–5.
41 Wolf H, Schaap AHP, Bruinse HW, Smolders-de Haas H, van Ertbruggen I, Treffers PE. Vaginal delivery compared with caesarean section in early preterm breech delivery: a comparison of long term outcome. Br J Obstet Gynaecol 1999; 106: 486–91.
42 Dietl J, Arnold H, Mentzel H, Hirsch HA. Effect of Cesarean section on outcome in high- and low-risk very preterm infants. Arch Gynecol Obstet 1989; 246: 91.
43 Rabe H, Reynolds GJ, Diaz-Rosello JL. Early versus delayed umbilical cord clamping in preterm infants. Cochrane Library 2009, vol. 1.

CHAPTER 22

Perinatal Care and Long-Term Implications

Janet E. Larson, Shobhana A. Desai & William McNett[1]
Division of Neonatology and [1]Department of Pediatrics, Nemours Pediatrics, Thomas Jefferson University, Philadelphia, USA

Key points

- Improved survival of premature infants (22–36 weeks) through technical advancement has resulted in new data regarding the consequences of prematurity.
- Immediate challenges facing the preterm infant include respiratory distress syndrome (RDS), patent ductus arteriosus (PDA), nutritional deficiency, intraventricular/periventricular hemorrhage (IVH/PVH), bacterial and fungal sepsis, and retinopathy of prematurity (ROP).
- Long term challenges facing the preterm infant include cerebral palsy, mental retardation, blindness, hearing loss and developmental disorders.
- Thirty percent to 50% of infants who are born at less than 25 weeks (or weighing less than 750 g at birth) have a moderate or severe disability.
- The risk for adverse outcomes is inversely related to gestational age. Other important prognostic factors are race, gender, antenatal corticosteroids, single vs multiple birth, fetal monitoring, willingness to perform Cesarean delivery, birth weight, and provision of life support to the neonate.
- Even infants born between 34 and 36 weeks (late preterm) demonstrate an increased incidence of cerebral palsy, developmental delay and mental retardation.
- No fetus should be delivered before 39 weeks unless indicated by accepted and evidence-based maternal or fetal indications.

Introduction

Neonatology is a field still in its infancy. Much of the early clinical effort in neonatology was aimed at improving survival of the preterm infant by managing the acute perinatal problem of lung immaturity. Indeed, **survival has improved over the last two decades and this trend is continuing** [1]. This decrease in mortality is **because of technical advances such as high-frequency oscillatory ventilation, surfactant therapy, and prenatal administration of corticosteroids**. Perinatal care systems aimed at

Preterm Birth. Edited by Vincenzo Berghella. © 2010 Blackwell Publishing

Table 22.1 Survival and selected major morbidities by gestational age at birth.
GA, gestational age. Chronic Lung Disease is defined as need for oxygen therapy at 36 weeks of postmenstrual age (Table 22.2). Severe intraventricular hemorrhage (IVH): grades III and IV (Table 22.3). Necrotizing enterocolitis includes medical and surgical. Severe ROP (retinopathy of prematurity) is defined as >grade 2.
Data from (with permission): Horbar JD, Carpenter JH, Kenny M, Eds. Vermont Oxford Network 2007 Very Low Birth Weight Summary. Vermont Oxford Network, Burlington, VT. 2008. Courtesy of Kevin Dysart, MD.

GA **(weeks)**	Survival **(%)**	Chronic lung disease **(%)**	Severe IVH **(%)**	Necrotizing enterocolitis **(%)**	Severe ROP **(%)**
<22	3.3	33.3	33.3	33.3	66.7
22	6.0	77.8	52.0	11.1	57.9
23	34.3	79.2	33.8	15.9	46.9
24	59.2	74.7	29.5	12.4	34.7
25	75.3	65.9	20.1	11.6	26.2
26	80.0	51.7	17.2	10.2	14.2
27	89.4	35.9	9.7	6.8	7.0
28	91.2	25.8	6.3	7.2	3.0
29	94.3	16.2	4.3	4.9	1.0
30	96.8	11.0	1.9	3.4	0.7
31	96.7	7.3	1.9	2.4	0.6
32	97.5	4.1	1.3	1.7	0.2
33	98.1	3.1	1.4	1.0	0.9
34	98.4	4.4	1.5	0.9	0.0
35	98.2	19.0	1.8	0.6	1.1
36	97.5	43.0	1.4	0.4	0.0
37	97.9		1.8	0.5	1.5
>37	98.0		1.5	0.3	0.2
All	95.4	17.3	5.3	1.5	7.2

stabilization in the immediate period, including **prenatal maternal transfer and regionalization**, have also decreased mortality rates [2].

However, as the field matures, new data regarding long-term consequences of prematurity have emerged, and many of these studies have focused on the adverse neurodevelopmental outcome of these children. No premature infant is immune to this risk; even late-preterm infants (born at 34–36 weeks gestation) have been shown to be adversely affected by their preterm birth (PTB) [3]. In all premature infants, **the risk for adverse neurodevelopmental outcomes is inversely related to gestational age** (Table 22.1). Other important prognostic factors are **race, gender, antenatal corticosteroids, single vs multiple birth, and birth weight** (www.nichd.nih.gov/neonatalestimates) [4]. Therefore, **the gestational age of the infant, their risk for adverse neurode-**

velopmental outcome, and decisions made regarding treatment in the perinatal period are inexorably linked.

Outcomes of infants born at the edge of viability (22–25 weeks gestation)

The **survival rate for infants increases each week** between 22 and 25 weeks gestation. However, the **incidence of moderate or severe neurodevelopmental disability** in surviving children remains discouragingly high (approximately 30–50%) and bears **no relation to gestational age at birth** during this short time period [1] (Table 22.1). Large studies in the United States and United Kingdom have used validated tools to measure neurodevelopmental outcome at 18–30 months of age. Approximately **30–50% of infants weighing less than 750g at birth (or who were born at less than 25 weeks gestation) had a moderate or severe disability**. Many infants had more than one disability that adversely affected their quality of life; these included **blindness, deafness and cerebral palsy**. While survival improved from 23 to 25 weeks gestation, the incidence of these disabilities did not decrease [1, 4, 5, 6].

In the United States these findings have prompted policy statements regarding the noninitiation and withdrawal of care [7]. The Committee on Fetus and Newborn of the American Academy of Pediatrics has recommended that **parents become active participants in the decision-making process in the treatment of these high-risk infants**. For the obstetrician, interventions such as fetal heart monitoring or Cesarean delivery for fetal indications need to be discussed in light of incidence of infant morbidity and mortality quoted by the neonatologist, and the consequent maternal wishes. **Fetal heart monitoring** of the periviable fetus improves outcomes (Chapter 21). **Willingness to perform Cesarean delivery** improves survival in fetuses at this gestational age [8]. **Provision of life support** improves survival in the infant [9]. Open conversations discussing the possibility of adverse outcomes are considered an integral part of the care of an infant and its family. Surveys by the Vermont Oxford Network from 1996 to 2000 reported that the mortality rate for infants with 401–500g birth weight was 83%; 52% of the infants died in the delivery room and it is thought that this high delivery room mortality was due to decisions made by the health care team in attendance in conjunction with family wishes [10]. For many parents, the survival of a severely handicapped child is the worst outcome. **The best and most common option is often to offer initially aggressive therapy to the family for the child** (Chapter 23). This therefore **includes maternal hospitalization, antenatal corticosteroids (Chapter 20), fetal monitoring,**

Cesarean if indicated, and provision of life support to the neonate. If 'trying everything possible' still is associated with devastating short-term outcomes (such as grade IV intraventricular hemorrhage), then withdrawal of care can be offered. Interestingly, **most neurologically-impaired neonatal intensive case unit (NICU) survivors judge their own quality of life to be acceptable** [11].

Challenges facing the very preterm infant (<32 weeks gestation)

Different challenges are faced by the medical team that treats infants who will live past the immediate perinatal period yet are still very immature. Preterm infants born at a gestational of less than 32 weeks face acute medical issues including **respiratory distress syndrome (RDS), patent ductus arteriosus (PDA), nutritional deficiency, intraventricular/periventricular hemorrhage (IVH/PVH), bacterial and fungal sepsis, and retinopathy of prematurity (ROP)**. The incidence of these complications is summarized in Table 22.1. Although the incidence of these problems occurs with less frequency, preterm infants between 32 and 34 weeks gestation may still have be faced with significant medical challenges during their hospital stay. Continuous reassessment of the child's condition/prognosis and open discussion with parents is a crucial part of their care [1]. Parents are often overwhelmed with the amount of information that they receive regarding their infant in the newborn period. The following conditions have the potential to affect long-term outcome and should be addressed clearly and repeatedly in conversations during the infant's hospital stay.

The clinical course of **RDS** has changed with the use of prenatal administration of steroids and use of artificial surfactant therapy. These treatments have resulted in a milder disease course. It should be emphasized to parents that while these therapies have reduced severity of the course of RDS, these new therapies do not necessarily obviate the need for long-term ventilation. Infants still succumb to chronic lung disease and pulmonary failure.

The development of **chronic lung disease (CLD, or bronchopulmonary dysplasia)** in very low birth weight infants [12] is multifactorial, but the greatest risk factor is decreased gestation at birth. Treatments aimed at reducing oxygen toxicity, blocking proinflammatory mediators, and decreasing ventilation pressure and duration have reduced the incidence and severity of CLD [13]. Infants with severe CLD (Table 22.2) are at higher risk for death and pulmonary infection during their hospital stay. They may have abnormal pulmonary function testing into late childhood, and are at increased risk for neurodevelopmental sequelae when

Table 22.2 Definition of chronic lung disease (bronchopulmonary dysplasia) for infants born at less than 32 weeks gestation [11].

None	No oxygen requirement at 28 days of life
Mild	Oxygen requirement at 28 days of life but no oxygen requirement by 36 weeks postmenstrual age
Moderate	Oxygen requirement at 28 days of life and oxygen requirement of <30% at 36 weeks postmenstrual age
Severe	Oxygen requirement and 28 days of life and oxygen requirement of >30% or positive pressure ventilation at 36 weeks postmenstrual age

compared with infants with mild or no CLD born at the same gestation [13–15]. Clinically, children may need supplemental oxygen with or without continued mechanical ventilation or continuous positive airway pressure (CPAP), bronchodilators, and/or diuretics. They are more susceptible to a reactive airway that is similar to asthma and may have poor respiratory health until school age [16].

Providing optimum **nutrition** to an immature gut is a significant immediate challenge in the premature infant. The goal to maintain an anabolic state with a growth velocity similar to *in utero* growth is often not met during the perinatal period. In addition, the inability to provide calcium to the infant at the same rate of *in utero* accretion often results in **osteopenia of prematurity**. The long-term consequences of these nutritional deficiencies are unknown. Children born with at a very low birth weight appear to have a relative growth deficiency that lasts into adulthood. While preterm infants have a period of catch-up growth once their conditions stabilize, it is incomplete. Although they seem to have adequate caloric intake, normal growth precursors, and lack of chronic conditions that would interfere with growth, **they remain lighter and shorter into adulthood** [17, 18].

Necrotizing enterocolitis (NEC) is a gastrointestinal disorder that occurs in 5–10% of infants of less than 1500 g birthweight. The pathogenesis of this multifactorial disease remains largely unknown [19]. Many risk factors, including ischemic injury, abnormal bacterial colonization, aggressive feeding practices, and activation of inflammatory cascades have been evaluated as possible etiologies. However, as with each of the adverse outcomes in prematurity, the main risk factor for development of NEC is decreasing gestational age. Recent new advances in the prevention of NEC have included the use of probiotics [20]. Besides a relative growth deficiency, these children are at risk for short gut and the need for supplemental feeds via gastrostomy tube once they are discharged from the hospital. In addition, infants with NEC have been shown to be at increased risk for subsequent neurodevelopmental disability [21].

Table 22.3 Gradation of germinal matrix and intraventricular hemorrhage in premature infants.

Grade I	Germinal matrix hemorrhage
Grade II	Intraventricular hemorrhage without ventricular dilation
Grade III	Intraventricular hemorrhage with acute ventricular dilation
Grade IV	Intraparenchymal hemorrhage

Because of their immature immune system, preterm infants are susceptible to both early and late onset infection and **sepsis** [22, 23]. Sepsis in these infants leads to an increased length of stay, mortality and risk for neurologic impairment [21, 24].

Infants are also susceptible to **germinal matrix/IVH** because of the high amount of vascularization that is occurring in the germinal matrix during brain development at 24–34 weeks gestation. Hemorrhage is diagnosed at the bedside by ultrasonogram and is graded by severity (Table 22.3). Serial ultrasounds are obtained to monitor for the associated condition of posthemorrhagic ventricular dilation, a conditioned caused by clots obstructing ventricular outflow. Severe hemorrhagic infarction predisposes the child to abnormalities in cognitive, visual and gross motor function [25]. **Periventricular leukomalacia (PVL)** is white matter injury that can be associated with injury in the cerebral cortex, thalamus, basal ganglia, brainstem and cerebellum [26]. The pathogenesis of PVL is related to immaturity, cerebral ischemia and inflammation [27]. Long-term sequelae of PVL include **cerebral palsy** and **cognitive defects (low IQ)** (Figure 22.1) [28]. Preterm birth is also associated with **school difficulties, behavioural problems, diminished long-term survival and reproduction** [29].

Even when a premature infant has no evidence of IVH or PVL during hospitalization, it is difficult to predict how that infant will do in terms of cognitive, motor, sensory and learning ability. Guiding principles in regards to neurodevelopmental outcomes associated with prematurity include the direct correlation of worsening debilitating outcomes associated with decreased gestational age, and that individual **problems such as cerebral palsy, mental retardation, blindness, hearing loss, and developmental disorders have the potential to be additive** [30]. Although many children born prematurely exhibit normal intelligence and development, children born with low birth weight are at increased risk for low IQ, attention-deficit hyperactivity disorder, anxiety, and autism when they reach school age [28, 31] (Figure 22.1). Many of these differences are subtle, including problems with visual processing and problem solving, auditory processing disorders, language disorders, behavioral issues and significantly reduced self-esteem [32–34].

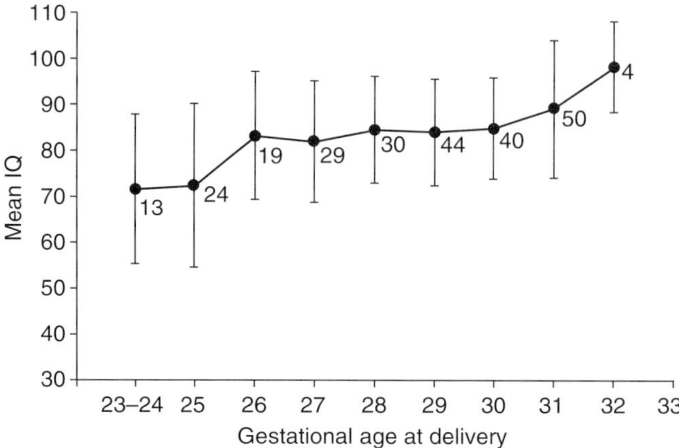

Figure 22.1 Mean intelligence quotient (IQ) score of children at age 6 years versus gestational age at delivery. The numbers represent the *n* for each gestational age, and the vertical lines represent the standard deviation. Reproduced from Andrews *et al.* [28] with permission from Elsevier.

Table 22.4 Selected short- and long-term complications in late-preterm infants [38].

Hypoglycemia
Temperature instability
Apnea
Respiratory distress
Hyperbilirubinemia
Feeding difficulties
Neonatal intensive care admission
Developmental delay
Cerebral palsy
Mental retardation

The premature infant is also at risk for both vision and hearing dysfunction. **ROP** results from neovascularization at the junction of the developing vascular and avascular retina. Laser therapy is used to prevent detachment of the retina and to preserve eyesight [35]. Laser therapy has improved long-term visual outcome but residual myopia, peripheral vision loss and possible blindness can occur despite therapy. Even if blindness is averted, the children born prematurely are still at a high risk of developing **myopia, amblyopia and strabismus** throughout their life-time.

Only a small amount of children that graduate from the NICU are affected by **hearing loss**, but infants are also at risk for problems with central auditory processing and discrimination. This may interfere with receptive and expressive language, and is associated with learning and behavior problems at school [32].

Complications in the late preterm infant (between 34 and 36 weeks gestation)

Until recently, infants born at 'near-term' were considered comparable to term infants and the two groups were combined in the study of outcomes [36]. **Infants born between 34 and 36 weeks gestation now comprise >70% of all preterm births**; this group accounts for much of the recent increase in PTB [3, 37, 38] (Chapter 4). **Even in this group, decreasing gestational age is associated with an increased incidence of cerebral palsy, developmental delay and mental retardation**. Children born late preterm were greater than three times as likely to have CP as those born at term. A modest association has been made for developmental delay and mental retardation [3]. Other complications in this age group are listed in Table 22.4. Therefore, **no fetus should be delivered before 39 weeks unless indicated by accepted and evidence-based maternal or fetal indications**.

Counseling parents in the perinatal period

The management of the premature fetus and then infant during the perinatal period should be a joint effort by the obstetrics and pediatrics teams. In many of these babies, the prognosis is uncertain and survival may be associated with a diminished quality of life for the child [6]. The care of these fetuses and infants benefits from **consistent and accurate information given to the parents** and they should be encouraged to participate actively in their child's care (Chapter 23). Counseling about potential survival, treatment options, and long–term outcome allows the family to have the information they need to participate in a plan of action that is medically sound and consistent with their goals [1].

References

1 MacDonald H. Perinatal care at the threshold of viability. Pediatrics 2002; 110: 1024–7.

2 Itabashi K, Horiuchi T, Kusuda S, *et al.* Mortality rates for extremely low birth weight infants born in Japan in 2005. Pediatrics 2009; 123: 445–50.

3 Petrini JR, Dias T, McCormick MC, Massolo ML, Green NS, Escobar GJ. Increased risk of adverse neurological development for late preterm infants. J Pediatr 2009; 154: 169–76.

4 Tyson JE, Parikh NA, Langer J, Green C, Higgins RD. Intensive care for extreme prematurity — moving beyond gestational age. N Eng J Med 2008; 358: 1672–81.

5 Vohr BR, Wright LL, Dusick AM, *et al.* Neurodevelopmental and functional outcomes of extremely low birth weight infants in the National Institute of Child Health and Human Development Neonatal Research Network, 1993–1994. Pediatrics 2000; 105: 1216–26.

6 Wood NS, Marlow N, Costeloe K, Gibson AT, Wilkinson AR. Neurologic and developmental disability after extremely preterm birth. EPICure Study Group. N Engl J Med 2000; 343: 378–84.

7 Bell EF. Noninitiation or withdrawal of intensive care for high-risk newborns. Pediatrics 2007; 119: 401–3.

8 Bottoms SF, Paul RH, Iams JD, *et al.* Obstetric determinants of neonatal survival: influence of willingness to perform Cesarean delivery on survival of extremely low-birth-weight infants. Am J Obstet Gynecol 1997; 176: 960–6.

9 Herbert-Jonat S, Schulze A, Kribs A, Roth B, Lindner W, Pohlandt F. Survival and major neonatal complications in infants born between 22 0/7 and 24 6/7 weeks of gestation (1999–2003). Am J Obstet Gynecol 2006; 195: 16–22.

10 Lucey JF, Rowan CA, Shiono P, *et al.* Fetal infants: the fate of 4172 infants with birth weights of 401 to 500 grams–the Vermont Oxford Network experience (1996–2000). Pediatrics 2004; 113: 1559–66.

11 Meadow W, Lantos J. Moral reflections on neonatal intensive care. Pediatrics 2009; 123: 595–7.

12 Northway WH Jr, Rosan RC, Porter DY. Pulmonary disease following respirator therapy of hyaline-membrane disease. Bronchopulmonary dysplasia. N Engl J Med 1967; 276: 357–68.

13 Geary C, Caskey M, Fonseca R, Malloy M. Decreased incidence of bronchopulmonary dysplasia after early management changes, including surfactant and nasal continuous positive airway pressure treatment at delivery, lowered oxygen saturation goals, and early amino acid administration: a historical cohort study. Pediatrics 2008; 121: 89–96.

14 Ehrenkranz RA, Walsh MC, Vohr BR, *et al.* Validation of the National Institutes of Health consensus definition of bronchopulmonary dysplasia. Pediatrics 2005; 116: 1353–60.

15 Vohr BR, Wright LL, Dusick AM, *et al.* Center differences and outcomes of extremely low birth weight infants. Pediatrics 2004; 113: 781–9.

16 Hennessy EM, Bracewell MA, Wood N, *et al.* Respiratory health in pre-school and school age children following extremely preterm birth. Arch Dis Child 2008; 93: 1037–43.

17 Euser AM, de Wit CC, Finken MJ, Rijken M, Wit JM. Growth of preterm born children. Horm Res 2008; 70: 319–28.

18 Farooqi A, Hägglöf B, Sedin G, Gothefors L, Serenius F. Growth in 10- to 12-year-old children born at 23 to 25 weeks' gestation in the 1990s: a Swedish national prospective follow-up study. Pediatrics 2006; 118: e1452–65.

19 Thompson AM, Bizzarro MJ. Necrotizing enterocolitis in newborns: pathogenesis, prevention and management. Drugs 2008; 68: 1227–38.

20 Alfaleh K, Bassler D. Probiotics for prevention of necrotizing enterocolitis in preterm infants. Cochrane Database Syst Rev, 2008; 1: p. CD005496.

21 Volpe JJ. Postnatal sepsis, necrotizing entercolitis, and the critical role of systemic inflammation in white matter injury in premature infants. J Pediatr 2008; 153: 160–3.
22 Stoll BJ, Hansen N, Fanaroff AA, *et al.* Late-onset sepsis in very low birth weight neonates: the experience of the NICHD Neonatal Research Network. Pediatrics 2002; 110: 285–91.
23 Stoll BJ, Hansen N, Fanaroff AA, *et al.* Changes in pathogens causing early-onset sepsis in very-low-birth-weight infants. N Engl J Med 2002; 347: 240–7.
24 Stoll BJ, Hansen NI, Adams-Chapman I, *et al.* Neurodevelopmental and growth impairment among extremely low-birth-weight infants with neonatal infection. JAMA 2004; 292: 2357–65.
25 Bassan H, Limperopoulos C, Visconti K, *et al.* Neurodevelopmental outcome in survivors of periventricular hemorrhagic infarction. Pediatrics 2007; 120: 785–92.
26 Volpe JJ. Brain injury in premature infants: a complex amalgam of destructive and developmental disturbances. Lancet Neurol 2009; 8: 110–24.
27 Khwaja O, Volpe JJ. Pathogenesis of cerebral white matter injury of prematurity. Arch Dis Child Fetal Neonatal Ed 2008; 93: F153–61.
28 Andrews WW, Cliver SP, Biasini F, *et al.* Early preterm birth: association between in utero exposure to acute inflammation and severe neurodevelopmental disability at 6 years of age. Am J Obstet Gynecol 2008; 4: 466–8.
29 Swamy GK, Ostbye T, Skjaerven R. Association of preterm birth with long-term survival, reproduction, and next-generation preterm birth. JAMA 2008; 299: 1429–36.
30 Doyle LW. Outcome at 5 years of age of children 23 to 27 weeks' gestation: refining the prognosis. Pediatrics 2001; 108: 134–41.
31 Hack M, Taylor HG, Schluchter M, Andreias L, Drotar D, Klein N. Behavioral outcomes of extremely low birth weight children at age 8 years. J Dev Behav Pediatr 2009; 30: 122–30.
32 Davis NM, Doyle LW, Ford GW, *et al.* Auditory function at 14 years of age of very-low-birthweight. Dev Med Child Neurol 2001; 43: 191–6.
33 Resnick MB, Gueorguieva RV, Carter RL, *et al.* The impact of low birth weight, perinatal conditions, and sociodemographic factors on educational outcome in kindergarten. Pediatrics 1999; 104: e74.
34 Rickards AL, Kelly EA, Doyle LW, Callanan C. Cognition, academic progress, behavior and self-concept at 14 years of very low birth weight children. J Dev Behav Pediatr 2001; 22: 11–8.
35 Yang CS, Wang AG, Sung CS, Hsu WM, Lee FL, Lee SM. Long-term visual outcomes of laser-treated threshold retinopathy of prematurity: a study of refractive status at 7 years. Eye 2009; 10: 1038.
36 Raju TN. The problem of late-preterm (near-term) births: a workshop summary. Pediatr Res 2006; 60: 775–6.
37 Davidoff MJ, Dias T, Damus K, *et al.* Changes in the gestational age distribution among U.S. singleton births: impact on rates of late preterm birth, 1992 to 2002. Semin Perinatol 2006; 30: 8–15.
38 Engle WA, Tomashek KM, Wallman C. 'Late-preterm' infants: a population at risk. Pediatrics 2007; 120: 1390–401.

CHAPTER 23

Ethical Issues Related to Preterm Birth

Frank A. Chervenak & Laurence B. McCullough[1]

Department of Obstetrics and Gyneology, Weill Cornell Medical College, New York Presbyterian Hospital, New York, USA and [1]Center for Medical Ethics and Health Policy, Baylor College of Medicine, Texas, USA

Key points

- The ethical concept of the fetus as a patient is an essential component of the management of preterm birth (PTB).
- The fetus is a patient when two conditions are met: (1) the fetus is presented to the physician or other healthcare professional; and (2) there exist medical interventions, whether diagnostic or therapeutic, that reliably can be expected to result in a greater balance of clinical goods over clinical harms for the child that the fetus is expected to become in the future.
- For the management of imminent PTB of a previable fetus there are two ethically justified options, because extrauterine survival is not possible: feticide followed by non-aggressive obstetric management; and non-aggressive obstetric management without feticide.
- After viability, aggressive obstetric management should be the rule in managing PTB.
- After viability, non-aggressive obstetric management and feticide are ethically justified depending on the presence and severity of fetal anomalies.

Introduction

In the past several decades important advances have occurred in the treatment of the fetus as a patient, with the goal of optimizing clinical outcomes. As a consequence, the ability to intervene and to improve outcomes of preterm births (PTB) has increased. Along with these significant clinical changes have come ethical challenges. Responsible clinical management of PTB should be based on the best available evidence and other chapters in this volume address and assess the evidence. **Responsible clinical**

Preterm Birth. Edited by Vincenzo Berghella. © 2010 Blackwell Publishing

management should also be based on the identification and management of the ethical issues that arise in PTB. In this chapter, we begin with definitions of ethics and medical ethics and then identify two relevant clinical ethical principles, beneficence and respect for autonomy. Using these ethical principles, we set out the ethical concept of the fetus as a patient. We then identify its clinical implications for the responsible management of PTB.

Ethics and medical ethics

Ethics is the disciplined study of morality. **Morality** concerns our actual judgments about what we ought to do and behaviors based on such judgments. Ethics seeks to continuously improve our moral judgments and behavior by subjecting them to critical scrutiny and argument.

Medical ethics is the **disciplined study of morality in medicine**. Medical ethics asks what ought to be the morality of physicians, of patients, of healthcare organizations, and of society regarding health policy. Ethical issues in PTB are largely in the first category. The professional obligations of physicians to pregnant and fetal patients will be the focus of this chapter.

Two ethical principles

Two ethical principles play a central role in the explication of the ethical concept of the fetus as a patient. The first is the ethical principle of **beneficence**, which takes a clinical perspective on the physician's obligation to protect and promote the health-related and other interests of the patient. The second is the ethical principle of respect for **autonomy**, which takes the pregnant woman's perspective on the physician's obligation to protect and promote the health-related and other interests of the patient [1, 2].

Beneficence obligates the obstetrician to seek the greater balance of clinical benefits over clinical harms for the pregnant and fetal patients in the clinical management of pregnancy. On the basis of rigorous clinical judgment, which should be shaped by current science and evidence-based reasoning, and a commitment to excellence in clinical practice, the obstetrician should identify those clinical strategies that are reliably expected to result in the greater balance of clinical benefits, i.e. the protection and promotion of health-related interests, over clinical harms, i.e. impairments of those interests.

Beneficence is the oldest ethical principle in the long global history of medical ethics. In Western medical ethics beneficence dates back to at least the time of Hippocrates [3]. The Hippocratic Oath is illustrative: it calls for physicians to act in ways that will 'benefit the sick according to my ability and judgment' [3].

The principle of beneficence should not be confused with the ethical principle of nonmaleficence. The latter ethical principle is also known as *Primum non nocere* or 'First, do no harm'. *Primum non nocere* appears neither in the Hippocratic Oath nor in any of the texts that accompany the Oath. The principle of beneficence, the obligation clinically to benefit patients and not simply to avoid harming them, was the primary consideration of the Hippocratic writers, as is clear from the language of the Oath. The primary emphasis is on beneficence: 'As to diseases, make a habit of two things — to help or to at least do no harm' [4]. The historical origins of *Primum non nocere* remain obscure.

Our point here is not just historical, but, more importantly, conceptual and clinical: if *Primum non nocere* were to become the primary ethical principle of obstetrics and perinatal medicine, then virtually all invasive aspects of obstetrics and neonatology would be unethical because of the risks they involve for the pregnant woman and newborn.

The patient's perspective on her own health-related and other interests must also be considered by the physician [1, 2]. The pregnant woman has her own values and beliefs, on the basis of which she is capable of making judgments about what will and will not protect and promote her health-related and other interests. All adult pregnant women should be presumed to possess the decision-making capacity to determine which clinical strategies are consistent with her interests and which are not, unless there is reliable clinical evidence of clinical deficits in her decision-making processes. In making decisions about their obstetric care pregnant women may utilize values and beliefs that go far beyond health-related interests, e.g. religious beliefs or beliefs about how many children she wants to have. As beneficence-based clinical judgment is limited by the competencies of medicine, it provides the physician no moral authority to assess the worth or meaning to the pregnant woman of her own non-health-related interests. Such are matters for the pregnant woman to determine for herself.

The ethical principle of respect for autonomy translates the patient's perspective into clinical practice. This principle obligates the physician to respect the integrity of the patient's values and beliefs, to respect her perspective on her interests, and to implement only those clinical strategies authorized by her as the result of the informed consent process. The informed process is typically understood to have three elements: (1) disclosure by the physician to the patient of adequate information about the patient's condition and its management; (2) understanding of that information by the patient; (3) a voluntary decision by the patient to authorize or refuse proposed management [1, 2, 5].

The ethical concept of the fetus as a patient

The obstetrician's perspective on the pregnant woman's health-related interests and the commitment to protect and promote her health-related interests creates beneficence-based obligations to her as a pregnant patient. At the same time, the woman's own perspective on her interests and the physician's commitment to respect her values and preferences creates autonomy-based obligations owed to her as a pregnant patient.

The fetus cannot meaningfully be said to possess values and beliefs, because its central nervous system is not sufficiently developed for it to be able to generate values and beliefs. There is therefore no basis for saying that a fetus has a perspective on its interests. There can, therefore, be no autonomy-based obligations to any fetus [1]. In other words, we cannot say with confidence that the fetus possesses independent moral status and generates its own rights. Despite this, the obstetrician has a perspective on the fetus's health-related interests and therefore can have beneficence-based obligations to the fetus, but only when the fetus is a patient. Because of its centrality for the ethical management of preterm pregnancies, the topic of the fetus as patient requires detailed consideration.

The major advantage of the beneficence-based ethical concept of the fetus as a patient is that the language of fetal rights has no meaning and, therefore, no application to the fetus in obstetric ethics. Thus, the ethical concept of the fetus as a patient can be understood and clinically applied without obstetricians having to become mired in current controversies about 'right to life'.

The authors have argued elsewhere that beneficence-based obligations to the fetus exist when the fetus can later, after birth, achieve independent moral status [1]. **The fetus is a patient** when two conditions are met: (1) the fetus is presented to the physician or other healthcare professional; and (2) there exist medical interventions, whether diagnostic or therapeutic, that reliably can be expected to result in a greater balance of clinical goods over clinical harms for the child that the fetus is expected to become in the future.

One link of a fetus to becoming a child is **viability**; the ability of the fetus to exist *ex utero* with full technological support as needed. Viability should not be viewed as an exclusively biological property of the fetus. Instead, viability must be understood in terms of both biological and technological factors. It is only by virtue of both factors that a viable fetus can exist *ex utero* and subsequently become a child and later achieve independent moral status. In countries with different levels of technological capacity, viability is a close correlate of access to technological capacity. When access to technology is present, viability occurs at approximately the end of 23–24 weeks of gestational age [6, 7]. The viable fetus therefore becomes a patient when a pregnant woman whose pregnancy has completed approximately 23–24 weeks presents for medical care.

The only link between the **previable fetus** and the child it is expected to become is the pregnant woman's autonomy. This is because technological factors cannot result in the previable fetus becoming a child: this is simply what previable means. When the fetus is previable, the link between a fetus and the child it can become can be established only by the pregnant woman's decision to confer the status of being a patient on her previable fetus. The previable fetus, therefore, has no claim to the status of being a patient independently of the pregnant woman's autonomy. The previable fetus becomes a patient when the pregnant woman confers this status on her fetus and she presents for medical care. The pregnant woman is free to withhold, confer, or, having once conferred, withdraw the status of being a patient on or from her previable fetus according to her own values and beliefs. The previable fetus is presented to the physician solely as a function of the pregnant woman's autonomy.

Implications for the clinical management of preterm delivery

The clinical management of PTB can either be aggressive or non-aggressive. By **aggressive obstetric management**, we mean optimizing perinatal outcome by utilizing effective antepartum and intrapartum diagnostic and therapeutic modalities, such as administration of steroids, inpatient fetal monitoring, ultrasound surveillance, Cesarean delivery, delivery in a tertiary center, and provision of life support (Chapter 22). By non-aggressive obstetric management, we mean that these modalities are not used and indications for clinical interventions are maternal [8]. The ethical concept of the fetus as a patient has implications for when non-aggressive obstetric management is ethically justified [1, 8].

Before viability, the fetus is a patient solely as a function of the pregnant woman's autonomous decision to confer this status. Before viability, she is also free to withhold this status or withdraw it after having earlier conferred it, especially in the context of an acute complication of pregnancy such as imminent preterm birth. The ethical implication for imminent PTB of a **previable fetus** is that there are **two options**, because extrauterine survival is not possible (Figure 23.1). The first is feticide followed by non-aggressive obstetric management, which is ethically permissible because the moral status of being a patient has been withdrawn. The other option is non-aggressive obstetric management without feticide. In explaining this option, the physician should make it clear that death cannot be guaranteed. These women should therefore be informed that, in the case of a

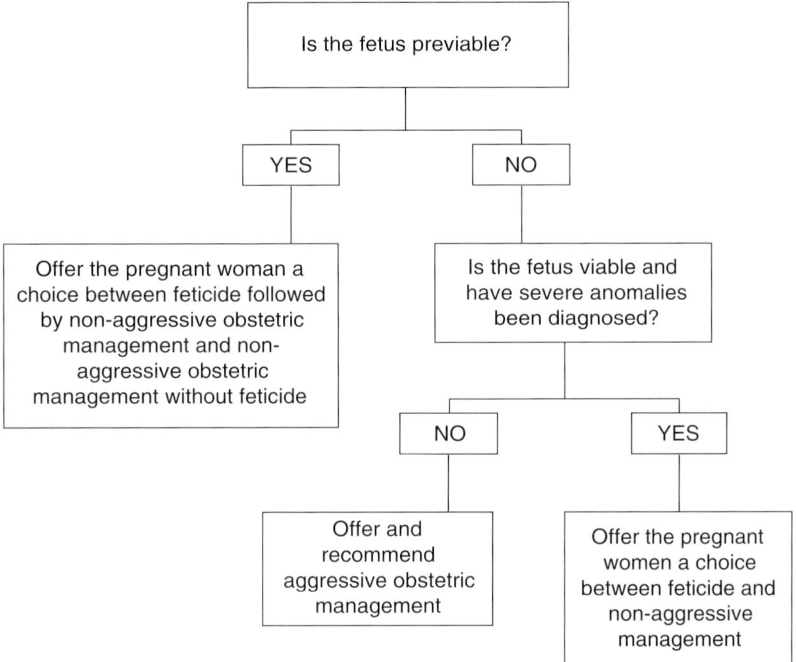

Figure 23.1 Algorithm for clinical management of imminent preterm birth.

live birth, neonatology justifiably may require intervention long enough to assess the newborn and make decisions about the appropriateness of resuscitation and transfer to the neonatal intensive care unit (NICU) and that these could indeed occur. For this second option, a request for Cesarean delivery should not be accepted, because it only subjects the pregnant women to clinical risk without altering the outcome for the previable fetus.

After viability, aggressive obstetric management should be the rule in managing PTB (Figure 23.1). However, non-aggressive obstetric management and feticide are ethically justified depending on the presence and severity of fetal anomalies. In all cases, the pregnant woman should be provided with a clear account of the nature and prognosis of the fetus' anomaly. The physician should make a reasonable effort to ensure that she understands this information, in the context of maximal psychosocial support from her spouse or partner, family members, and others, as she selects.

Non-aggressive obstetric management of a viable fetus is ethically justified when: (1) there is a very high probability, but sometimes less than complete certainty, about the diagnosis of a fetal anomaly and; (2) there is a very high probability of death or irreversible deficit of cognitive developmental capacity as an outcome of the anomaly diagnosed [1, 8–10]. In such circumstances, feticide may be considered to avoid severe morbidity in a dying neonatal patient.

The informed consent process when these two criteria are met justifiably focuses exclusively on beneficence-based and autonomy-based obligations to the pregnant woman. The physician should explain that clinical management recommendations will be based on protecting the pregnant woman's health. In particular, Cesarean delivery will not be offered for non-reassuring fetal testing or other fetal indications. In addition, the physician, in coordination with neonatology, should recommend against resuscitation and transfer of a liveborn infant to the NICU. In the case of live birth when these two criteria are met, only palliative care should be provided.

Some women will want to have the opportunity to have their child born alive, to help with their grieving process. In such a setting, **Cesarean delivery may be considered for maternal psychosocial indications**, rather than fetal indications, followed by palliative care of the live born neonate. Obviously, **neonatology should be included in preparing this plan of management** (Chapter 22).

The distinction between pre-viable and viable fetuses, in the range of 23 completed weeks, without anomalies is sometimes not clear. The recent publication by Tyson *et al.* [6] about neonatal viability may have some application in obstetric clinical judgment and refine traditional obstetric thinking that has defined viability solely on the basis of gestational age.

Conclusion

Ethics is an essential component of the clinical management of PTB. This is because the responsible management of PTB requires attention to ethical issues concerning the justification of non-aggressive obstetric management and feticide. Utilizing the clinical ethical concept of the fetus as a patient, we have defined ethically justified clinical criteria that can be used to support non-aggressive obstetric management of PTB and feticide in limited circumstances and their implications for the informed consent process.

References

1 McCullough LB, Chervenak FA. Ethics in Obstetrics and Gynecology. New York: Oxford University Press. 1994.
2 Beauchamp TL, Childress JF. Principles of Biomedical Ethics, 5th edn. New York: Oxford University Press, 2001.

3 Temkin O, Temkin CL, Edelstein L. Ancient Medicine. Baltimore: Johns Hopkins University Press, 1967: 3.
4 Hippocrates. Epidemics i:xi. W.H.S. Jones, trans. Loeb Classical Library, vol. 147. Cambridge: Harvard University Press, 1923.
5 Faden RR, Beauchamp TL. A History and Theory of Informed Consent. New York: Oxford University Press, 1986.
6 Tyson JE, Parikh NA, Langer J, *et al.* Intensive care for extreme prematurity — moving beyond gestational age. N Engl J Med 2008; 358: 1672–1.
7 Chervenak FA, McCullough LB, Levene MI. An ethically justified, clinically comprehensive approach to peri-viability: gynaecological, obstetric, perinatal and neonatal dimensions. J Obstet Gynaecol 2007; 27: 3–7.
8 Chervenak FA, McCullough LB. Nonaggressive obstetric management: an option for some fetal anomalies during the third trimester. JAMA 1989; 261: 3439–40.
9 Chervenak FA, McCullough LB, Campbell S. Is third trimester abortion justified? Br J Obstet Gynaecol 1995; 102: 434–5.
10 Chervenak FA, McCullough LB, Campbell S. Third trimester abortion: is compassion enough? Br J Obstet Gynaecol 1999; 106: 293–6.

CHAPTER 24

Future Research

Catherine Y. Spong

Pregnancy and Perinatology Branch, Eunice Kennedy Shriver National Institute of Child Health and Human Development, National Institutes of Health, Maryland, USA

Key points

- Preterm birth (PTB) is a public health priority affecting over half a million births in the United States each year.
- A 2006 report from the Institutes of Medicine provided an extensive review and analysis of prematurity including research needs, implications, economic impact and a summary of the evidence to date.
- The United States Surgeon General held a conference on the Prevention of Preterm Birth in 2008 highlighting the problem and developed a research and action agenda.
- Basic science and pathophysiologic studies are needed to understand the mechanism of PTB; epidemiologic research and work to understand the significant disparities are critically needed.
- Optimal strategies for prevention and treatment will likely be those tailored to the underlying pathophysiology, which rely on the careful identification and classification of PTB.
- Testing of proven therapies for other at risk groups to identify which subgroups may benefit is essential, rather than extrapolating to treat all at risk women. Clinical trials also need to address all at risk groups, including women traditionally considered 'low risk'.
- Research on how to implement research findings and practice change will facilitate incorporation of advances.

Preterm birth (PTB) is a public health priority, affecting over half a million births in the United States each year. In 2007, one of every eight babies was born preterm [1] (Chapter 4). Over the last decade the PTB rate increased more than 16%, rising 36% since 1980. Factors related to the increase include the rise in multiple gestations, the use of artificial reproductive technologies, the increase in maternal age and the rise in late preterm infants (those born between 34 and 37 weeks); however, the relative contributions are not clear (Chapter 4). The impact of prematurity is dramatic, as it has surpassed birth defects as the leading cause of death in the first month of life and can result in lifelong health complications including cerebral palsy and mental retardation. For those infants born low birthweight, a common condition in preterm infants, they have an increased risk of heart disease including myocardial infarction and stroke in adult life (Chapters 1 and 22).

Research in PTB has demonstrated the multifaceted complex nature of this condition and includes work in basic science, clinical trials, role of environment, disparities, genetics and epigenetics among others. **A 2006 report from the Institutes of Medicine provided an extensive review and analysis of prematurity including research needs, implications, economic impact and a summary of the evidence to date** [2]. Using this as a foundation, in 2008, the **United States Surgeon General** held a **conference on the Prevention of Preterm Birth**, bringing together experts to increase awareness, review key findings and establish an agenda. Workgroups of experts developed agendas focusing on biomedical research, epidemiological research, psychosocial and behavioral factors in PTB, professional education and training, outreach and communication and quality of care and health services [3].

Much work lies ahead to understand and ultimately prevent PTB. **Basic and mechanistic studies are needed** to understand the mechanism of PTB, including the relative contributions to the etiology of the **role of infection, inflammation, abnormal implantation and placentation, genetics, epigenetics and gene-environment interactions** (Chapters 2 and 5). In addition, a thorough understanding of the normal physiology of placentation and labor may provide insights. Utilization of the advances from other fields using **genomics, proteomics, and metabolomics** may help to identify why specific subgroups are at risk and what constellation of factors ultimately lead to PTB. **Combining these findings with exposure history** including sociodemographics, lifestyle factors, stress and disparities may delineate and identify **predictors of PTB**. Studies of families at high risk for PTB and family linkage could help to identify not only novel genes but also exposures.

Epidemiologic research especially focusing on the continued large disparity in PTB among racial and ethnic groups is well characterized yet poorly understood. Investigations into these **disparities** will require multidisciplinary efforts using novel approaches and will likely need to incorporate demographic, social, environmental, nutritional, genetic, biologic and clinical factors. Some of these studies may be accomplished using large ongoing studies, such as the National Children's Study and the Community Child Health Research Network; others may be possible using provider-networks such as Kaiser and Obstetrix/Pediatrix. However, the latter will be limited by the insured populations they cover. Enhanced clinical understanding of the heterogeneity of PTB from the very preterm to the dramatic rise in late PTBs and the relative contributions of factors to the specific etiologies will be needed to provide data for potential interventions and practice changes.

Clinical research needed includes **identifying markers** that can predict who is at risk to deliver preterm, identification and management of preterm labor, preventative therapies for both high and low risk women, and management of the preterm infant. With the identification of markers, the ultimate goal is to identify and test potential **interventions**. The heterogeneity of PTB is a limiting factor. **The optimal strategies for prevention and treatment will likely be those tailored to the underlying pathophysiology, which rely on the careful identification and classification of PTB. Testing of proven therapies for other at risk groups to identify which subgroups may benefit is critical, rather than extrapolating to treat all at risk women**. For example, preventative progesterone supplementation appears to be beneficial in women with a prior spontaneous PTB, but not in women with multiple gestations. Current work is evaluating its effectiveness in women with a shortened cervix. Similarly the utility of cerclage in the prevention of PTB has had mixed results, depending on the characteristics of the population studied. Designing trials that test specific subgroups may allow faster identification of therapies.

Clinical trials also need to address all at risk groups, including women traditionally considered 'low risk' — those women without medical complications who are in their first pregnancy. This subgroup comprises around 40% of pregnant women in the United States. A recent national registry study showed that the rate of PTB among low risk primiparas increased 50% in the past decade. At least 12% of nulliparous women in the United States will have a PTB, and complications during the first pregnancy impact subsequent pregnancies. Because nulliparas are a large proportion of pregnant women, understanding the mechanism for future prevention of PTB and other related adverse pregnancy outcomes will have a significant public health impact.

Advances also are needed on **understanding how to implement change** by providing interventions that are known to improve pregnancy outcome including preventing PTB. Although cigarette smoking is associated with PTB and low birth weight, optimal strategies for pregnant women to stop smoking are not well defined. **Societal change** to discourage and decrease smoking in reproductive age women would improve the health of the nation, yet is not readily accepted. In fact in some locations, smoking rates are rising in this group. Improving **preconception health and nutrition**, especially supplementation of reproductive age women with folic acid and B12, may improve pregnancy outcome on a societal level. Similarly, given the effect of obesity on medical conditions and pregnancy outcome, research on how to optimize the weight of reproductive age women is urgently needed. Finally, the ability to implement successful interventions, such as progesterone, to high risk women requires both research on optimal implementation as well as an available, accessible source of the medication.

Based on the input from the Institute of Medicine's report, the summary from the Surgeon General's meeting on Preventing Preterm Birth, as well as numerous workshops and available literature, there is a solid foundation of research needed to understand and hopefully ultimately prevent PTB. **Numerous funding sources, including federal, public and private dollars are available.** The National Institutes of Health, Center for Disease Control, March of Dimes and Burroughs Wellcome Fund all have established interest in supporting research to prevent prematurity and its sequelae. Advances in this area have the potential for remarkable impact on the outcome of the pregnancy, subsequent pregnancies for the mother and child, as well as ultimately the health of the world.

References

1 Hamilton BE, Martin JA, Ventura SJ. Births: preliminary data for 2006. Natl Vital Stat Rep 2007; 56: 1–18.

2 Behrman RE, Stith Butler A, Eds. Institute of Medicine, Committee on Understanding Preterm Birth and Assuring Healthy Outcomes, Board on Health Sciences Policy. Preterm Birth: Causes, Consequences, and Prevention. Washington, DC: The National Academies Press, 2007 (released July 2006).

3 Ashton DM, Lawrence HC, Adams NL, Fleischman AR. Surgeon General's Conference on the Prevention of Preterm Birth. Obstet Gynecol 2009; 13: 925–30.

Index

Note: page numbers in *italics* refer to figures; those in **bold** to tables.